Control of Arthropod Pests of Livestock:

A Review of Technology

Authors

Roger O. Drummond, Ph.D.
Laboratory Director
United States Livestock Insects Laboratory
Agricultural Research Service
United States Department of Agriculture
Kerrville, Texas

John E. George, Ph.D.
Research Leader
United States Livestock Insects Laboratory
Agricultural Research Service
United States Department of Agriculture
Kerrville, Texas

Sidney E. Kunz, Ph.D.
Research Leader
United States Livestock Insects Laboratory
Agricultural Research Service
United States Department of Agriculture
Kerrville, Texas

CRC Press, Inc.
Boca Raton, Florida

Library of Congress Cataloging-in-Publication Data

Drummond, Roger O., 1931-
    Control of arthropod pests of livestock.

    Includes bibliographies and index.
    1. Arthropod pests--Control. 2. Veterinary
entomology. I. George, John E., 1935-   . II. Kunz,
Sidney E., 1935-   . III. Title.
SF810.A3D78 1988   636.089′6968   87-11740
ISBN 0-8493-6860-X

International Standard Book Number 0-8493-6860-X

Library of Congress Card Number 87-11740
Printed in the United States

FOREWORD

The reader will find that this book specifically reviews the materials and methods used to control arthropod pests of livestock. The authors have assumed that the reader already has considerable knowledge about the life history and biology of arthropod pests found on livestock or in their environment. Such information is available from a variety of sources, including state extension bulletins, federal publications, and recent general books, such as *Livestock Entomology,*[1] *Fundamentals of Applied Entomology,*[2] and *Medical and Veterinary Entomology.*[3] Except for *Livestock Entomology,* these books do not present details of the technologies used to control these pests. *Livestock Entomology* contains a chapter on general principles of control, and most chapters have a short section on control of the specific arthropod pests addressed in the chapter.

After we were approached by CRC Press to write a book on the control of arthropod pests of livestock, we gave considerable thought to the subject. Has a book been written on that topic? What would be the value of such a book? How would such a book be received? Who would be interested? We noted that *Insect Control by Chemicals*[4] has an excellent, detailed chapter (with 242 references) on the use of chemicals, especially chlorinated hydrocarbon insecticides, to control arthropod pests of man and animals through the 1940s. There has not been a book that broadly focused on the control of arthropod pests of livestock. *Mammalian Diseases and Arachnids, Volume II*[5] contains a chapter on the biology and control of acarine parasites of domestic animals. *Parasites, Pests and Predators*[6] contains 9 brief chapters on the general aspects of arthropod parasites of livestock and their control. *Chemotherapy of Parasitic Diseases*[7] contains 7 chapters that present information on the current use of drugs to control arthropod parasites of veterinary and medical importance. We decided to write this book in the belief that there should be a place where the broad and diverse history of the details of the materials and methods used to control arthropod pests of livestock is documented. We did not want to write a "how to" book or one that focused only on recent advancements in the field. We hope that this book achieves our goal.

This book is written by specialists for specialists in veterinary entomology who wish to become more fully aware of the information found in the large body of literature that is available on control technology. We decided to focus on the literature on technology used or developed in the United States and Canada through 1985. We realize the shortcomings of this approach, but recognize that the world literature on control technology is many times greater than that available for North America. Also, we believe that the history of changes in materials and methods used to control arthropod pests of livestock in North America is similar to and reflects the history of those changes that occurred on a world-wide basis. Nevertheless, where necessary or appropriate to supplement or complement the literature in North America, we have cited literature outside of North America.

In our literature review, we decided that we would include as many pertinent references as possible, but would generally restrict them to those published in refereed journals available in most large libraries. We have also cited a number of older U.S. Department of Agriculture (USDA) publications — Farmers' Bulletins, Miscellaneous Publications of the Bureau of Animal Industry, Bureau of Entomology, etc. — that provide an unique broad-based history of changes in control technology that is evident in the several revisions of many of these publications through the years. We have made limited use of State Agricultural Experiment Station Bulletins because they often deal with state problems, are usually not of a general nature, and may not be readily available. Also, we have generally not used mimeographed, limited-distribution publications or articles found in non-refereed publications, especially *Insecticide and Acaricide Tests,* published by the Entomological Society of America since 1976, and Pesticide Research Reports, published by Agriculture Canada since 1967. However, if an article was of specific interest we have cited it, but generally we have only summarized these reports so that the reader will be aware of the materials and methods used.

This book deals mostly with chemicals and their application to livestock. When available, we have used the common names of chemicals, as published by the Entomological Society of America.[8] Chemicals without common names are listed by name or number. An appendix contains a list of the organic chemicals reviewed in this book and presents the chemical nomenclature for chemicals without common names. We have not presented details of dosages or concentrations of the chemicals discussed. We believe that these details are not necessary, when our purpose is to document that the chemical was tested or used for a specific purpose and was or was not effective. We have also emphasized the testing or evaluation of materials and methods in the field. Where we have cited laboratory studies, generally, these studies have used animals as part of their testing procedure.

Although the major theme of this book is the use of insecticides and acaricides to control arthropod pests of livestock, we have included chapters on other materials, methods, and techniques that have been used in place of chemicals or in conjunction with chemicals to control certain arthropod pests.

Throughout this book we have used the approved common names of insects and acarines as published by the Entomological Society of America.[9] In each chapter, whenever an approved common name is used for the first time that name precedes the scientific name and is marked with a ◆.

We hope that this book satisfies the need to have detailed documentation of the developments and the changes in the technologies used to control arthropod pests of livestock. The reader wishing to know currently approved and recommended treatments for the control of arthropod pests of livestock must check with local state authorities. Mention of a proprietary product in this book does not constitute an endorsement or a recommendation for its use by USDA, nor does it imply registration under FIFRA as amended.

Because R. O. Drummond had more time to devote to this book project, he drafted the chapters after gathering and reviewing the literature. The other authors reviewed the drafts, edited them and suggested changes that were incorporated into subsequent drafts. Mrs. Geneva Alexander (R.O.D.'s secretary) typed all of the drafts. She did an exceptional job by making extensive changes in drafts in very short periods of time. Without her speed and skills, this book would not have been attempted or finished by the deadline. Miss Margarita Carreon provided a great deal of help when we needed extra assistance. Rolando Garza also helped with certain aspects of the manuscript.

Each chapter was sent to a number of specialists for peer review. We wish to acknowledge and thank the following persons who reviewed chapters: Drs. J. R. Anderson, R. C. Axtell, D. R. Barnard, W. N. Beesley, R. A. Bram, A. B. Broce, S. J. Brown, R. C. Bushland, J. F. Butler, R. L. Byford, J. B. Campbell, W. F. Chamberlain, W. C. Clymer, L. M. Cooksey, M. M. Crystal, D. A. Dame, R. B. Davey, J. A. DeVaney, J. H. Drudge, Mr. E. P. Duren, Mr. W. F. Fisher, Drs. G. I. Garris, G. P. Georghiou, W. J. Gladney, O. H. Graham, F. S. Guillot, R. D. Hall, R. L. Harris, T. L. Harvey, C. E. Hoelscher, A. Hogg, J. A. Hogsette, F. R. Holbrook, Mr. H. W. Homan, Drs. M. A. Khan, D. L. Kline, F. W. Knapp, H. G. Koch, L. E. LaChance, J. L. Lancaster, Jr., J. E. Lloyd, E. C. Loomis, M. J. McGowan, L. Meek, J. A. Meyer, J. A. Miller, R. W. Miller, Mr. W. V. Miller, Drs. R. D. Moon, N. O. Morgan, G. A. Mount, M. S. Mulla, B. A. Mullens, W. A. Nelson, M. P. Nolan, Jr., R. S. Patterson, J. L. Peterson, R. E. Pfadt, F. W. Plapp, Jr., J. H. Pruett, Jr., J. E. Roberts, R. H. Roberts, J. P. Roth, R. T. Roush, D. A. Rutz, E. W. Saadi, Mr. C. D. Schmidt, Drs. E. F. Schmidtmann, P. J. Scholl, K. A. Schwinghammer, D. C. Sheppard, J. W. Snow, D. E. Sonenshine, R. K. Strickland, G. D. Thomas, E. C. Turner, Jr., S. K. Wikel, D. R. Williams, R. E. Williams, D. D. Wilson, Mr. F. C. Wright and Dr. R. E. Wright.

June 1986

REFERENCES

1. **Williams, R. E., Hall, R. D., Broce, A. B., and Scholl, P. J., Eds.**, *Livestock Entomology*, John Wiley & Sons, New York, 1985.
2. **Pfadt, R. E., Ed.**, *Fundamentals of Applied Entomology*, 4th ed., Macmillan, New York, 1985.
3. **Kettle, D. W.**, *Medical and Veterinary Entomology*, John Wiley & Sons, New York, 1985.
4. **Brown, A. W. A.**, *Insect Control by Chemicals*, John Wiley & Sons, New York, 1951.
5. **Nutting, W. B. Ed.**, *Mammalian Diseases and Arachnids, Vol II*, CRC Press, Boca Raton, Fla., 1984.
6. **Gaffar, S. M., Howard, W. E., and Marsh, R. E., Eds.**, *Parasites, Pests and Predators*, Elsevier Press, Amsterdam, 1985.
7. **Campbell, W. D. and Rew, R. S., Eds.**, *Chemotherapy of Parasitic Diseases*, Plenum Press, New York, 1986.
8. **Larson, L. L., Kenaga, E. E., and Morgan, R. W.**, *Commercial and Experimental Organic Insecticides*, (1985 Revision), Entomological Society of America, College Park, Md., 1985.
9. **Werner, F. G.**, *Common Names of Insects and Related Organisms*, 1982, Entomological Society of America, College Park, Md., 1982.

THE AUTHORS

Roger O. Drummond, Ph.D., retired from the Agricultural Research Service of the U.S. Department of Agriculture (USDA) in October 1986 after a 30-year career of research and administration. After receiving his Ph.D. degree in Acarology from the University of Maryland, he accepted a position at the U.S. Livestock Insects Laboratory in Kerrville, Texas, where he spent his career. He has published more than 200 papers on his research on tick biology and control and on the use of animal systemic insecticides to control cattle grub larvae and other arthropod pests of livestock. He served as Investigations Leader and Research Leader of the laboratory and was Laboratory Director from 1977 until his retirement.

Dr. Drummond is recoginzed nationally and internationally for his research. He has served on several Food and Agriculture Organization of the United Nations (FAO) expert committees on ticks and tick-borne diseases. He has served on the editorial boards of several journals and has held several offices in the Entomological Society of America. He is a member of a number of other professional societies and is a member of the American Registry of Professional Entomologists. Dr. Drummond now is a collaborator with the U.S. Livestock Insects Laboratory and also is a consultant to several international organizations and corporations.

John E. George, Ph.D., is currently the Research Leader of the Tick Research Unit of the U.S. Livestock Insects Laboratory (U.S. Department of Agriculture [USDA] Agricultural Research Service), in Kerrville, Texas. The mission of the Tick Research Unit is to develop new and improved methods for controlling ticks affecting livestock, humans, and wildlife. Dr. George's general research interests are the control of ticks on cattle and the behavioral ecology of ticks. His current research includes the characterization of the spectrum of resistance in strains of *Boophilus microplus* resistant to organophosphorus acaricides, evaluation of a sterile hybrid male *Boophilus* eradication method, and studies of the effects of photoperiod on tick oviposition, development, behavior.

Dr. George is a member of the Entomological Society of America and is past President of the Southwestern Branch of the society. He received his doctoral degree in entomology from the University of Kansas. After a year of postdoctoral training in medical virology at the University of Maryland School of Medicine, he investigated arboviral diseases in humans at the University of Maryland's International Center for Medical Research and Training (ICMRT) in Lahore, Pakistan. He held faculty positions in biology at Texas Tech University and Gerogia Southern College before joining the Agricultural Research Service.

Sidney E. Kunz, Ph.D., is Director of the U.S. Livestock Insects Laboratory, Agricultural Research Service, U.S. Department of Agriculture, Kerrville, Texas.

Dr. Kunz has had 20 years of research experience in the area of livestock entomology and has published extensively on the biology and ecology of the horn fly, stable fly, and turkey chigger. Dr. Kunz's research took him to Mauritius for 2 years with the Food and Agriculture Organization of the United Nations (FAO) in 1973 to 1974 to conduct stable fly research. He has also traveled to Africa on tsetse fly consultantships in Tanzania and Somalia and to Australia to participate in Commonwealth Scientific and Industrial Research Organization (CSIRO) buffalo fly and bush fly research reviews.

Dr. Kunz received his B.S. and M.S. degrees from Texas A & M University and Ph.D. from Oklahoma State University. Dr. Kunz is a member of a number of entomology organizations and is past President of the American Registry of Professional Entomologists.

TABLE OF CONTENTS

Chapter 1

EFFECTS OF ARTHROPOD PESTS ON LIVESTOCK PRODUCTION*

I. INTRODUCTION

It is important that, at the beginning, we review our knowledge of the losses in livestock production due to infestations by arthropod pests. There are complex interrelations between animal breed, environment, nutrition, innate resistance, stress, diseases, internal parasites, and arthropod pests. Generally, our knowledge of production losses in livestock due to arthropod pests is fragmentary and incomplete in that there have been few controlled studies with livestock in which the only variable has been the presence or absence of a specific arthropod pest. Specific studies have determined losses in production of milk, meat, eggs, wool, and other animal products that were the direct result of the infestation of animals by an arthropod pest.

Despite the fact that there have been few controlled studies to determine production losses due to arthropod pests, there have been a number of publications that have presented estimates of losses in income to livestock producers as a result of arthropod pests on their animals. In the U.S., early U.S. Department of Agriculture (USDA) reports often listed estimated losses as a result of infestation by the pest(s) that was the subject of the publication. In 1930, a limited USDA report[1] estimated annual losses in livestock production to screwworms, cattle grubs, and flies to be an estimated $99.0 million. The first broad-based USDA report on losses in 1938[2] estimated that annual losses, including some costs of technologies used to control the pests, in livestock production due to ticks, screwworms, cattle grubs, stable flies, horn flies, black flies, buffalo gnats, goat lice, and poultry pests totaled $168.8 million. The 1942 *U.S. Dep. Agric. Yearbook of Agriculture*[3] reported that annual losses in livestock production due to arthropod pests were $166.9 million. In 1954, USDA publication[4] ARS-20-1 estimated that the annual losses in livestock production as a result of arthropod pests were $507.7 million or about 9.7% of the value of livestock production for 1942 to 1951. In 1965, *U.S. Dep. Agric. Agricultural Handbook* No. 291[5] estimated that annual losses for 1951 to 1960 were $877.8 million. More recently, Drummond et al.[6] estimated that annual losses in production due to arthropod pests for cattle were $2260.6 million; for sheep and goats, $54.4 million; for swine, $231.6 million, and for poultry, $499.0 million. The total estimated loss of $3045.6 million did not include losses in value of horses or of the costs to control arthropod pests of livestock. In general, these estimates were highly extrapolated figures that used as their basis limited data on specific pests and livestock that were obtained under specific circumstances.

In his review of effects of arthropods on domestic livestock production, Steelman[7] emphasized the need for quantitative data on losses in animal production due to arthropods in order to rationally develop integrated pest management systems to control specific, economically important pests. Economic thresholds are necessary to be able to determine when the costs of treatment are justified in relation to the losses in production as a result of arthropod infestation.[8] Several review articles focus on the effect that arthropods and arthropod-borne diseases have on livestock production throughout the world.[9-16]

The rest of this chapter will list and review some of the key papers that provide estimates and/or specific data on the losses in production of livestock due to arthropod pests. The outline of this chapter will follow the general outline of the book. We have not included

---

* Common names of insects and acarines, as listed in *Common Names of Insects and Related Organisms* (published by the Entomological Society of America), are marked with a ♦ the first time they are cited preceding the scientific name.

data on losses as a result of infestation of livestock by the screwworm◆, *Cochliomyia hominivorax* (Coquerel), because an infestation of screwworm larvae, if not treated, can lead to the death of the animal. Also, data are not available on losses in horse "production" due to arthropods, for the value of horses is different from that of livestock.

II. EFFECTS OF ARTHROPOD PESTS ON PRODUCTION OF CATTLE

A. Horn Flies

In their critical review of the effect of the horn fly◆, *Haematobia irritans* (Linnaeus), on production of cattle, Palmer and Bay[17] stated: "Although the horn fly is often described as a 'serious pest' of the cattle industry, data presently available do not satisfactorily justify this claim". Many early reports on the effects of "biting" flies on milk production or on weight gain did not differentiate between the effects of horn flies, the stable fly◆, *Stomoxys calcitrans* (Linnaeus), the house fly◆, *Musca domestica* Linnaeus, horse flies, deer flies, and a number of "small" biting flies. An excellent review of early research on the control of flies, the economics of production losses to flies, and the use of fly sprays was presented by Decker,[18,19] who concluded "that under normal field conditions, biting flies do adversely affect both milk and meat production."

1. Mixed Species of Flies

After the review by Decker,[18,19] there continued to be research on the control of biting flies with daily or weekly applications of toxicant-repellent mixtures and the effects these treatments had on milk production and weight gains. Weekly application of a toxicant-repellent mixture controlled biting flies and provided a 4 to 14% increase in milk production.[20,21] Effects on milk production of controlling biting flies were much less evident in dairy herds that were provided adequate pasture and supplemental feed.[22] Beef cattle treated daily with toxicant-repellent mixtures to control mixed species of biting flies gained 4.6 to 9.7% more than untreated animals.[23,24]

2. Field Tests with Horn Flies

In pioneering research with DDT sprays and dips to control horn flies on range cattle, Laake[25] reported the treated cattle gained an average of 22 kg more than untreated animals during a 3.5- to 5-month period.

Daily spraying of dairy cattle with a toxicant-repellent mixture significantly reduced the horn fly population but did not affect milk production.[26]

Calves treated three times with coumaphos sprays, which controlled horn flies, had smaller weight gains than untreated, infested calves. This loss was apparently the result of subclinical toxicity of the coumaphos, for the substitution of DDT for coumaphos allowed for an immediate weight gain.[27] Horn flies reduced the growth rates of cattle, especially during a period of increase in the abundance of flies, but the subclinical toxicity of coumaphos lessened the growth rate advantage provided by the control of horn flies.[28]

There was no consistent relationship between partial control of horn flies and average daily gain of treated and untreated calves.[29] Partial control of horn flies on cows did not affect the weights of calves nursing on these cows.[30] Insecticide dust bag treatments controlled horn flies, and treated yearlings gained an average of 1.6 to 6.9 kg per animal more than untreated cattle over a 2.5- to 3-month period.[31]

Weekly spraying of steers on summer pastures with a toxicant-repellent mixture provided excellent control of horn flies and fair to good control of horse flies. Although treated steers gained 0.09 to 0.1 kg/day per animal more than untreated cattle, and when cattle were later placed in a feedlot, the treated steers had higher daily gains and required less feed than untreated steers, the differences were not statistically significant.[32]

Calves weaned from cows which were forced to use insecticide dust bags to control horn flies weighed significantly more (5.9 kg per animal) than calves from untreated cows.[33] The treating of cows with one or two insecticide-impregnated ear tags controlled horn flies, and the weaning weights of calves were 1.5 to 6.6 kg greater than weights of calves from untagged cows.[34]

In a 6-year study, weights of treated steers averaged 8 kg greater than weights of untreated steers during grazing periods, and there was an additional 2-kg advantage during a feedlot phase.[35] Steers treated with one or two insecticide-impregnated ear tags per animal gained an average of 8.8 kg per animal more than untreated steers.[36] Treated steers spent less time walking and resting than untreated steers and had decreased frequency of tail switching.[37] These activity differences may account for reduced weight gain. Steers treated with two insecticide-impregnated ear tags weighed ca. 18% greater than steers infested with horn flies.[38]

In tests with steers or cows each treated with two insecticide-impregnated ear tags, treated steers gained ca. 11 to 14% more than untreated steers, and calves weaned from treated cows averaged 7.4 kg heavier at weaning than calves from untreated cows.[39] Treating cows with two insecticide-impregnated ear tags per animal controlled horn flies, and the calves weaned from treated cows averaged 5.6 kg heavier than calves from untreated cows.[40]

Canadian studies showed that low infestations of only 60 to 70 horn flies per animal reduced weight gains of yearlings by 17 to 22%, and high infestations of 200 flies per animal reduced the growth rate by 45%. There is a host-parasite regulation range (the injury threshold) of 12 to 230 flies per animal which breaks down when fly numbers exceed the higher figure.[41,42] These data were used by Klein and Gordon[43] to determine an economic threshold, which ranged from 10 to 230 flies per animal, depending upon soil, cattle prices, and insecticide application. In most years, fly populations exceeded the economic threshold.

3. Cattle Specifically Infested with Horn Flies

Dairy cows held in screened stalls were infested daily with horn flies, and the loss in milk production was only 1.4%.[44] In recent studies with steers held in large screened cages and exposed to measured populations of horn flies, the average daily gain of unexposed steers was 0.16 kg/day greater than fly-infested animals, but there was no difference in feed conversion values.[45]

4. Overview

Early trials to determine if horn flies affected weight gains or milk production of cattle were complicated by the presence of several species of biting flies on cattle. Data obtained in tests in which horn flies were controlled throughout an entire horn fly season with insecticides in dust bags or ear tags show that control of horn flies provides for weight gains that were greater than those of untreated cattle. In addition, the treating of cows allowed for the weaning of calves that were heavier than calves from untreated cows. Recent research in Canada on injury and economic thresholds of horn flies should provide a stimulus for additional research to determine these factors for cattle exposed to incremental populations of horn flies. Additional data are needed from specific tests with cattle maintained under controlled conditions in which the only variable is different populations of horn flies.

B. Stable Flies

There is a considerable amount of information available on the effects of stable flies on the production of dairy and beef cattle. Most early studies, which focused on the increases in milk flow as the result of controlling or repelling "flies" from dairy cattle, did not differentiate between the abundance of stable flies, house flies, or horn flies, and did not have sufficient numbers of cattle or comparable untreated herds for proper analysis of results.

However, some of these trials were conducted when stable flies were the predominant species. More recent studies have been conducted with cattle maintained under controlled conditions and exposed to specific infestations of stable flies.

1. Field Studies

Daily application of a repellent to dairy cows did not affect yeilds of milk and butterfat during 2-week treatment periods.[46] In a switch-back test, dairy cows sprayed daily with a homemade repellent had milk yields of about 4% greater than unsprayed cows.[47] Shaw and Atkeson[48] reviewed earlier research on the effects of flies and the spraying of cattle on milk production and concluded from their tests that neither infestation by stable flies nor spraying cows twice daily with an "acceptable" spray depressed milk production.

Dairy cows infested with stable flies and horn flies were sprayed daily, and, despite heterogeneity in fly counts, there was a significant negative correlation of -0.82 between numbers of flies and changes in milk production. Herds treated with toxicants maintained higher milk production than herds treated with repellents.[49] Daily treatment of dairy cows with a variety of sprays showed that there was a significant correlation of 0.9 between numbers of stable flies and percent monthly loss in butterfat production. Because depressed production extended for months beyond the fly season, an increase in production of 10 to 20% could result from the control of stable flies.[50] Recently, weight losses of 2.3 to 3.5 kg per animal in feedlots were recorded as a result of stable fly infestations.[51]

2. Cattle Specifically Infested with Stable Flies

Dairy cows, held in a screen-enclosed shed and infested with stable flies, had a 9% reduction in milk production, but spraying of the cows with an insecticidal spray caused an additional loss in production.[44] However, spraying cows daily caused a greater reduction in production than the reduction as a result of infestation with large numbers of house flies.[52] Petroleum oil sprays as well as infestations of stable flies caused an increase in body temperatures and respiration rates of dairy cows and heifers.[53]

Stanchioned dairy cows held in controlled-environment chambers were exposed to 600 to 1600 stable flies per day, and the flies had no effect on milk production when cows had free access to a high-energy ration.[54] In contrast, crossbred beef calves held in screened enclosures and exposed to stable flies had average weight gains reduced by 0.9 kg/day and feed efficiency reduced by 12.9% for 100 days on a growing ration, and weight gains reduced by 0.22 kg/day and feed efficiency by 10.9% for 100 days on a finishing ration.[55]

3. Overview

Field studies have provided evidence of an inverse relationship between the numbers of stable flies on dairy cattle and milk production. Also, feedlot cattle infested with stable flies gained less weight than uninfested cattle.

Critical tests with cattle held under controlled conditions showed that stanchioned dairy cows with free access to high-energy rations did not experience a reduction in milk production as a result of stable fly infestations. However, in other controlled studies, stable flies affected weight gains and the feed efficiency of beef calves. Additional controlled-environment trials are needed to determine the effects of different levels of stable fly populations on the production of dairy and beef cattle on diets with different energy levels.

C. Small Biting and Nuisance Flies

There are very few reports that contain any general information, much less data, on the effects of most "small" biting and nuisance flies on cattle production. Several publications have presented data on the effects of mosquitoes and black flies on cattle production.

1. Mosquitoes

Although we do not specifically address the control of mosquitoes in this book, some effects of mosquitoes on cattle production have been documented. An outbreak of *Psorophora columbiae* Dyar and Knab in Florida killed cattle as a result of blood loss.[56] As a result of a massive outbreak of the salt marsh mosquito♦, *Aedes sollicitans* (Walker), in Texas and Louisiana, cattle deaths and production losses were estimated to be in excess of $430,000.[57] Sanders et al.[58] noted that pastures along the Gulf Coast of Texas were not grazed during the summer months because of high populations of salt marsh mosquitoes. In Texas, massive *A. sollicitans* populations caused the death of cattle by exsanguination.[59]

Steelman et al.[60-62] conclusively demonstrated that in southern Louisiana, attacks by mosquitoes, *Psorophora confinnis* (Lynch-Arribalzaga), the common malaria mosquito♦, *Anopheles quadrimaculatus* Say, and *A. crucians* Wiedemann caused significant and economically damaging reductions in weight gains of feedlot steers. Also, Brahman steers or crossbred Brahman × Hereford steers were less affected by mosquito attacks than Hereford steers.

The controlled feeding of the yellow fever mosquito♦, *Aedes aegypti* Linnaeus, or of *A. triseriatus* on cattle did not affect the quality of the hide and leather at the sites where the mosquitoes had fed.[63]

2. Black Flies

In Canada, there is considerable evidence that massive outbreaks of black flies, especially *Simulium arcticum* Malloch, cause the death of cattle and other livestock as a result of acute toxemia from large numbers of flies extensively feeding on the animals.[64] In a study of a series of economic outbreaks of black flies, Rempel and Arnason[65] described weather conditions, the breeding situation and feeding habits of flies, and the clinical symptoms of attack. Death was due to shock and loss of blood, but not suffocation. A review of Simuliidae in Canada[66] discussed outbreaks of *S. arcticum* and noted that numbers of this species had declined as a result of changing river conditions and that a new species, *S. luggeri,* was becoming more prevalent.

In field experiments, a pouron of phosmet reduced harassment of cattle by *S. arcticum* for 5 to 6 weeks and, during the protection period, the treated cattle gained more weight than untreated cattle, but untreated cattle made compensatory weight gains after the end of the black fly season.[67] Phosmet pouron decreased the incidence of clinical toxicosis to *S. arcticum* and also allowed for a general increase in weight gains during the black fly season.[68] In California, an outbreak of *S. trivittatum* caused a 10% reduction in milk flow during the period of high fly activity, but milk flow recovered to pre-outbreak levels after the end of the outbreak.[69]

3. Overview

Although there is little information available on the effects that small biting and nuisance flies have on cattle production, it is apparent that the consequences of attacks by large populations can be significant. Massive, transient populations of mosquitoes have been shown to cause exsanguination and death losses of cattle. In Louisiana, large numbers of mosquitoes feeding on feedlot cattle caused decreased weight gains. The breed of cattle exposed to these attacks can be a mitigating factor in the degree of damage experienced, for Brahman cattle were less affected by mosquito feeding than Hereford cattle.

The massive populations of black flies that attack cattle in areas of Canada can cause production losses as a result of decreased grazing by cattle and acute toxemia from the flies feeding on the animals. These losses can be prevented or reduced by treating cattle with phosmet pouron. Usually, cattle make compensatory gains after the outbreak of flies has ended.

D. Horse Flies and Deer Flies

There are few data on the effect that the large variety of horse flies and deer flies which attack cattle in North America have on the economics of the production of cattle. Controlling horse flies can increase weight gains of beef cattle and butterfat production in dairy cattle. Horse flies feeding on the animals have been shown to cause some damage to hides and quality of leather and a measurable blood loss in cattle. Horse flies have been recognized as vectors of a number of disease organisms that affect cattle and other livestock.

1. Meat and Milk Production

Controlling *Tabanus sulcifrons* Macquart and a few less-prevalent tabanid species with a daily application of synergized pyrethrins caused a significant increase in butterfat production of dairy cattle and an increase in weight gain of 9 to 13 kg per head of beef cattle over 38 days. There was a significant negative correlation of -0.75 between butterfat production and numbers of horse flies.[70] In further tests, mixtures of repellents and toxicants, applied with a treadle sprayer, reduced populations of *T. sulcifrons* and increased milk production. There was a significant negative correlation of -0.98 between numbers of flies and milk production, and animal routine affected both the repellency and milk production response.[71]

Yearling Hereford heifers were held in screened pens and others in open pens so that they were exposed to attack by *Tabanus abactor* Philip, *T. atratus* Fabricius, *T. equalis* Hine, *T. mularis* Stone, *T. subsimilis* Bellardi, and *T. sulcifrons*. Average daily gain of heifers exposed to flies (66 to 90 flies per day per animal) was 0.09 kg per animal less than that of protected heifers, and feed efficiency of exposed heifers was 16.9% less than protected heifers.[72] The potential annual loss was estimated to be >$10.00 per animal.

2. Damage to Hide and Leather

Leather from hides of cattle exposed to natural populations of *Hybomitra lasiophthalma* (Macquardt) and *T. quinquevittatus* Weidemann contained shallow grain pits and translucent pinholes in areas where tabanids ordinarily feed. Thus, the grain spotting was attributed to the flies feeding on the animals.[63]

3. Blood Loss

T. sulcifrons feeding on the animals could cause blood loss of 115 cm³/day under favorable conditions for fly populations.[73] Hollander and Wright[74] estimated that, during periods of peak activity, tabanids could cause blood loss of over 200 cm³ per animal per day, and they noted a need for an energy-use index to relate energy lost by cattle in avoiding tabanids to production loss.

4. Transmission of Disease Agents

In an excellent review of the Tabanidae as vectors of animal disease agents, Krinsky[75] presented evidence that tabanids were biological or mechanical vectors of viruses, bacteria, protozoa, and helminths. Of particular interest to cattle production in North America is the mechanical transmission of anaplasmosis by tabanids.[76]

5. Overview

Only limited data are available on the effects of horse flies and deer flies on cattle production. Early field studies showed that there was a highly significant inverse relationship between butterfat production and numbers of horse flies on dairy cattle. Recent field tests showed that horse flies feeding on cattle adversely affected weight gains and feed efficiency of beef cattle. Similar tests are needed with lactating dairy cows. More highly controlled trials with artificially infested cattle await a technique to rear large numbers of tabanids in the laboratory. There is little known about losses in production as a result of the disease agents that are transmitted by tabanids.

E. Face Flies

Although the face fly[*], *Musca autumnalis* DeGeer, was recently introduced into North America, it has received considerable attention as a pest of economic importance. During their spread across Canada and the U.S. in the 1950s and 1960s, whenever face flies were found for the first time in an area, cattle owners were aware that their animals (1) had an increased incidence of eye disorders, (2) were often seen "fighting flies", and (3) were not grazing normally.[76] However, there were no data on the economic aspects of the infestation of face flies. Subsequently, there have been data collected that show that face flies can damage eyes of cattle by their feeding activity alone and are also vectors of diseases and parasites of the eyes of cattle.

1. Nuisance Feeding

Calves exposed for only 8 days to face flies, which were not contaminated with *Moraxella bovis* (Hauduroy), the etiological agent of pinkeye, had eyes that showed mild signs of keratoconjunctivitis as a result of face-fly feeding.[78] In a closely controlled test with cattle held in screened pens, a lacrimation eye score was used to assess the damage of face flies, and an economic injury level of only one face fly per eye per month was proposed.[79] Populations of 12 to 13 face flies per face had no effect on feed consumption, feed efficiency, or average daily gain of Hereford heifers that were held in screened pens. No pinkeye was seen, although some irritation of the eyes was noted.[80]

As few as 10 to 11 face flies per animal reduced grazing time by ca. 20 to 25 min/day, but had no effect on grazing patterns or weight gains of Holstein heifers.[81] Field populations of face flies did not affect percentage of milkfat, protein, or nonfat solids, silage consumption or conversion, nor average milk weight of lactating Holstein cows.[82]

2. Transmission of Infectious Bovine Keratoconjunctivitis (IBK or Pinkeye)

Pinkeye can cause significantly lower weight gains in calves both before and after weaning.[83] Pinkeye was a problem to cattle producers before the appearance of face flies, but the presence of a fly that feeds around the eyes, and an increase in the incidence of pinkeye in herds infested with face flies, suggested that this species might be a carrier of the disease organism.[84] *M. bovis* was recovered from the external surfaces of face flies exposed to lacrimal exudates of infected cattle.[85] In contrast, although face flies were found to carry *M. bovis*, they did not appear to be important as disseminators of pinkeye in the cattle herds studied.[86] Cattle protected from face flies had fewer cases of pinkeye, and there was a highly significant correlation between numbers of face flies on cattle and numbers of new isolates of *M. bovis* from cattle.[87] *M. bovis* was recovered from the crops of female face flies which had fed on the eyes of infected cattle.[88]

In a thorough review of the face fly-pinkeye relationship, Hall[89] concluded that data were available that incriminated the face fly as a vector of *M. bovis*, and control of the species could be justified as part of a program to manage pinkeye. Face fly control was one of the aspects of a practical pinkeye control program.[90]

3. Transmission of Eyeworms, Thelazia spp.

Although face flies were known to be intermediate hosts of larvae of eyeworms, *Thelazia* spp., in Europe, no infestations had been reported from face flies in the U.S. until 1971 when Chitwood and Stoffolano[91] indentified *Thelazia* larvae in a sample of face flies from Massachusetts. Subsequently, additional larvae were recovered from other pools of face flies.[92] The eyeworms, *T. gulosa* Railliet and Henry and *T. skrjabini* Ershov, were recovered from cattle,[93] and *T. lacrymalis* (Gurlt) was recovered from horses.[94] Although >12% of cattle eyes were infested with eyeworms, the infestations were generally subclinical.[95] Parasitism rates of face flies with eyeworm larvae ranged from 0.4 to 13.2%.[96] As yet, there are not data on economic effects of thelaziosis on cattle production.

4. Overview

Face flies can cause lacrimation and eye lesions in cattle because of their feeding activity; however, their appearance on grazing cattle did not affect weight gains of dairy heifers or beef cattle or milk production of dairy cows. Although face flies can cause irritation to the eyes of cattle, their presence, in the absence of pinkeye, does not appear to warrant treatment nor present an economic problem to cattle owners. However, face flies are proven vectors of *Moraxella bovis,* the etiological agent of keratoconjunctivitis (IBK or pinkeye), which can be a serious problem in cattle herds. Thus, control of face flies is warranted as a part of a pinkeye prevention and management program. Although face flies can harbor and presumably transmit eyeworms, the economic aspects of that parasite are yet unknown.

F. Cattle Grubs

The common cattle grub♦, *Hypoderma lineatum* (Villers), and the northern cattle grub♦, *H. bovis* (Linnaeus), have long been recognized as arthropods that are of economic importance to the production of cattle. Early publications generally listed dollar estimates of losses caused by the different stages of the life cycle. Later, some data were obtained on the effect on weight gains when rotenone treatments were used to control cattle grub larvae in warbles in the backs of cattle. The advent of animal systemic insecticides allowed for specific studies on increases in production and decreases in losses in hide and carcass value as a result of the elimination of cattle grubs from cattle.

1. Early Estimates of Losses

In the U.S., in 1896, Osborn[97] listed three distinct ways in which infestations of cattle grubs caused losses in the production of cattle: (1) losses in value of hides as the result of holes caused by cattle grub larvae, (2) losses in milk and beef supply as a result of cattle running from the egg-laying activities of heel flies, and (3) losses in meat and milk production as a result of the presence of larvae in the backs of cattle. Generally, during the "grubby season" from January to June, more than half of the hides were depreciated in value as a result of holes caused by cattle grub larvae. He estimated annual losses due to cattle grubs of $90 million.

The annual loss in Canada in 1912 in the value of hides alone as the result of holes caused by cattle grub larvae was estimated to be between 25 and 30% of the value of uninfested hides.[98] In 1926, Bishopp et al.[99] estimated that annual losses were $50 million. The initial edition[100] of *U.S. Dep. Agric. Farmers' Bulletin* No. 1596 in 1929 estimated losses from $50 to 100 million annually. Losses in Canada in 1936 were estimated to be from $7 to 14 million annually.[101] The 1949 issue[102] of Bulletin No. 1596 still listed losses to cattle grubs of $50 to 100 million annually.

2. Weight Gains in Response to Control of Cattle Grub Larvae with Rotenone

When cattle grub larvae in warbles in feedlot cattle were controlled with rotenone, treated cattle gained from 0.05 to 0.19 kg/day per animal more than untreated cattle.[103] Over a 6-month period, uninfested steers gained an average of 61 kg and infested steers gained an average of 42 kg even though rotenone and nicotine-sulfur dusts killed cattle grub larvae in the backs of the infested cattle.[104] Feeder calves were treated monthly with rotenone to control cattle grub larvae, and the treated calves gained 2.1 to 5.3 kg more weight than untreated calves, but these differences were not statistically significant.[105]

3. Weight Gains after Treatment with Animal Systemic Insecticides

An opportunity to determine if the presence of cattle grub larvae in backs of cattle affected cattle production came with the advent of animal systemic insecticides that, when given to cattle after the end of the heel-fly season, prevented the appearance of cattle grub larvae in the backs of cattle.

Feedlot calves in which cattle grub larvae were controlled gained an average of 8.6 kg per animal more than untreated calves and also had better feed conversion.[106] With cattle on differing feed and protein supplements, no differences in weight gains could be related to the control of cattle grub larvae.[107] Although treated steers on winter rations had fewer cattle grub larvae in their backs than untreated steers, there were no differences in average weight gains; however, controlling cattle grub larvae in heifers on fattening rations caused a significant increase of 12 kg in average weight gains of treated cattle over those of untreated cattle.[108] Controlling cattle grub larvae in heifers or cows on a maintenance ration did not cause a significant difference in weight gains.[109] Control of cattle grub larvae in calves on a fattening ration or on a wintering ration did not affect weight gain significantly.[110,111] When ronnel was available for free-choice administration in a salt-bonemeal mixture, there was a sixfold variation in consumption of the treated mineral. Low consumption did not control cattle grub larvae and high consumption reduced weight gains in treated calves.[112] In a summary of 32 tests with feedlot cattle, Norris and Howe[113] reported increased weight gains in treated cattle in 9 of 12 trials when cattle were treated before November 1 and in 9 of 20 trials when cattle were treated after November 1 when cattle grub larvae were in their backs. Although cattle grub larvae were controlled, there was not a consistent relationship between control of larvae and gaining ability of calves held in a drylot.[114,115]

Control of cattle grub larvae in feedlot cattle did not affect weight gain, feed efficiency, dressing percentage, or carcass grade of cattle at slaughter.[116] When cattle grub larvae already in the backs of feedlot cattle were controlled, there was no difference in average daily gain, but hide damage and carcass trim at slaughter were less with treated cattle than with untreated cattle.[117]

Controlling cattle grub larvae in steers fed on grass hay did not cause a difference in weight gain between treated and untreated cattle. Also, there was no relationship between weight gains and numbers of cattle grub larvae, which ranged from 1 to >36 per animal, that appeared in the animal's back.[118] A variety of systemic treatments controlled cattle grub larvae but had no effect on weight gains of calves on grass hay ration[119] in a drylot[120,121] or on pasture.[122] Although cattle grub larvae were controlled, there was no consistent effect on average daily gain from treatment to weaning or in a feedlot after weaning.[123,124]

In a major study on the effects of the control of cattle grub larvae in feedlot cattle, Ludwig and Bucek[125] recorded significant increases in average daily gain of treated cattle and significant decreases in losses due to trimming of carcasses of treated cattle. In other feedlot trials, control of cattle grub larvae did not affect average daily gain or feed conversion.[126,127] When cattle grub larvae as well as certain roundworms were controlled in feedlot calves, the average daily gain and feed conversion were greater for treated calves than for untreated calves.[128]

As the result of a program for the area-wide control of cattle grubs in Canada,[129] treated cattle sold for $0.01 to 0.02 per kilogram more than untreated cattle, and numbers of hides with zero to four grub holes increased dramatically, thus avoiding the $0.02 per kilogram reduction in value of the hides. Also, the ranchers noted a dramatic decrease in gadding in the spring. In a specific study to determine the economics of cattle grub control in Canada, Rich[130] determined that losses at slaughter as a result of cattle grub damage ranged from $0.55 to 2.10 per carcass if animals were slaughtered when cattle grub larvae were in their backs. Unfortunately, there was no mechanism to return the profit from the treatment which accrued to the abattoir to the applicator of the treatment. In contrast, the average daily gain of treated, nursing calves from treatment date to weaning was greater than that of untreated calves in 2 of 3 years of testing, but treatment did not affect weights at any of the postweaning weighings.[131] Thus, the rancher would benefit from the preweaning gains if calves were sold at weaning.

Cattle grub larvae were controlled in a large number of feeder calves, and treated calves had a significantly higher gain of 5.4 kg per calf than untreated calves.[132] In contrast, in a series of 19 tests, there was no significant difference between average daily weight gains of treated and untreated calves on a wintering ration.[133] Controlling cattle grub larvae in steers on a fattening diet caused a significant increase of 13.4 to 29.9 kg per animal in weight gain of treated steers over untreated steers.[134]

4. Overview

Historically, cattle grubs/heel flies have been recognized as economically important pests of cattle. Losses in production as a result of the gadding of cattle by heel flies, the losses in value of hides with holes in them, and the downgrading of carcasses because of the presence of cattle grub larvae were obvious, although specific data on these losses were lacking.

Animal systemic insecticides, which prevented cattle grub larvae from appearing in the backs of cattle, allowed for the accumulation of data on the effects of these larvae on cattle production. Data on weight gains show that controlling cattle grub larvae in cattle held on maintenance rations has little or no effect on weight gains. However, cattle in feedlots gain more and that gain will be added more efficiently when cattle do not have cattle grub larvae in their backs. Losses occur if cattle have cattle grub larvae in their backs at slaughter. Economic benefits in terms of increased weight gains in feedlots or decreased losses as a result of fewer holes in hides or little or no trim of carcasses at slaughter experienced at the feedlot, the tannery, or the abattoir are not realized by the producer, who treated the calves with systemics. The producer will benefit as a result of decreased losses due to less gadding of cattle if there were few or no heel flies present on pasture the year following the use of systemics.

G. Lice

Early *U.S. Dep. Agric. Farmers' Bulletins*[135] listed effects of lice on cattle production as irritation, raw skin, hairless areas, lower vitality, unthrifty condition, decreased milk flow, stunted growth, and increased death rate. Heavier infestations were usually found on underfed and poorly housed animals and were first noticed on the weak and unthrifty animals, especially younger and older animals. Infestation was more common in winter when hair coats were long and diets were poor. These early publications did not present data on the effect of lice on productivity. Matthysse[136] stated that lice, especially high populations of the cattle biting louse♦, *Bovicola bovis* (Linnaeus), on dairy cattle, lowered milk production of cows and weight gains of heifers, but did not present data on losses.

1. Shortnosed Cattle Louse

One effect of sucking lice, especially as a result of heavy infestations of the shortnosed cattle louse♦, *Haematopinus eurysternus* (Nitzsch), on cattle, was anemia.[137] Red blood cell volume was reduced by 9 to 30%, but increased rapidly when lice were controlled. Cattle infested with *H. eurysternus* were anemic, unthrifty, lacked vigor, and had erythrocyte count and hemoglobin content about 50% of those of louse-free animals.[138]

Control of light to heavy populations of lice, principally *H. eurysternus,* on feeder heifers did not affect weight gains in a 42-day trial, and thus Scharff[139] concluded that control of sucking and biting lice on all but 5% of cattle was not of economic benefit, but that louse-prone or "carrier" cattle should be treated and/or eliminated from the herd. In contrast, Collins and Dewhirst[140] showed that heavy or moderate infestations of *H. eurysternus,* found on ca. 12% of cattle, can cause anemia and a significant increase in weight loss of range cattle without supplemental feed through the winter. Heifers were more affected by moderate infestations than bulls. There was a statistically significant negative correlation between numbers of *H. eurysternus* and average daily gain and final weight of steers,[141] and the type of ration appeared to influence the degree of louse infestation.

2. Mixed Infestations of Lice

As part of a large-scale field test with cattle primarily infested with *H. eurysternus, B. bovis,* and the longnosed cattle louse[*], *Linognathus vituli* (Linnaeus), in one trial, treated range cows gained an average of 34 kg per animal more than untreated cows.[142] In Canada, controlling mixed infestations of sucking and biting lice on cattle on different diets did not result in a significant difference between average weight gains of treated and untreated cattle.[143] In the U.S., in a series of tests with heifers infested with *L. vituli, B. bovis,* and *Solenopotes capillatus* Enderlein, the little blue louse,[144] there were significant differences in weight gains between heavily infested cattle and uninfested cattle, but not cattle with light to moderate or moderate to heavy infestations. There were no significant differences in feed consumption or feed efficiency between infested and louse-free cattle.

3. Overview

The only louse that appears to affect the production of cattle is the shortnosed cattle louse. Heavy infestations may cause anemia, and effects of the lice are particularly evident when cattle are stressed by less than adequate diets. Heavily infested cattle should be eliminated from the herd. There are complex interrelationships between nutrition and the effects of lice (and other arthropod pests as well) on productivity of cattle. Animals on a moderate to high plane of nutrition appear to be less affected by lice than animals on a poor level of nutrition. There is a need for additional data on the effects of biting lice and longnosed sucking lice on beef and dairy cattle that are maintained on different dietary levels.

H. Mites

Although only limited amounts of data are available on the effects of mites on cattle production, it appears that cattle production is affected only by infestations of the cattle follicle mite[*], *Demodex bovis* (Stiles), and the sheep scab mite[*], *Psoroptes ovis* (Hering). Infestations of *Demodex* and *Psoroptes* affect the quality of the leather, and *Psoroptes* infestations cause weight losses and other growth effects.

1. Damage to Hides and Leather

Early (1931) microscopic studies[145] of hides from cattle with demodectic mange showed that the mites damaged leather, but at that time there were no estimates of losses to the hides and leather industry from that damage. The pimple-like defects caused by demodectic mange in cattle, first seen in hides after the hair has been removed, resulted in coarse and scarred grain, weak leather, and holes in split leather. In 1954, these defects caused an estimated loss of $5 million per year.[146] Light infestations of demodectic mange caused little damage in finished leather, but a heavy infestation caused defects which made leather practically valueless. Leather damage was of more importance than the clinical manifestations of the infestation, which are often not detected.[147] Demodectic lesions were found in 7.7% of calf hides and more than 24% of cattle hides in Canada and caused serious leather defects.[148] Incidental infestation of cattle with demodectic mange mites causes a moderate to severe damage to the grain of leather.[63]

Psoroptes ovis infestation caused hyperkeratosis of cattle hides, and leather from untreated cattle was severely downgraded because of rough, uneven appearance due to papillation. Leather from a treated animal (mites were eradicated 24 days prior to slaughter) showed marked improvement, but the value of this leather was not equal to the value of leather from uninfested cattle.[149]

2. Weight Gains

Early USDA Farmers' Bulletins on scabies in cattle presented figures on estimated losses in production as a result of scab, especially psoroptic scab, but contained no specific data on losses documented by experimentation. In a study of case histories of five epizootics of *P. ovis* in feedlot cattle,[150] there was a decrease of 21.5% in feed consumption and a weight loss of 68 kg per infested animal. After elimination of infestation, an additional feeding time of 100 days was needed to restore cattle to marketable weights. Other losses included increased respiratory problems, injuries, treatment expense, and intangible losses, such as restricted markets and costs of quarantine procedures. In a drylot trial with calves exposed to *P. ovis*,[151] highly susceptible calves had to be removed from the test after 2 months because of life-threatening infestations. Weight gains of moderately susceptible, infested calves were 25%, and of refractory, infested calves were 63% of the weight gains of uninfested calves. There was a significant relationship between average subjective ratings of the amount of psoroptic scab and cumulative weight gains of steer calves. When scab infestations were classified as high, cumulative weight gains decreased significantly.[152] Treating of infested calves allowed for an immediate decrease in scab rating and an increase in weight gain. Infestations of *P. ovis* caused significant increases in total protein, α-, β-, and γ-globulin, and significant reduction in total cholesterol of infested calves.[153] In carefully controlled studies, infested cattle had significantly lower daily weight gains and gain to feed ratios than uninfested calves, and there was a significant relationship between extent of body area infested with mites and reduction in daily weight gain.[154]

3. Overview

Both *P. ovis* and *D. bovis* infestions cause defects in the leather of cattle. The hyperkeratosis caused by *P. ovis* and the pimple-like defects caused by *D. bovis* cause severe downgrading of leather. Additional studies are needed to further quantify the relationship between infestations of both species and defects found in hides and leather.

Psoroptes ovis infestation of cattle, if uncontrolled, can cause loss in condition and weight and can lead to the death of animals. Recent controlled studies showed that infested cattle had lowered weight gain and feed efficiency. There is little doubt that this arthropod is of economic significance, especially in feedlots and other crowded conditions.

I. Ticks

In the U.S., there are a few published reports on the effects of ticks on economics of cattle production. Early publications focused on the importance of the cattle tick♦, *Boophilus annulatus* (Say), that led to the eradication campaign. This species not only affected production of cattle when ticks were found in large numbers, but also the tick was the vector of babesiosis, a disease that was often fatal to cattle that had not become immune as calves. None of the other North American tick pests of livestock are vectors of major diseases of cattle; thus, their economic impact is the result of the effect that they have on weight gain, on damage to cattle hides, and as the cause of tick paralysis.

1. Cattle Tick

Cows were infested with larval cattle ticks and some cows, though previously exposed to cattle ticks and cattle fever, became sick with cattle fever. Some cows became more heavily infested than others; milk production of tick-infested cows was only ca. 67% of that of the uninfested cows and weight gain of tick-infested cows was 40% less than that of tick-free cows.[155] Although spraying dairy cows with arsenic caused a temporary reduction in milk flow of 6% for 5 days following treatment, at the end of a 152-day test the cows lightly infested with cattle ticks produced ca. 19% less and heavily infested cows produced ca. 42% less milk than tick-free cows.[156]

2. Lone Star Tick

Hereford steers, placed on pastures infested with the lone star tick♦, *Amblyomma amer-*

icanum (Linnaeus), were sprayed monthly to control ticks. These cattle gained 4 kg per animal more than untreated steers.[157] In a recent series of controlled experiments to determine the effects of *A. americanum* on the average daily gain of pre-weaner Angus calves, the injury threshold (the level of infestation that causes a significant injury) was estimated to be 15 feeding females per calf.[158] The economic threshold (the level at which cost of treatment is justified to prevent a loss) was estimated to range from 26 to 38 feeding female ticks per calf per day, depending upon the cost of the treatment.[159]

The lone star tick is not only an economically important pest of cattle, but also massive infestations cause gross tissue damage around the eyes and head and can lead to the death of fawns of the white-tailed deer, *Odocoileus virginianus*.[160] In addition, lone star ticks are a major problem in some recreational and tourist areas. The economic threshold of only 0.65 ticks per hour collected at CO_2-baited sites was suggested for general use to determine the need for tick management activities in recreational areas.[161]

3. Gulf Coast Tick

Infestations of the Gulf Coast tick♦, *A. maculatum* Koch, found in states along the Gulf Coast and through Oklahoma, can damage the ears of cattle, which results in a condition known as "gotch ear". These damaged ears were attractive sites for oviposition of the screwworm fly♦, *Cochliomyia hominivorax* (Coquerel), and resulted in a decreased value of cattle at sales.[162]

The effect of the Gulf Coast tick on weight gains of Hereford steers in a drylot for 7 weeks was 24 kg per animal with highly infested animals and 14 kg per animal with lightly infested cattle.[163] Tick-infested Hereford steers in drylot gained 27 kg less than uninfested steers, but tick infestation did not affect weight gains of Brahman steers.[164] Tick-infested Hereford steers on native grass pasture during the 8-week tick season gained an average of ca. 10 kg less per animal than uninfested cattle.[165]

4. Damage to Hides and Leather

Severe damage to the grain of leather was noted as a result of the infestation of cattle with ticks.[63] There was no difference in the damage caused by infestations of the lone star tick, the cayenne tick♦, *A. cajennense* (Fabricius), the Gulf Coast tick, and the American dog tick♦, *Dermacentor variabilis* (Say). Feeding lesions were not healed by 9 weeks after the ticks had fed.

5. Tick Paralysis

The subject of tick paralysis of livestock (also humans and pets) in North America was thoroughly reviewed by Gregson.[166] He recorded that paralysis in livestock was most prevalent in the northwestern part of the continent and was associated with the feeding of the Rocky Mountain wood tick♦, *Dermacentor andersoni* Stiles. Other species of ticks that can cause tick paralysis are the Pacific coast tick♦, *D. occidentalis* Marx, and *D. variabilis*. Paralysis can be rapidly reversed by the treating of cattle with acaricides to kill the attached ticks.

6. Overview

The losses in cattle production because of massive infestations of cattle ticks or the transmission of babesiosis by cattle ticks were eliminated with the eradication of cattle ticks from the U.S. The injury threshold of Lone Star ticks was only 15 feeding females per calf, and 26 to 38 feeding females per calf was the economic threshold. Lone star ticks affect the well-being of wildlife and are such a nuisance to humans that the threshold for the need to control lone star ticks at recreational areas is less than 1 tick per hour collected at CO_2 traps.

The Gulf Coast tick feeding on the ears of cattle causes a decrease in weight gains of cattle and a condition known as "gotch ear". It is reported that "gotch eared" cattle are of less value at sale than cattle with normal ears, but there are no quantitative data available to support that contention.

Preliminary tests show that the tissue destruction at the attachment sites of ticks causes severe damage to the grain of leather. Additional information is needed to determine the extent of that relationship. Although tick paralysis of cattle and other livestock is considered a problem, there are little data on losses in cattle as a result of paralysis.

III. EFFECTS OF ARTHROPOD PESTS ON PRODUCTION OF SHEEP AND GOATS

Sheep and goats are parasitized by a variety of arthropod pests that live continuously on or in sheep and goats or are found intermittently feeding on the animals. Limited data have been obtained on specific responses of sheep to these various pests in North America, and some data have been obtained with these same pests in other countries.

A. Sheep Keds and Lice
1. Production Losses due to Sheep Keds

U.S. Dep. Agric. Farmers' Bulletin No. 798, in 1917,[167] stated that the sheep ked*, *Melophagus ovinus* (Linnaeus), reduced vitality, stunted growth, and damaged wool, and estimated losses at $0.25 per lamb and $0.20 per ewe.

Several specific studies, designed to evaluate the effect of keds on weight gains and wool production in feeder lambs, showed that keds had no significant effect on either factor.[168-170] In South Africa,[171] keds did not affect body weight or quantity of scoured wool of Merino sheep on a good diet, but with sheep on a poor diet, keds caused a 20% death loss and 10% reduction in the value of wool. In Canada, ked-free lambs on an alfalfa hay diet gained 3.5 kg per animal more than infested lambs, and the difference was only 1.5 kg per animal when lambs were fed a high-energy ration, but neither difference was statistically significant.[172] However, ked-resistant yearling ewes produced ca. 11% less clean wool than ked-free ewes.

2. Keds as the Cause of Cockle

"Cockle", which consists of dense brownish nodules found in the grain layer of sheepskin, seriously downgrades both grain and suede leather. The feeding of keds is the cause of "cockle",[173] and such damage need not be confused with "seedy" or "ticky" defects caused by sharp seeds and awns of grasses.[174] Lambs on an alfalfa hay diet[175] had a statistically significant, 9% lower carcass weight as a result of ked infestation; however, greater losses of 29% were recorded for wool yield and quality, and greatest losses of 47% were recorded as a result of downgrading of hides for suede because of "cockle".

3. Biting Lice

Control of a biting louse, *Bovicola limbata*, on Angora goats[176] did not increase weight gains or weights of fleeces. In New Zealand, moderate numbers of the sheep biting louse*, *Bovicola ovis* (Schrank), did not affect weight gains of infested sheep, nor fleece weight, but quality of the fleece was lowered.[177] In Australia, sheep biting lice did not affect live weight gain of Merino sheep but lowered production of clean wool by 0.3 to 0.8 kg per sheep, and infested wool yielded, at processing, 4.8 to 7.2% less of the top wool and short fibers than uninfested wool.[178]

B. Sheep Scab Mite and Other Mite Pests

Sheep scab, caused by the sheep scab mite*, *Psoroptes ovis* (Hering), a very important ectoparasite of sheep throughout the world, has been eradicated in the U.S.[179] As early as 1898, the USDA Bureau of Animal Industry Bulletin No. 21[180] listed losses in wool production, general unthriftiness, and death of sheep as a result of scab and called for its eradication from the U.S. Because this pest is so obviously injurious to sheep and wool production, there appears to be little experimental data on losses as a result of *P. ovis* infestation. Recent studies in the U.K. showed that untreated, infested sheep had a 30% loss in weight gain over 14 weeks, plus a loss of 0.2 kg of wool per sheep and the fleece that remained was ragged and stained.[181]

Although rarely found in the U.S., in Australia, *Psorergates ovis* Womersley causes fleece derangement in fine-wooled Merino sheep, which can lead to severe and extensive fleece damage and discoloration.[182] Infestations of the goat follicle mite♦, *Demodex caprae* Railliet, especially in the nodular form, caused holes and white spots in leather from goats in India.[183] Occasionally, infestations of *Psoroptes cuniculi* Delafond or *D. caprae* require treatment of dairy goats in the U.S.[184]

C. Myiasis-Producing Flies

No specific data are available on losses in sheep and goat production in the U.S. as a result of infestations by larvae of blow flies or fleece worms. Generally, infestations are scattered and limited, but large numbers of sheep and goats can be infested and should be treated.

In constrast, in Australia,[185] an analysis of production costs of the sheep industry in 1962 to 1963 concluded that annual direct losses, in terms of death, wool losses, and value depreciation, plus costs of control measures, were 9.9 million pounds for blow flies alone. Costs of control only of keds, biting lice, and itch mite were 4.7 million pounds; this estimate did not include production losses of fleece damage, loss of wool rubbed off sheep, unthriftiness, and loss of body condition. These estimates, updated[186] in 1969 to 1970, showed that losses had increased to 28.0 million Australian dollars for blow flies and 9.4 million Australian dollars for other external parasites. By 1975 to 1976, estimated costs and losses for blow flies alone increased to 44.3 million Australian dollars.[187]

In the U.S., nuisance flies that congregated on exudates from shearing cuts on recently sheared lambs were controlled,[188] and the treated lambs gained significantly more weight than untreated lambs.

D. Sheep Bot Larvae

Although the sheep bot fly♦, *Oestrus ovis* Linnaeus, has been recognized for centuries as a parasite of sheep, little experimental data exist on the effect of larvae of this pest on productivity of sheep. In a feedlot and pasture experiment in which lambs were freed of *O. ovis* larvae,[189] there were no significant differences in growth curves, weight gains, and carcass evaluations between treated and untreated lambs. In Russia,[190] control of *O. ovis* larvae allowed treated lambs to gain 19 g/day more than untreated lambs and to produce an average of 117 g more wool. Treated sheep averaged 3.2 kg more weight and 200 g more wool than untreated sheep.[191]

In South Africa, control of sheep bot fly larvae[192] allowed for increased weight gains in treated lambs of 1.5 to 1.9 kg per animal greater than infested sheep. Control of *O. ovis*, nematodes, and cestodes by treatment at specific intervals or "strategically" allowed for greater live weight gains and wool production in treated lambs than in untreated lambs.[193]

E. Overview

There are some overseas data that show that keds and lice are an economic problem for sheep raisers, but critical tests are needed for the U.S. and Canada. There is no doubt that keds are the cause of "cockle", a serious defect in the leather of sheep, and control of keds can be justified by prevention of this loss alone.

The eradication of *Psoroptes ovis* from sheep in the U.S. eliminated the losses from this very destructive and economically important pest. Other mite pests appear to be of little economic significance. However, additional data need to be obtained on the effects of demodicosis on leather from goats.

If sheep or goats become infested with fleece worms or wool maggots they must be treated in order to prevent production losses. These infestations can be kept to a minimum by appropriate ranching operations. There are no data in the U.S. on the economic consequences as the result of these infestations.

The only data obtained in the U.S. showed that infestations of sheep bot fly larvae did not affect production of sheep. There are enough foreign data that show there is an economic aspect to the infestation, but much more data from carefully controlled tests are needed in order to accurately define the extent of loss caused by sheep bot larvae on production of sheep.

IV. EFFECTS OF ARTHROPOD PESTS ON PRODUCTION OF SWINE

In the U.S., there are few reported specific studies to determine the effects of infestation of the hog louse♦, *Haematopinus suis* (Linnaeus), the itch mite♦, *Sarcoptes scabiei* (De Geer), and other arthropods on the economics of swine production. Hog lice cause discomfort in swine, and infested animals scratch themselves on any stationary object. Such scratching leads to thick, cracked, and tender skin and arrested growth and unthrifty feed conversion. Lice also can transmit the virus of swine pox and the staphylococcus infection that often accompanies the skin lesions. Lice are potential vectors of hog cholera (eradicated from the U.S.) and eperythrozoonosis. High infestations of lice cause a skin condition that makes hair removal difficult at slaughter. It is interesting that in spite of all the statements above, we can find no trials in the literature that present specific data on the physiological or economic effects of parasitism of swine by the hog louse.

General effects of infestation of swine with itch mites include intense itching and scratching, urticaria, pruritis, and rough, thickened, encrusted, dry, reddened skin that may become raw, cracked, and heavily folded. Production responses in swine include loss of condition, decreased growth rates, decrease in feed efficiency, emaciation, stunting, and even death.

A number of the early USDA publications only present figures on estimated losses due to lice and mites. However, critical controlled studies conducted in the U.K., Australia, and, most recently, in the U.S. have quantitated the effect of itch mites on swine production.

A. Estimates of Losses to Lice and Itch Mites

U.S. Dep. Agric. Farmers' Bulletin No. 1085 in 1920[194] estimated that hog lice caused a 2 to 6% loss in market value of infested swine. The 1942 *U.S. Dep. Agric. Yearbook of Agriculture*[195] noted that there were no specific data on losses in swine production to mange mites, but estimated losses at about $2 per animal in infested herds plus losses at slaughter and of hide value.

B. Controlled Clinical Trials with Itch Mites

Magee[196] controlled mange and found no difference in weight gains between treated and untreated swine, but related the lack of a difference to a high plane of nutrition of the animals and development of resistance of the infested swine to the mites. In South Australia, where sarcoptic mange of swine is a notifiable disease, losses of 500,000 Australian dollars per year were the result of chronic mange, mite hypersensitivity, condemnation at slaughter, rejection at markets, and costs of control treatments.[197] Yeoman[198] reviewed earlier studies and considered sarcoptic mange of swine a major depressant on productivity and warned of losses not only from chronic mange, with its classical symptoms and mite isolations, but also from mite hypersensitivity.

In Ireland, artificial infestation of portions of litters of piglets with *S. scabiei* did not cause a statistically significant reduction in growth rate or feed efficiency. However, sarcoptic mange could stress swine so that other factors or coexistent diseases would cause the production effects observed by earlier workers.[199] In contrast, treatment of infested swine with an insecticide to eliminate *S. scabiei* allowed for a highly statistically significant improvement (ca. 20%) in weight gains of treated swine.[200]

In Australia, mite-infested pigs had growth rates depressed by 9.2 to 12.5% and feed efficiency depressed by 9.4 to 12.5%. The loss was closely related to the intensity of a generalized hypersensitivity reaction to mange mites rather than to the extent of classical lesions.[201] Control of sarcoptic mange on fattening swine allowed for an increased weight gain of 2.3 to 7% and increased feed efficiency of ca. 10%.[202] Control of sarcoptic mange in sows significantly increased average daily weight gain and weights of piglets at weaning by ca. 9%.[203,204] Elimination of *S. scabiei* caused a significant increase in average weight gain of castrated males, but not females, and the feed efficiency was greater in treated than untreated animals.[205]

In the U.S., even with modern pork production systems, including confinement production, hog lice and itch mites were found on 12 to 41% of swine examined.[206] Results of recent trials in the U.S. indicate that control of sarcoptic mange on swine allowed for a weight gain of 2.4 to 5 kg per animal, a 5.6 to 14.3% increase in feed efficiency, 7 to 14 days earlier maturity of feeder pigs, 0.5 to 2.1 more pigs weaned per litter, a 5.6 to 6.2% decrease in death loss to weaning, and a 8.9 kg per litter increase in weaning weight.[207]

C. Biting and Nuisance Flies

Feeder pigs exposed to house flies and stable flies, in a controlled test, gained an average of 1.8 kg per pig less than fly-free pigs over 84- and 98-day feeding trials.[208] This difference was not statistically significant; however, the populations of house flies and stable flies may have been below the economic threshold level. There were no differences in feed efficiencies.

D. Overview

There are no specific data that show that the hog louse causes economic losses in the production of swine. There is a need for controlled trials with louse-infested swine to determine if diet and nutrition levels affect the influence that lice may have on productivity. There are adequate data available to prove that infestations of itch mites affect weight gains, feed efficiency, maturity of feeder pigs, and death losses. Certainly, these losses can be prevented by eliminating the itch mite from swine herds and then keeping the herds free of this pest.

V. EFFECTS OF ARTHROPOD PESTS ON PRODUCTION OF POULTRY

Poultry are infested with a variety of lice, mites, fleas, ticks, bed bugs, flies, and other arthropod pests. For most pests, quantitative data on effects of infestation on production are lacking. For example, the chicken mite◆, *Dermanyssus gallinae* (De Geer), was described in *U.S. Dep. Agric. Farmers' Bulletin* No. 801 in 1917[209] as a pest that, in heavily infested coops, can cause weakening of hens, anemia, loss of egg or chick production, or death of hens. In *U.S. Dep. Agric. Farmers' Bulletin* No. 1070 in 1919,[210] the fowl tick◆, *Argas persicus* (Oken), was reported to cause weakness in poultry, anemia, reduction in egg production and growth, and death of poultry. With appearance of modern, confined techniques of rearing poultry, infestations of these once common pests are rare and usually limited to small flocks of chickens maintained for personal use.

There is limited information on the effects of certain arthropod pests on poultry production in terms of weight gain, egg production, and other parameters.

A. Biting Lice

Data presented on the effects of "body" lice on production of eggs[211] indicated no significant difference in production between hens with heavy, moderate, light, or no infestation. In contrast, moderate infestations of the chicken body louse*, *Menacanthus stramineus* (Nitzsch), caused a 11.7% reduction in egg production, an increased mortality of 3.7% and decreased weight gains.[212] There were statistically significant decreases in egg production, especially during weeks 10 to 14 of the laying period as a result of chicken body louse infestation.[213] Chicken body louse infestation of hens did not affect egg production nor weight gains of broilers, which were marketed before lice could reach deleterious populations.[214] Artificial infestations of caged laying hens with the chicken body louse significantly reduced egg production, hen weights, and feed efficiency. All these decreases were correlated with the density of the louse population.[215]

B. Northern Fowl Mite

The northern fowl mite*, *Ornithonyssus sylviarum* (Canestrini & Fanzago), first found on poultry in the U.S. in 1917,[216] has subsequently become the most important arthropod pest of poultry held under modern, high-density poultry production conditions. Cameron[217] reviewed the early literature on the economic significance of the northern fowl mite and noted death, loss of blood, reduced egg production, secondary infection of mite "bites", and an intrinsic variability of infestation on different chickens. Noting that there were no data on the specific effects of infestation of northern fowl mites on the well being of poultry or on egg production, Loomis et al.[218] infested caged laying hens with northern fowl mites and determined that egg production or blood parameters were not affected by heavy infestations of mites. In other tests, roosters were more affected than hens as a result of mite infestation, and there was a 9.8% decrease in egg production of hens; this decrease was especially evident with hens on a lower protein diet.[219] Insecticide treatment to control northern fowl mites was recommended, for the costs of control were much lower than losses in egg production. The infestation of roosters by the northern fowl mite caused ca. 4% loss in weight gain and a decrease in seminal fluid and serum testosterone levels.[220]

A national survey indicated that the northern fowl mite was considered by the poultry producers and extension specialists as the most important arthropod pest of the poultry industry.[221] Controlling northern fowl mites on hens by clipping feathers in the vent area significantly reduced populations of the northern fowl mite but did not cause a significant increase in egg production. Egg production of infested, unclipped hens was significantly less (7.6%) than egg production of uninfested hens; there was no effect of infestation on egg weight, hen weight or feed consumption.[222] Northern fowl mites did not affect egg production, and heavier hens had more mites than lighter ones.[223] Although shells of eggs laid by mite-infested hens were significantly thicker than those laid by uninfested hens, both figures were within the normal biological range.[224] Dipping hens in acaricides eliminated northern fowl mites and prevented decreases in egg production, but had no effect on body weight or feed consumption.[225] Controlling northern fowl mites did not affect feed consumption, egg weight, or feed efficiency, but significantly increased egg mass (gram of egg per hen per day).[226] Northern fowl mite infestations of broiler-breeder flocks caused a loss of 7.7 eggs per hen and a decrease in feed efficiency.[227] Controlling northern fowl mites did not significantly affect egg weight or percentage egg production, although both were higher with treated hens.[228]

C. Turkey Chigger on Turkey Production

The turkey chigger*, *Neoschongastia americana* (Hirst), found in heavy clay soils in southern and western states, attaches to turkeys in clumps that cause lesions on the skin of turkeys.[229] If turkeys are slaughtered before or after the chigger season, such lesions are not a problem. However, modern turkey production allows for slaughter throughout the year, and the presence of these lesions causes a downgrading of the turkey carcass because of the trimming of the skin necessary to remove the lesion.[230] The treating of soil controlled chiggers and decreased losses from \$0.55 to 1.10 per turkey.[231,232] Turkeys on a 10-year-old range averaged significantly more lesions than turkeys on a new range.[233]

D. Biting of Black Flies on Egg Production

An outbreak of a black fly, *Simulium meridionale* Riley, caused a decrease in egg production of caged layers of greater than 60% during the period when large numbers of flies were feeding on the hens.[234] In Jasper County, South Carolina, annual death loss to *Leucocytozoon* disease in turkeys, transmitted by black flies, was estimated to be 5% of the production.[235]

E. Overview

As a result of modern systems of poultry production, domestic fowl are seldom infested with lice, the chicken mite, the fowl tick, or other "classic" pests. In contrast, modern systems are ideal for the development of high populations of the northern fowl mite. Infested hens lay significantly fewer eggs than uninfested hens. There are also lesser effects on weight gains, feed conversion, and other aspects of poultry production as a result of infestations of northern fowl mites.

The turkey chigger is an economic problem if turkeys are processed when they have feeding lesions on their skin. These areas must be trimmed and the trimming causes a downgrading of the carcass. Controlling the chiggers prevents this loss.

Massive numbers of black flies feeding on chickens caused a decrease in egg production. The transmission of *Leucocytozoon* disease by black flies is an economic problem in certain areas of South Carolina.

REFERENCES

1. **Hyslop, J. A.,** An estimate of the damage by some of the more important insect pests in the United States, Bur. Entomol. Plant Quaran. E-286, U.S. Department of Agriculture, Washington, D.C., 1930.
2. **Hyslop, J. A.,** Losses occasioned by insects, mites, and ticks in the United States, Bur. Entomol. Plant Quaran., E-444, U.S. Department of Agriculture, Washington, D.C., 1938.
3. **Mohler, J. R., Wight, A. E., MacKellar, W. M., and Bishopp, F. C.,** Losses caused by animal diseases and parasites, *U.S. Dep. Agric. Yearb. Agric.,* 109, 1942.
4. U.S. Department of Agriculture, Losses in agriculture, a preliminary appraisal for review, ARS-20-1, U.S. Department of Agriculture, Washington, D.C., 1954.
5. U.S. Department of Agriculture, Losses in agriculture, *U.S. Dep. Agric. Agric. Handb.,* 291, 1965.
6. **Drummond, R. O., Lambert, G., Smalley, H. E., Jr., and Terrill, C. E.,** Estimated losses of livestock to pests, in *CRC Handbook of Pest Management in Agriculture,* Vol. 1, Pimentel, D., Ed., CRC Press, Boca Raton, Fla., 1981, 111.
7. **Steelman, C. D.,** Effects of external and internal arthropod parasites on domestic livestock production, *Annu. Rev. Entomol.,* 21, 155, 1976.
8. **Geier, P. W.,** The concept of pest management — economic threshold levels of losses, *Prot. Ecol.,* 4, 239, 1982.
9. **Gibson, T. E.,** The cost of animal parasites, *Span,* 7, 2, 1964.
10. **Snelson, J. T.,** Animal ectoparasites and disease vectors causing major reductions in world food supplies, *FAO Plant Prot. Bull.,* 23, 103, 1975.
11. **Jacobs, D. E.,** Pest control in livestock production, in *Pesticides and Human Welfare,* Gunn, D. L. and Stevens, J. G. R., Eds., Oxford University Press, Oxford, England, 1976, 103.
12. **Pritchard, W. R.,** Animal disease constraints to world food production, *Theriogenology,* 6, 305, 1976.
13. **Griffiths, R. B.,** The relevance of parasitology to human welfare today — veterinary aspects, *Br. Soc. Parasitol.,* 16, 41, 1977.

14. **Drummond, R. O., Bram, R. A., and Konnerup, N.,** Animal pests and world food production, in *World Food, Pest Losses, and the Environment,* Pimentel, D., Ed., Westview Press, Boulder, Colo., 1978, 63.

15. **Fallis, A. M.,** Arthropods as pests and vectors of disease, *Vet. Parasitol.,* 6, 47, 1980.

16. **Wharton, R. H. and Norris, K. R.,** Control of parasitic arthropods, *Vet. Parasitol.,* 6, 135, 1980.

17. **Palmer, W. A. and Bay, D. E.,** A review of the economic importance of the horn fly, *Haematobia irritans irritans* (L.), *Prot. Ecol.,* 3, 237, 1981.

18. **Decker, G. C.,** Fly control on livestock — does it pay? I, *Soap Chem. Spec.,* 21, 142, 1955.

19. **Decker, G. C.,** Fly control on livestock — does it pay? II, *Soap Chem. Spec.,* 21, 151, 1955.

20. **Granett, P. and Hansens, E. J.,** The effect of biting fly control on milk production, *J. Econ. Entomol.,* 49, 465, 1956.

21. **Granett, P. and Hansens, E. J.,** Further observations on the effect of biting fly control on milk production on cattle, *J. Econ. Entomol.,* 50, 332, 1957.

22. **Cheng, T. and Kesler, E. M.,** A three-year study on the effect of fly control on milk production by selected and randomized dairy herds, *J. Econ. Entomol.,* 54, 751, 1961.

23. **Cheng, T.,** The effect of biting fly control on weight gain in beef cattle, *J. Econ. Entomol.,* 51, 275, 1958.

24. **Cutkomp, L. K. and Harvey, A. L.,** The weight responses of beef cattle in relation to control of horn and stable flies, *J. Econ. Entomol.,* 51, 72, 1958.

25. **Laake, E. W.,** DDT for the control of the horn fly in Kansas, *J. Econ. Entomol.,* 39, 65, 1946.

26. **Neel, W. W.,** The effectiveness of new repellents for the control of horn flies on dairy cattle, *J. Econ. Entomol.,* 50, 502, 1957.

27. **Haufe, W. O. and Thompson, C. O. M.,** Weight changes in cattle on dry range in relation to chemical treatments for fly control, *Can. J. Anim. Sci.,* 44, 272, 1964.

28. **Haufe, W. O.,** Interaction of pesticidal toxicity, parasites, and reversible anticholinesterase activity as stresses on growth rate in cattle infested with horn flies *Haematobia irritans* L., *Toxicol. Appl. Pharmacol.,* 25, 130, 1973.

29. **Khan, M. A. and Lawson, J. E.,** Summer treatments for cattle grub control and their effects on horn flies and cattle weight gains, *Can. J. Anim. Sci.,* 45, 43, 1965.

30. **Essig, H. W. and Pund, W. A.,** Horn fly control in beef cattle, *Feedstuffs,* 37, 34, 1965.

31. **Duren, E. and O'Keeffe, L. E.,** Horn fly control with dust bags: Effect on weight gains, *Anim. Nutr. Health,* 27, 3, 1972.

32. **Roberts, R. H. and Pund, W. A.,** Control of biting flies on beef steers: Effect on performance in pasture and feedlot *J. Econ. Entomol.,* 67, 232, 1974.

33. **Campbell, J. B.,** Effect of horn fly control on cows as expressed by increased weaning weights of calves, *J. Econ. Entomol.,* 69, 711, 1976.

34. **Huston, J. E., Wilson, N. L., and Bales, K. W.,** Effect of stirofos-impregnated ear tags on horn fly numbers and weight changes in beef cattle, *Texas Agric. Exp. Stat. Misc. Publ.,* 1429, 1979.

35. **Harvey, T. L. and Brethour, J. R.,** Effect of horn flies on weight gains of beef cattle, *J. Econ. Entomol.,* 72, 516, 1979.

36. **Harvey, T. L. and Brethour, J. R.,** Control of horn fly, *Haematobia irritans* (L.) (Diptera: Muscidae) on cattle by partial herd treatment with fenvalerate-impregnated ear tags, *Prot. Ecol.,* 2, 313, 1981.

37. **Harvey, T. L. and Launchbaugh, J. L.,** Effect of horn flies on behavior of cattle, *J. Econ. Entomol.,* 75, 25, 1982.

38. **Haufe, W. O.,** Growth of range cattle protected from horn flies *(Haematobia irritans)* by ear tags impregnated with fenvalerate, *Can. J. Anim. Sci.,* 62, 567, 1982.

39. **Kunz, S. E., Miller, J. A., Sims, P. L., and Meyerhoeffer, D. C.,** Economics of controlling horn flies (Diptera: Muscidae) in range cattle management, *J. Econ. Entomol.,* 77, 657, 1984.

40. **Quisenberry, S. S. and Strohbehn, D. R.,** Horn fly (Diptera: Muscidae) control on beef cows with permethrin-impregnated ear tags and effect on subsequent calf weight gains, *J. Econ. Entomol.,* 77, 422, 1984.

41. **Haufe, W. O.,** Reduced productivity of beef cattle infested with horn flies, in *Research Highlights — 1978,* Croome, G. C. R. and Holmes, N. O., Eds., Agriculture Canada Research Station, Lethbridge, Alberta, Canada, 1979, 61.

42. **Haufe, W. O.,** Efficiency of horn fly control and production of beef cattle on pasture, in *Research Highlights — 1980,* Croome, G. C. R. and Atkinson, T. G., Eds., Agriculture Canada Research Station, Lethbridge, Alberta, Canada, 1981, 49.

43. **Klein, K. K. and Gordon, D. V.,** Economic threshold for horn fly control in Alberta, in *Research Highlights — 1980,* Croome, G. C. R. and Atkinson, T. G., Eds., Agriculture Canada Research Station, Lethbridge, Alberta, Canada, 1981, 47.

44. **Freeborn, S. B., Regan, W. M., and Folger, A. H.,** The relation of flies and fly sprays to milk production, *J. Econ. Entomol.,* 18, 779, 1925.

45. **Kinzer, H. G., Houghton, W. E., Reeves, J. M., Kunz, S. E., Wallace, J. D., and Urquhart, N. S.,** Influence of horn flies on weight loss in cattle with notes on prevention of loss by insecticide treatment, *Southwest. Entomol.,* 9, 212, 1984.

46. **Eckles, C. H.,** Test of a fly repellant, *Univ. Mo. Agric. Exp. Stat. Bull. No. 68,* 1905.

47. **Baker, A. W. and College, O. A.,** The effect of stable and horn fly attacks on milk production, *Annu. Rep. Entomol. Soc. Ont.* 30, 91, 1918.

48. **Shaw, A. O. and Atkeson, F. W.,** Effect of spraying cows with repellent type sprays as measured by milk production, *Dairy Sci.,* 26, 179, 1943.

49. **Bruce, W. N. and Decker, G. C.,** Fly control and milk flow, *J. Econ. Entomol.,* 40, 530, 1947.

50. **Bruce, W. N. and Decker, G. C.,** The relationship of stable fly abundance to milk production in dairy cattle, *J. Econ. Entomol.,* 51, 269, 1958.

51. **Berry, I. L., Stage, D. A., and Campbell, J. B.,** Populations and economic impacts of stable flies on cattle, *Trans. Am. Assoc. Agric. Eng.,* 26, 873, 1983.

52. **Freeborn, S. B., Regan, W. M., and Folger, A. H.,** The relation of flies and fly sprays to milk production, *J. Econ. Entomol.,* 21, 494, 1928.

53. **Melvin, R.,** Physiological studies on the effect of flies and fly sprays on cattle, *J. Econ. Entomol.,* 25, 1151, 1932.

54. **Miller, R. W., Pickens, L. G., Morgan, N. O., Thimijan, R. W., and Wilson, R. L.,** Effect of stable flies on feed intake and milk production of dairy cows, *J. Econ. Entomol.,* 66, 711, 1973.

55. **Campbell, J. B., White, R. G., Wright, J. E., Crookshank, R., and Clanton, D. C.,** Effects of stable flies on weight gains and feed efficiency of calves on growing or finishing rations. *J. Econ. Entomol.,* 70, 592, 1977.

56. **Bishopp, F. C.,** Mosquitoes kill live stock, *Science,* 77, 115, 1933.

57. **Hoffman, R. A. and McDuffie, W. C.,** The 1962 Gulf Coast mosquito problem and the associated losses in livestock, in Proc. 50th Annu. Meet. N.J. Mosq. Exterm. Assoc. and 19th Annu. Meet. Am. Mosq. Control Assoc., 421, 1963.

58. **Sanders, D. P., Riewe, M. E., and McNeill, J. C.,** Salt marsh mosquito control in relation to beef cattle production: a preliminary report, *Mosq. News,* 28, 311, 1968.

59. **Abbitt, B. and Abbitt, L. G.,** Fatal exsanguination of cattle attributed to an attack of salt marsh mosquitoes *(Aedes sollicitans), J. Am. Vet. Med. Assoc.,* 179, 1397, 1981.

60. **Steelman, C. D., White, T. W., and Schilling, P. E.,** Effects of mosquitoes on the average daily gain of feedlot steers in southern Louisiana, *J. Econ. Entomol.,* 65, 462, 1972.

61. **Steelman, C. D., White, T. W., and Schilling, P. E.,** Effects of mosquitoes on the average daily gain of Hereford and Brahman breed steers in southern Louisiana, *J. Econ. Entomol.,* 66, 1081, 1973.

62. **Steelman, C. D., White, T. W., and Schilling, P. E.,** Efficacy of Brahman characters in reducing weight loss of steers exposed to mosquito attack, *J. Econ. Entomol.,* 69, 499, 1976.

63. **Everett, A. L., Miller, R. W., Gladney, W. J., and Hannigan, M. V.,** Effects of some important ectoparasites on the grain quality of cattlehide leather, *J. Am. Leather Chem. Assoc.,* 72, 6, 1977.

64. **Millar, J. L. and Rempel, J. G.,** Live stock losses in Saskatchewan due to blackflies, *Can. J. Comp. Med. Vet. Sci.* 8, 334, 1944.

65. **Rempel, J. G. and Arnason, A. P.,** An account of three successive outbreaks of the black fly, *Simulium arcticum,* a serious livestock pest in Saskatchewan, *Sci. Agric.,* 27, 428, 1947.

66. **Fredeen, F. J. H.,** A review of the economic importance of black flies (Simuliidae) in Canada, *Quaest. Entomol.,* 13, 219, 1977.

67. **Khan, M. A.,** Protection of pastured cattle from black flies (Diptera: Simuliidae): improved weight gains following a dermal application of phosmet, *Vet. Parasitol.,* 8, 327, 1981.

68. **Khan, M. A. and Kozub, G. C.,** Response of Angus, Charolais, and Hereford bulls to black flies (*Simulium* spp.), with and without phosmet treatment, *Can. J. Anim. Sci.,* 65, 269, 1985.

69. **Anderson, J. R. and Voskuil, G. H.,** A reduction in milk production caused by the feeding of blackflies (Diptera:Simuliidae) on dairy cattle in California, with notes on the feeding activity on other animals, *Mosq. News,* 23, 126, 1963.

70. **Bruce, W. N. and Decker, G. C.,** Tabanid control on dairy and beef cattle with synergized pyrethrins, *J. Econ. Entomol.,* 44, 154, 1951.

71. **Bruce, W. N. and Decker, G. C.,** Factors affecting the performance of treadle sprayers, *J. Econ. Entomol.,* 48, 167, 1955.

72. **Perich, M. J., Wright, R. E., and Lusby, K. S.,** Impact of horse flies (Diptera: Tabanidae) on beef cattle, *J. Econ. Entomol.,* 79, 128, 1986.

73. **Tashiro, H. and Schwardt, H. H.,** Biology of the major species of horse flies of central New York, *J. Econ. Entomol.,* 42, 269, 1949.

74. **Hollander, A. L. and Wright, R. E.,** Impact of tabanids on cattle: blood meal size and preferred feeding sites, *J. Econ. Entomol.,* 73, 431, 1980.

75. **Krinsky, W. L.**, Animal disease agents transmitted by horse flies and deer flies (Diptera: Tabanidae), *J. Med. Entomol.*, 13, 225, 1976.

76. **Hawkins, J. A., Love, J. H., and Hidalgo, R. J.**, Mechanical transmission of anaplasmosis by tabanids (Diptera: Tabanidae), *Am. J. Vet. Res.*, 43, 732, 1982.

77. **Teskey, H. J.**, On the behavior and ecology of the face fly, *Musca autumnalis* (Diptera: Muscidae), *Can. Entomol.*, 101, 561, 1969.

78. **Brown, J. F. and Adkins, T. R., Jr.**, Relationship of feeding activity of face fly (*Musca autumnalis* DeGeer) to production of keratoconjunctivitis in calves, *Am. J. Vet. Res.*, 33, 2551, 1972.

79. **Shugart, J. I., Campbell, J. B., Hudson, D. B., Hibbs, C. M., White, R. G., and Clanton, D. C.**, Ability of the face fly to cause damage to eyes of cattle, *J. Econ. Entomol.*, 72, 633, 1979.

80. **Arends, J. J., Wright, R. E., Lusby, K. S., and McNew, R. W.**, Effect of face flies (Diptera: Muscidae) on weight gains and feed efficiency in beef heifers, *J. Econ. Entomol.*, 75, 794, 1982.

81. **Schmidtmann, E. T., Valla, M. E., and Chase, L. E.**, Effect of face flies on grazing time and weight gain in dairy heifers, *J. Econ. Entomol.*, 74, 33, 1981.

82. **Schmidtmann, E. T., Berkebile, D., Miller, R. W., and Douglass, L. W.**, The face fly (Diptera: Muscidae): effect on Holstein milk secretion, *J. Econ. Entomol.*, 77, 1200, 1984.

83. **Thrift, F. A. and Overfield, J. R.**, Impact of pinkeye (infectious bovine kerato-conjunctivitis) on weaning and postweaning performance of Hereford calves, *J. Anim. Sci.*, 38, 1179, 1974.

84. **Cheng, T.**, Frequency of pinkeye incidence in cattle in relation to face fly abundance, *J. Econ. Entomol.*, 60, 598, 1967.

85. **Steve, P. C. and Lilly, J. H.**, Investigations on transmissability of *Moraxella bovis* by the face fly, *J. Econ. Entomol.*, 58, 444, 1965.

86. **Berkebile, D. R., Hall, R. D., and Webber, J. J.**, Field association of female face flies with *Moraxella bovis*, an etiological agent of bovine pinkeye, *J. Econ. Entomol.*, 74, 475, 1981.

87. **Gerhardt, R. R., Allen, J. W., Greene, W. H., and Smith, P. C.**, The role of face flies in an episode of infectious bovine keratoconjunctivitis, *J. Am. Vet. Med. Assoc.*, 180, 156, 1982.

88. **Glass, H. W., Jr. and Gerhardt, R. R.**, Recovery of *Moraxella bovis* (Hauduroy) from the crops of face flies (Diptera: Muscidae) fed on the eyes of cattle with infectious bovine keratoconjunctivitis, *J. Econ. Entomol.*, 76, 532, 1983.

89. **Hall, R. D.**, Relationship of the face fly (Diptera: Muscidae) to pinkeye in cattle: a review and synthesis of the relevant literature, *J. Med. Entomol.*, 21, 361, 1984.

90. **Troutt, H. F. and Schurig, G.**, Part 2: Infectious bovine keratoconjunctivitis "Pinkeye", *Anim. Nutr. Health*, 40, 14, 1985.

91. **Chitwood, M. B. and Stoffolano, J. G.**, First report of *Thelazia* sp. (Nematoda) in the face fly, *Musca autumnalis*, in North America, *J. Parasitol.*, 57, 1363, 1971.

92. **Branch, G. J. and Stoffolano, J. G., Jr.**, Face fly: invertebrate vector and host of a mammalian eye worm in Massachusetts, *J. Econ. Entomol.*, 67, 304, 1974.

93. **Lyons, E. T. and Drudge, J. H.**, Two eyeworms, *Thelazia gulosa* and *Thelazia skrjabini*, in cattle in Kentucky, *J. Parasitol.*, 61, 1119, 1975.

94. **Lyons, E. T. and Drudge, J. H.**, Occurrence of the eyeworm, *Thelazia lacrymalis*, in horses in Kentucky, *J. Parasitol.*, 61, 1122, 1975.

95. **Geden, C. J. and Stoffolano, J. G., Jr.**, Bovine thelaziasis in Massachusetts, *Cornell Vet.*, 70, 344, 1980.

96. **Geden, C. J. and Stoffolano, J. G., Jr.**, Geographic range and temporal patterns of parasitization of *Musca autumnalis* (Diptera: Muscidae) by *Thelazia* sp. (Nematoda: Spirurata) in Massachusetts, with observations on *Musca domestica* (Diptera: Muscidae) as an unsuitable intermediate host, *J. Med. Entomol.*, 18, 449, 1981.

97. **Osborn, H.**, Insects affecting domestic animals: an account of the species of importance in North America, with mention of related forms occurring on other animals, *U.S. Dep. Agric. Div. Entomol. Bull. No. 5*, 1896.

98. **Hadwen, S.**, Warble flies, the economic aspect and a contribution on the biology, *Can. Dep. Agric. Bull.*, 16, 1912.

99. **Bishopp, F. C., Laake, E. W., Brundrett, H. M., and Wells, R. W.**, The cattle grubs or ox warbles, their biologies and suggestions for control, *U.S. Dep. Agric. Bull.*, 1369, 1926.

100. **Bishopp, F. C., Laake, E. W., and Wells, R. W.**, Cattle grubs or heel flies with suggestions for their control, *U.S. Dep. Agric. Farmers' Bull.*, 1596, 1929.

101. **Gibson, A. and Twinn, C. R.**, Warble fly control in Canada, *Sci. Agric.*, 17, 179, 1936.

102. **Bishopp, F. C., Laake, E. W., and Wells, R. W.**, Cattle grubs or heel flies with suggestions for their control, *U.S. Dep. Agric. Farmers' Bull.*, 1596, 1949.

103. **Gunderson, H.**, Effect of cattle grub treatment on weight gains in beef cattle, *J. Econ. Entomol.*, 38, 398, 1945.

104. **Munro, J. A., Aanestad, A., and Knapp, R.,** Reveal definite figures on weight loss due to grubs, *West. Live Stock,* 32, 64, 1947.

105. **Raun, E. S.,** Weight gains in feeder calves treated with low pressure rotenone sprays to control cattle grubs, *J. Econ. Entomol.,* 48, 604, 1955.

106. **Raun, E. S. and Herrick, J. B.,** Clinical test of the efficacy of Dow ET-57 for grub control in cattle, *J. Econ. Entomol.,* 50, 832, 1957.

107. **Knapp, F. W., Terhaar, C. J., and Roan, C. C.,** Field studies with feed and bolus formulations of Dow ET-57 for control of cattle grubs, *J. Econ. Entomol.,* 51, 119, 1958.

108. **Turner, E. C., Jr. and Gaines, J. A.,** Systemic insecticides for control of cattle grubs in Virginia, *J. Econ. Entomol.,* 51, 582, 1958.

109. **Neel, W. W.,** Field tests with systemic insecticides for the control of cattle grubs, *J. Econ. Entomol.,* 51, 793, 1958.

110. **Jones, C. M. and Matsushima, J.,** Effects of ronnel on control of cattle grubs and weight gains of beef cattle, *J. Econ. Entomol.,* 52, 488, 1959.

111. **Kohler, P. H., Rogoff, W. M., and Duxbury, R.,** Continuous individual feeding of systemic insecticides for cattle grub control, *J. Econ. Entomol.,* 52, 1222, 1959.

112. **Rogoff, W. M. and Kohler, P. H.,** Free-choice administration of ronnel in a mineral mixture for the control of cattle grubs, *J. Econ. Entomol.,* 52, 958, 1959.

113. **Norris, M. G. and Howe, R. G.,** Weight gains and cattle grub control in cattle treated with trolene, *Down Earth,* 15, 4, 1959.

114. **Rogoff, W. M., Kohler, P. H., and Duxbury, R. N.,** The *in vivo* activity of several systemic insecticides against cattle grubs in South Dakota, *J. Econ. Entomol.,* 53, 183, 1960.

115. **Rogoff, W. M. and Kohler, P. H.,** Effectiveness of Ruelene applied as localized ''pour-on'' and as spray for cattle grub control, *J. Econ. Entomol.,* 53, 814, 1960.

116. **Raun, E. S. and Herrick, J. B.,** Organophosphate systemics as sprays and feed additives for cattle grub control, *J. Econ. Entomol.,* 53, 125, 1960.

117. **Thurber, H. E. and Peterson, G. D., Jr.,** Feed lot tests with ronnel for control of cattle grubs, *J. Econ. Entomol.,* 53, 339, 1960.

118. **Marquardt, W. C., Lovelace, S. A., and Fritts, D. H.,** Spray treatment of calves with Bayer 21/199 for control of cattle grubs and lice in Montana, *J. Am. Vet. Med. Assoc.,* 137, 589, 1960.

119. **Marquardt, W. C. and Lovelace, S. A.,** A comparison of dimethoate administered as an injection and in supplemental feed for control of cattle grubs, *J. Econ. Entomol.,* 54, 252, 1961.

120. **Kohler, P. H. and Rogoff, W. M.,** Control of cattle grubs by pour-on, injection, and spray, *J. Econ. Entomol.,* 55, 540, 1962.

121. **Marquardt, W. C. and Hawkins, W. W., Jr.,** Control of cattle grubs by the intramuscular injection of Bayer 29493 or CL 38023, *Cornell Vet.,* 52, 228, 1962.

122. **Neel, W. W., Blount, C. L., and Kilby, W. W.,** Systemic insecticides applied as a topical pour-on and as an oral drench for cattle grub control, *J. Econ. Entomol.,* 56, 101, 1963.

123. **Khan, M. A. and Lawson, J. E.,** Summer treatments for cattle grub control and their effects on horn flies and cattle weight gains, *Can. J. Anim. Sci.,* 45, 43, 1965.

124. **Knapp, F. W., Bradley, N. W., and Templeton, W. C., Jr.,** Effect of ronnel mineral block (Rid-Ezy®) on control of cattle grubs and weight gain of beef cattle, *J. Econ. Entomol.,* 60, 1455, 1967.

125. **Ludwig, P. D. and Bucek, O. C.,** Cattle grub control is of economic importance, *Pract. Vet.,* 38, 32, 1966.

126. **Cox, D. D., Allen, A. D., and Maurer, E. M.,** Control of cattle grubs with organic phosphorus compounds administered in feed, *J. Econ. Entomol.,* 60, 105, 1967.

127. **Cox, D. D., Mullee, M. T., and Allen, A. D.,** Cattle grub control with feed additives (coumaphos and fenthion) and pour-ons (fenthion and trichlorfon), *J. Econ. Entomol.,* 60, 522, 1967.

128. **Landram, J. F., Ludwig, P. D., Bucek, O. C., Swart, R. W., and McGregor, W. S.,** The effect on cattle grubs, internal parasites, and weight gains in feedlot cattle treated topically with crufomate, *Pract. Nutr.,* 3, 9, 1969.

129. **Khan, M. A.** Extermination of cattle grubs (*Hypoderma* spp.) on a regional basis, *Vet. Rec.,* 83, 97, 1968.

130. **Rich, G. B.,** The economics of systemic insecticide treatment for reduction of slaughter trim loss caused by cattle grubs, *Hypoderma* spp., *Can. J. Anim. Sci.,* 50, 301, 1970.

131. **Collins, R. C. and Dewhirst, L. W.,** The cattle grub problem in Arizona. II. Phenology of common cattle grub infestations and their effects on weight gains of preweaning calves, *J. Econ. Entomol.,* 64, 1467, 1971.

132. **Campbell, J. B., Woods, W., Hagen, A. F., and Howe, E. C.,** Cattle grub insecticide efficacy and effects on weight-gain performance on feeder calves in Nebraska, *J. Econ. Entomol.,* 66, 429, 1973.

133. **Smith, D. L.,** Weight gain in calves in response to control of cattle grubs with insecticides, *Man. Entomol.,* 10, 5, 1976.

134. **Khan, M. A. and Kozub, G. C.,** Systemic control of cattle grubs (*Hypoderma* spp.) in steers treated with Warbex® and weight gains associated with grub control, *Can. J. Comp. Med.,* 45, 15, 1981.

135. **Imes, M.,** Cattle lice and how to eradicate them, *U.S. Dep. Agric. Farmers' Bull.,* 909, 1918.

136. **Matthysse, J. G.,** Cattle lice, their biology and control, *Cornell Univ. Agric. Exp. Sta. Bull.,* 832, 1946.

137. **Peterson, H. O., Roberts, I. H., Becklund, W. W., and Kemper, H. E.,** Anemia in cattle caused by heavy infestations of the blood-sucking louse, *Haematopinus eurysternus, J. Am. Vet. Med. Assoc.,* 122, 373, 1953.

138. **Shemanchuk, J. A., Haufe, W. O., and Thompson, C. O. M.,** Anemia in range cattle heavily infested with the short-nosed sucking louse, *Haematopinus eurysternus* (N.) (Anoplura: Haematopinidae), *Can. J. Comp. Med.,* 24, 158, 1960.

139. **Scharff, D. K.,** An investigation of the cattle louse problem, *J. Econ. Entomol.,* 55, 684, 1962.

140. **Collins, R. C. and Dewhirst, L. W.,** Some effects of the sucking louse, *Haematopinus eurysternus,* on cattle on unsupplemented range, *J. Am Vet. Med. Assoc.,* 146, 129, 1965.

141. **Ely, D. G. and Harvey, T. L.,** Relation of ration to short-nosed cattle louse infestations, *J. Econ. Entomol.,* 62, 341, 1969.

142. **Snipes, B. T.,** Beef cattle freed of lice in one treatment control, *Agric. Chem.,* 3, 30, 1948.

143. **Madder, D. J. and Surgeoner, G. A.,** Effect of permethrin, cypermethrin and chlorpyrifos on louse populations of beef cattle, *Proc. Entomol. Soc. Ontario,* 110, 29, 1979.

144. **Gibney, V. J., Campbell, J. B., Boxler, D. J., Clanton, D. C., and Deutscher, G. H.,** Effects of various infestation levels of cattle lice (Mallophaga: Trichodectidae and Anoplura: Haematopinidae) on feed efficiency and weight gains of beef heifers, *J. Econ. Entomol.,* 78, 1304, 1985.

145. **O'Flaherty, F. and Roddy, W.,** A microscopic study of the effect of follicular mange on skins, hides, and leather, *J. Am. Leather Chem. Assoc.,* 26, 394, 1931.

146. **O'Flaherty, F.,** Mange diseases causing millions of dollars in hide damage, *Leather Shoes,* 141, 13, 1954.

147. **Smith, H. J.,** Bovine demodicidosis.III. Its effect on hides and leather, *Can. J. Comp. Med.* 25, 243, 1961.

148. **Smith, H. J.,** Bovine demodicidosis-lesions and the resulting damage to hides and leather, *Wiad. Parazytol.,* 13, 4, 1967.

149. **Buechler, P. R., Hannigan, M. V., Carroll, R. J., Dahms, M. P., Feairheller, S. H., Meleney, W. P., and Wright, F. C.,** Studies of hyperkeratosis of cattlehides attributable to psoroptic scabies, *J. Am. Leather Chem. Assoc.,* 79, 416, 1984.

150. **Tobin, W. C.,** Cattle scabies can be costly, *J. Am. Vet. Med. Assoc.,* 141, 845, 1962.

151. **Meleney, W. P. and Fisher, W. F.,** The effect of exposure to mites, *Psoroptes ovis* (Acarina: Psoroptidae), on calves of varying susceptibility to common scabies, *Proc. U.S. Anim. Health Assoc.,* 340, 1979.

152. **Fisher, W. F. and Wright, F. C.,** Effects of the sheep scab mite on cumulative weight gains in cattle, *J. Econ. Entomol.,* 74, 234, 1981.

153. **Fisher, W. F. and Crookshank, H. R.,** Effects of *Psoroptes ovis* (Acarina: Psoroptidae) on certain biochemical constituents of cattle serum, *Vet. Parasitol.,* 11, 241, 1982.

154. **Cole, N. A., Guillot, F. S., and Purdy, C. W.,** Influence of *Psoroptes ovis* (Hering) (Acari: Psoroptidae) on the performance of beef steers, *J. Econ. Entomol.,* 77, 390, 1984.

155. **Woodward, T. E., Turner, W. F., and Curtice, C.,** The effect of the cattle tick upon the milk production of dairy cows, *U.S. Dep. Agric. Bull.,* 147, 1915.

156. **McClain, J. H.,** Eradication of the cattle tick necessary for profitable dairying, *U.S. Dep. Agric. Farmers' Bull.,* 639, 1914.

157. **Lancaster, J. L., Jr., Brown, C. J., and Honea, R. S.,** Steers gained more when ticks were controlled, *Arkansas Farm Res.,* 4, 6, 1955.

158. **Barnard, D. R.,** Injury thresholds and production loss functions for the lone star tick, *Amblyomma americanum* (Acari: Ixodidae), on pastured, preweaner beef cattle, *Bos taurus, J. Econ. Entomol.,* 78, 852, 1985.

159. **Barnard, D. R., Ervin, R. T., and Epplin, F. M.,** Production system-based model for defining economic thresholds in preweaner beef cattle, *Bos taurus,* infested with the lone star tick, *Amblyomma americanum* (Acari: Ixodidae), *J. Econ. Entomol.,* 79, 141, 1986.

160. **Bolte, J. R., Hair, J. A., and Fletcher, J.,** White-tailed deer mortality following tissue destruction induced by lone star ticks, *J. Wildl. Manag.,* 34, 546, 1970.

161. **Mount, G. A. and Dunn, J. E.,** Economic thresholds for lone star ticks (Acari: Ixodidae) in recreational areas based on a relationship between CO_2 and human subject sampling, *J. Econ. Entomol.,* 76, 327, 1983.

162. **Gladney, W. J., Price, M. A., and Graham, O. H.,** Field tests of insecticides for control of the Gulf Coast tick on cattle, *J. Med. Entomol.,* 13, 579, 1977.

163. **Williams, R. E., Hair, J. A., and Buckner, R. G.,** Effects of the Gulf Coast tick on blood composition and weights of drylot Hereford steers, *J. Econ. Entomol.,* 70, 229, 1977.

164. **Stacey, B. R., Williams, R. E., Buckner, R. G., and Hair, J. A.,** Changes in weight and blood composition of Hereford and Brahman steers in drylot and infested with adult Gulf Coast ticks, *J. Econ. Entomol.*, 71, 967, 1978.

165. **Williams, R. E., Hair, J. A., and McNew, R. W.,** Effects of Gulf Coast ticks on blood composition and weights of pastured Hereford steers, *J. Parsitol.*, 64, 336, 1978.

166. **Gregson, J. D.,** Tick paralysis an appraisal of natural and experimental data, *Can. Dept. Agric. Monogr.*, 9, 1973.

167. **Imes, M.,** The sheep tick and its eradication by dipping, *U.S. Dep. Agric. Farmers' Bull.*, 798, 1917.

168. **Muma, M. H., Hill, R. E., Hixson, E., and Harris, L.,** Control of sheep-ticks on feeder lambs, *J. Econ. Entomol.*, 45, 833, 1952.

169. **Pfadt, R. E., Paules, L. H., and DeFoliart, G. R.,** Effect of the sheep ked on weight gains of feeder lambs, *J. Econ. Entomol.*, 46, 95, 1953.

170. **Whiting, F., Nelson, W. A., Slen, S. B., and Bezeau, L. M.,** The effects of the sheep ked (*Melophagus ovinus* L.) on feeder lambs, *Can. J. Agric. Sci.*, 34, 70, 1954.

171. **Bosman, W. W., Botha, M. L., and Louw, D. J.,** Effect of the ked on Merino sheep, *Union S. Afr. Dept. Agric. Sci. Bull.*, 281, 1950.

172. **Nelson, W. A. and Slen, S. B.,** Weight gains and wool growth in sheep infested with the sheep ked *Melophagus ovinus*, *Exp. Parasitol.*, 22, 223, 1968.

173. **Everett, A. L., Roberts, I. H., Willard, H. J., Apodaca, S. A., Bitcover, E. H., and Naghski, J.,** The cause of cockle, a seasonal sheepskin defect, identified by infesting a test flock with keds (*Melophagus ovinus*), *J. Am. Leather Chem. Assoc.*, 64, 460, 1969.

174. **Everett, A. L. and Bitcover, E. H.,** The common origin of the seedy and ticky defects of sheepskin, *J. Am. Leather Chem. Assoc.*, 65, 402, 1970.

175. **Everett, A. L., Roberts, I. H., and Naghski, J.,** Reduction in leather value and yields of meat and wool from sheep infested with keds, *J. Am. Leather Chem. Assoc.*, 66, 118, 1971.

176. **Taylor, C. A., Stewart, J. R., and Shelton, M.,** Evaluation of an insecticide for control of goat lice, *Tex. Agric. Exp. Stn. Prog. Rep.*, 33, 46, 1974.

177. **Kettle, P. R. and Pearce, D. M.,** Effect of the sheep body louse (*Damalinia ovis*) on host weight gain and fleece value, *N.Z. J. Exp. Agric.*, 2, 219, 1974.

178. **Wilkinson, F. C., de Chaneet, G. C., and Beetson, B. R.,** Growth of populations of lice, *Damalinia ovis*, on sheep and their effects on production and processing performance of wool, *Vet. Parasitol.*, 9, 243, 1982.

179. **Graham, O. H. and Hourrigan, J. L.,** Eradication programs for the arthropod parasites of livestock, *J. Med. Entomol.*, 13, 629, 1977.

180. **Salmon, D. E. and Stiles, C. W.,** Sheep scab: its nature and treatment, *U.S. Dep. Agric. Bur. Anim. Ind. Bull.*, 21, 1898.

181. **Kirkwood, A. C.,** Effect of *Psoroptes ovis* on the weight of sheep, *Vet. Rec.*, 107, 469, 1980.

182. **Sinclair, A. N.,** Fleece derangement of Merino sheep infested the by itch mite *Psorergates ovis*, *N.Z. Vet. J.*, 24, 149, 1976.

183. **Bhaskaran, R., Divakaran, S., and Barat, S. K.,** Demodicosis in goats, cattle and sheep and its influence on leather, *J. Am. Leather Chem. Assoc.*, 63, 512, 1968.

184. **Schillhorn van Veen, T. W. and Williams, J. F.,** Some typical parasitic diseases of the goat, *Mod. Vet. Pract.*, 61, 847, 1980.

185. **Cumming, J. N.,** An estimate of costs to the sheep industry due to blowflies and parasites, *Q. Rev. Agric. Econ.*, 197, 1964.

186. **Patrick, H. L.,** Blowflies and Parasites: costs to the sheep industry 1969—70, *Wool Econ. Res. Rep. No. 22*, Canberra, Australia, 1972.

187. **Brideoake, B. R.,** The estimated cost of blowfly control in the Australian sheep industry: 1969—70 to 1975—76, Symposium and Workshop on Flystrike in Sheep, New South Wales Department of Agriculture, Sydney, Aust., 1979.

188. **Campbell, J. B. and Doane, T. H.,** Weight gain response and efficacy of washing and various insecticide treatments for prevention of flies feeding on shear wounds of summer shorn lambs, *J. Econ. Entomol.*, 70, 132, 1977.

189. **Buchanan, R. S., Dewhirst, L. W., and Ware, G. W.,** The importance of sheep bot fly larvae and their control with systemic insecticides in Arizona, *J. Econ. Entomol.*, 62, 675, 1969.

190. **Ponomarev, I. A.,** Effect of peroral treatment of sheep with trichlorfon for the control of *Oestrus ovis* infestation on productivity and reproductive functions, *Nauchn. Tr. Stavrop. Skhaist. Inst.*, 39, 45, 1976.

191. **Bukshtynov, V. I.,** Economic losses from *Oestrus ovis* infestation in sheep, and the cost of treatment, *Veterinariia*, 8, 43, 1980.

192. **Horak, I. G. and Snijders, A. J.,** The effect of *Oestrus ovis* infestation on Merino lambs, *Vet. Rec.*, 94, 12, 1974.

193. **Horak, I. G., Honer, M. R., and Schroder, J.,** Live mass gains and wool production of Merino sheep: three treatment programmes for parasite control, *J. S. Afr. Vet. Assoc.,* 47, 247, 1976.

194. **Imes, M.,** Hog lice and hog mange methods of control and eradication, *U.S. Dep. Agric. Farmers' Bull.,* 1085, 1920.

195. **Imes, M.,** Mange of swine, *U.S. Dep. Agric. Year. Agric.,* 734, 1942.

196. **Magee, J. C.,** Studies on *Sarcoptes scabiei* on swine in Iowa, in *Proc. North Cent. Branch Entomol. Soc. Am.,* 29, 125, 1974.

197. **Dobson, K. J. and Cargill, C. F.,** Epidemiology and economic consequences of sarcoptic mange in pigs, *Proc. 2nd Int. Symp. Vet. Epidemiol. Econ.,* 401, 1979.

198. **Yeoman, G. H.,** Pig mange: new concepts in control, *Vet. Ann.,* 24, 132, 1984.

199. **Sheahan, B. J.,** Experimental *Sarcoptes scabiei* infection in pigs: clinical signs and significance of infection, *Vet. Rec.,* 94, 202, 1974.

200. **Sheahan, B. J., O'Connor, P. J., and Kelly, E. P.,** Improved weight gains in pigs following treatment for sarcoptic mange, *Vet. Rec.,* 95, 169, 1974.

201. **Cargill, C. F. and Dobson, K. J.,** Experimental *Sarcoptes scabiei* infestation in pigs. II. Effects on production, *Vet. Rec.,* 104, 33, 1979.

202. **Larsen, L. P. and Storm, H. P.,** The influence of mange on feed consumption and weight gain in fattening pigs, *Vet. Med. Rev.,* 1, 98, 1981.

203. **Hewett, G. R. and Heard, T. W.,** Phosmet for the systemic control of pig mange, *Vet. Rec.,* 111, 558, 1982.

204. **Heard, T. W.,** *Sarcoptes scabei* var *suis,* its epidemiology and control in U.K. pig herds, *Proc. Pig Vet. Soc.,* 10, 89, 1983.

205. **Alva, R., Wallace, D. H., Benz, G. W., Foster, A. G., and Brokken, E. S.,** The effects of Ivermectin on the productivity of pigs naturally infested with *Sarcopes scabiei* var. *suis, Proc. 8th Int. Pig Vet. Cong.,* 207, 1984.

206. **Williams, R. E.,** External swine parasites lice and mite infestations still a common problem, *Anim. Nutr. Health,* 36, 16, 1981.

207. **Holscher, K.,** Mange and lice control on swine, *Farm Supplier,* 60, 38, 1986.

208. **Campbell, J. B., Boxler, D. J., Danielson, D. M., and Crenshaw, M. A.,** Effects of house and stable flies on weight gain and feed efficiency by feeder pigs, *Southwest Entomol.,* 9, 273, 1984.

209. **Bishopp, F. C. and Wood, H. P.,** Mites and lice on poultry, *U.S. Dep. Agric. Farmers' Bull.,* 801, 1917.

210. **Bishopp, F. C.,** The fowl tick and how premises may be freed from it, *U.S. Dep. Agric. Farmers' Bull.,* 1070, 1919.

211. **Warren, D. C., Eaton, R., and Smith, H.,** Influence of infestations of body lice on egg production in the hen, *Poultry Sci.,* 27, 641, 1948.

212. **Edgar, S. A. and King, D. F.,** Effect of the body louse, *Eomenacanthus stramineus,* on mature chickens, *Poultry Sci.,* 29, 214, 1950.

213. **Gless, E. E. and Raun, E. S.,** Effects of chicken body louse infestation on egg production, *J. Econ. Entomol.,* 52, 358, 1959.

214. **Stockdale, H. J. and Raun, E. S.,** Economic importance of the chicken body louse, *J. Econ. Entomol.,* 53, 421, 1960.

215. **DeVaney, J. A.,** Effects of the chicken body louse, *Menacanthus stramineus,* on caged layers, *Poultry Sci.,* 55, 430, 1976.

216. **Wood, H. P.,** Tropical fowl mite in the United States with notes on life history and control, *U.S. Dep. Agric. Dept. Circ.,* 79, 1920.

217. **Cameron, D.,** The northern fowl mite (*Liponyssus sylviarum* C. & F., 1877), *Can. J. Res.,* 16, 230, 1938.

218. **Loomis, E. C., Bramhall, E. L., Allen, J. A., Ernst, R. A., and Dunning, L. L.,** Effects of the northern fowl mite on white leghorn chickens, *J. Econ. Entomol.,* 63, 1885, 1970.

219. **Matthysse, J. G., Jones, C. J., and Purnasiri, A.,** Development of northern fowl mite populations on chickens, effects on the host, and immunology, *Search Agric.,* 4, 1, 1974.

220. **DeVaney, J. A., Elissalde, M. H., Steel, E. G., Hogan, B. F., and Petersen, H. D.,** Effect of the northern fowl mite, *Ornithonyssus sylviarum* (Canestrini and Fanzago) on white leghorn roosters, *Poultry Sci.,* 56, 1585, 1977.

221. **DeVaney, J. A.,** A survey of poultry ectoparasite problems and their research in the United States, *Poultry Sci.,* 57, 1217, 1978.

222. **DeVaney, J. A. and Beerwinkle, K. R.,** A nonchemical method of controlling the northern fowl mite, *Ornithonyssus sylviarum* (Canestrini and Fanzago), on caged white leghorn hens, *Poultry Sci.,* 59, 1226, 1980.

223. **Eklund, J., Loomis, E., and Abplanalp, H.,** Genetic resistance of white leghorn chickens to infestation by the northern fowl mite, *Ornithonyssus sylviarum, Arch. Geflugelk.,* 44, 195, 1980.

224. **DeVaney, J. A.,** Effects of the northern fowl mite, *Ornithonyssus sylviarum* (Canestrini and Fanzago), on egg quality of white leghorn hens, *Poultry Sci.,* 60, 2200, 1981.

225. **DeVaney, J. A., Beerwinkle, K. R., and Ivie, G. W.,** Residual activity of selected pesticides on laying hens treated for northern fowl mite control by dipping, *Poultry Sci.,* 61, 1630, 1982.
226. **Hall, R. D., Vandepopuliere, J. M., Fischer, F. J., Lyons, J. J., and Doisy, K. E.,** Comparative efficacy of plastic strips impregnated with permethrin and permethrin dust for northern fowl mite control on caged laying hens, *Poultry Sci.,* 62, 612, 1983.
227. **Arends, J. J., Robertson, S. H., and Payne, C. S.,** Impact of northern fowl mite on broiler breeder flocks in North Carolina, *Poultry Sci.,* 63, 1457, 1984.
228. **Hall, R. D., Vandepopuliere, J. M., Jaynes, W., and Fischer, F. J.,** Prophylactic efficiency and longevity of polyvinyl chloride strips containing permethrin for control of northern fowl mites (Acari: Macronyssidae) on caged chickens, *J. Econ. Entomol.,* 77, 1224, 1984.
229. **Mullen, M. A. and Paul, J. J.,** Observations on lesions caused by the chigger, *Neoschoengastia americana* (Hirst) (Acarina: Trombiculidae) on turkeys, *J. Ga. Entomol. Soc.,* 3, 170, 1968.
230. **Kunz, S. E., Price, M. A., and Graham, O. H.,** Biology and economic importance of the chigger *Neoschongastia americana* on turkeys, *J. Econ. Entomol.,* 62, 872, 1969.
231. **Price, M. A., Kunz, S. E., and Matter, J. J.,** Use of Dursban® to control *Neoschongastia americana,* a turkey chigger, in experimental pens, *J. Econ. Entomol.,* 63, 377, 1970.
232. **Kunz, S. E., Price, M. A., and Everett, R. E.,** Large-scale testing of chlorpyrifos for control of *Neoschongastia americana* on turkeys, *J. Econ. Entomol.,* 65, 1207, 1972.
233. **Cunningham, J. R., Kunz, S. E., and Price, M. A.,** Effects of selected environmental factors on damaging populations of *Neoschongastia americana, J. Econ. Entomol.,* 69, 161, 1976.
234. **Edgar, S. A.,** A field study of the effect of black fly bites on egg production of laying hens, *Poultry Sci.,* 32, 779, 1953.
235. **Jones, C. M. and Richey, D. J.,** Biology of the black flies in Jasper County, South Carolina, and some relationships to a *Leucocytozoon* disease of turkeys, *J. Econ. Entomol.,* 49, 121, 1956.

Chapter 2

CONTROL OF HORN FLIES ON CATTLE*

I. INTRODUCTION

The major arthropod pest of pastured cattle in the U.S. and Canada is the horn fly,♦ *Haematobia irritans* (Linnaeus), an obligate blood-sucking parasite. Adults may feed 24 to 38 times per day. Populations of adults on cattle may exceed 1000 flies per animal. Mating takes place on the host, and gravid females leave hosts only to lay eggs in crevices and cracks of freshly deposited manure. Eggs hatch in 10 to 18 hr, and larvae develop in 3 to 5 days in undisturbed manure pats. Pupation takes place in and under manure pats. Control measures can be directed toward the adult stage on cattle or the larval stage found in manure. The literature on the biology and control of this species, which has had several different scientific names through the years, is voluminous. Morgan and Thomas[1] listed 1130 references in their annotated bibliography; Supplement I[2] to that bibliography contained an additional 402 references. Thus, we can only present highlights of the dynamics of changes and new developments in the technologies used to control horn flies. References cited will be key papers that represent changes or improvements in control technologies.

II. DERMAL TREATMENTS

A. Early Treatment Technology

Bruce[3] reviewed the early literature on the horn fly and gave a brief history of the appearance of the horn fly in the U.S., which occurred around 1885, when it was then called *H. serrata* Robineau-Desvoidy. Measures used before 1900[4,5] to control adults included treating cattle with repellents (such as fish oil, tar, carbolic acid, or axle grease) or with toxicants (such as kerosene or tobacco emulsions, or tobacco and creosote dusts). A cattle fly trap was used to collect flies which were attracted to light after leaving cattle as the animals passed through a darkened passage. Horn fly larvae were controlled by treating manure with lime or by destroying and drying manure pats. United States Department of Agriculture (USDA) Bureau of Entomology Circular No. 115 in 1910[6] listed most of the earlier treatments and noted that fitting dipping vats with splash boards would redirect the liquids that ordinarily splash out of dipping vats back onto the cattle and thus the liquids killed the flies trying to escape from the cattle. The 1912 *U.S. Dep. Agric. Yearbook of Agriculture*[7] described the horn fly, then called *Lyperosia irritans* Linnaeus, as "one of the most widespread and injurious insects in this country", and listed manure spreading, use of repellents, and splashing of liquids from dipping vats onto cattle as control measures. An emulsion of pine-tar creosote sprayed daily onto dairy cattle controlled horn flies.[8] Pyrethrins dusts were more effective than rotenone dusts for the control of horn flies and other flies affecting cattle, and the observed repellent action was actually the result of a rapid toxic effect of the insecticides.[9]

Control measures changed little for 30 years, as illustrated in the 1940 USDA Leaflet No. 205[10] which still listed destruction of manure pats, spraying of cattle with toxicants, especially those which contain pyrethrins, but not repellents (which were impractical or undesirable), the use of splash boards on dipping vats, and cattle fly traps as the current

* Common names of insects and acarines, as listed in *Common Names of Insects and Related Organisms* (published by the Entomological Society of America), are marked with a ♦ the first time they are cited preceding the scientific name.

control technologies. A new, practical cattle fly trap, a modified version of previous traps, consisted of a darkened tunnel with screened sides exposed to light to attract flies and contained strips of cloth to brush flies off the cattle. These traps reduced horn fly populations once cattle were trained to use them.[11]

B. Organochlorine Treatments

1. Sprays, Dips, and Dusts

The control of horn flies on range cattle was revolutionized after World War II with the advent of sprays or dips of DDT which controlled horn flies for 2 to 4 weeks or longer.[12-15] Sprays of benzene hexachloride (BHC) were as effective as sprays of DDT.[16] Sprays of toxaphene and chlordane were slightly more effective than DDT and methoxychlor, while TDE sprays were slightly less effective.[17-20] Even though ca. 25,000 cattle were treated one to four times during the summer with DDT in a 186,000-ha area in Kansas, horn flies were not eradicated from cattle in the area.[21]

The presence of residues of chlorinated hydrocarbon insecticides in the milk of dairy cows treated with DDT, TDE, and chlordane[22] prompted the removal of their use on dairy cows and in dairy barns. Sprays of methoxychlor, toxaphene, and lindane were as effective as DDT, but pyrethrins plus piperonyl butoxide provided less than half the residual protection of DDT.[23,24] The addition of fused bentonite sulfur increased the residual protection period of sprays of methoxychlor, lindane, and synergized pyrethrins.[25] The 1952 *U.S. Dep. Agric. Yearbook of Agriculture*[26] recommended sprays of DDT, TDE, toxaphene, and methoxychlor for the control of horn flies on beef cattle. Only methoxychlor and synergized pyrethrins were approved for use on dairy cattle. Hand dusting of dairy cattle with ca. 15 g of methoxychlor wettable powder or dusting cattle with DDT wettable powder with a hand-operated rotary duster controlled horn flies for 3 weeks.[27,28]

2. Automatic Sprayers

In the 1950s there was considerable interest in the development and use of automatic sprayers to apply small amounts of mixtures of insecticides and repellents to dairy or beef cattle daily or more often to control biting flies. The first sprayer[29] applied synergized pyrethrins to cattle as they stepped on a treadle which activated the spray applicator. A similar sprayer[30] applied methoxychlor, synergized pyrethrins, cyclethrin, and several repellents to beef cattle two to four times per day, and the treatment controlled several species of biting flies. Methoxychlor and pyrethrins with or without repellents applied by an electric-eye-controlled automatic sprayer[31] controlled several species of biting flies. Most mechanical automatic sprayers require continual maintenance and care, and such sprayers were never used widely in the U.S.

3. Backrubbers and Dustrubbers

Rogoff and Moxon[32] developed the cable-type backrubber so that cattle could treat themselves to control flies. The backrubber was constructed of burlap sacking wrapped around a cable or chain suspended between two posts. The burlap was treated with insecticides in oil which were transferred to cattle as the cattle rubbed against the burlap. DDT was more effective than methoxychlor, toxaphene, or lindane. Such backrubbers were less effective than sprays of DDT in large, brushy, rough pastures with large water areas, where cattle had alternative rubbing surfaces.[33] DDT or chlordane in backrubbers controlled horn flies, but not horse flies, deer flies, mosquitoes, or the stable fly*, *Stomoxys calcitrans* (Linnaeus).[27] Backrubbers charged with DDT, methoxychlor, malathion, or Perthane® controlled horn flies, and the addition of butoxy polypropylene glycol to DDT and methoxychlor slightly increased their effectiveness.[34] Methods and materials used to control horn flies on dairy cattle were reviewed by Knipling and McDuffie.[35]

Dusting cattle by hand or with a rotary duster was adapted to a self-treatment method for use by cattle when toxaphene, chlordane, methoxychlor, or coumaphos dusts were placed inside burlap bags and the bags wrapped around wire in a form similar to cable-type back-rubbers.[36] Insecticides in these dustrubbers controlled horn flies on beef and dairy cattle that used them either by free choice or were forced to use them daily. Rotenone or methoxychlor dust in dustrubbers were more effective than malathion or deet dust.[37]

C. Organophosphorus Treatments

1. Sprays, Dips, and Dusts

Toward the end of the 1950s, organophosphorus insecticides were tested and developed as treatments applied to livestock for the control of a variety of arthropods, including horn flies. Effective spray treatments included carbaryl (a carbamate), dioxathion, coumaphos, and ronnel.[38,39] Ronnel was also effective as a backrubber treatment.[40] Both ronnel and coumaphos were more effective than toxaphene as backrubber treatments.[41] Ronnel, coumaphos, and diazinon sprayed into barns controlled horn flies for several weeks on dairy cattle brought into the barns for milking and feeding.[42] Dusts of diazinon and azinphosmethyl were generally more effective than sprays of diazinon, dimethoate, crufomate, and coumaphos.[43] Sprays of carbaryl, fenthion, and crotoxyphos and backrubber treatment of crotoxyphos controlled horn flies.[44]

Noting that male horn flies tend to frequent the feet and lower legs of cattle, Witherspoon and Burns[45] controlled horn flies and reduced male to female ratios and percentages of females inseminated by applying crotoxyphos sprays only to the lower parts of the legs of cattle.

2. Pouron Application

The pouron technique, developed to apply systemics to cattle to control cattle grubs, was first used by Rogoff and Kohler[46] to apply insecticides to cattle to control horn flies. A treatment of 100 mℓ of concentrated emulsions of toxaphene or crufomate poured along the backline of cattle was more effective in terms of reducting horn fly numbers and lengthening the duration of effectiveness than equal or greater amounts of these insecticides applied as whole body sprays. Pourons of coumaphos, crufomate, and trichlorfon were generally more effective than spray applications.[43] Pourons of the organochlorine insecticides, DDT and toxaphene, also controlled horn flies.[47]

3. Automatic Sprayers

Because certain organophosphorus insecticides were effective at very low concentrations and were approved for use on dairy cattle, interest was renewed in daily treatment of dairy cattle with low volumes of these insecticides, especially crotoxyphos, by means of cow-activated automatic sprayers. Crotoxyphos, synergized pyrethrins, and dichlorvos applied daily with a photocell-activated automatic sprayer controlled horn flies.[44] Excellent control of horn flies, but not other biting flies, was obtained[48] with one or two daily treatments of 50 to 150 mℓ per cow of crotoxyphos applied by a sprayer activated by a step-on switch.[49] Crotoxyphos or malathion applied at a rate of 1 mℓ per application by an improved sprayer[50,51] provided excellent control of horn flies on cattle forced to use the sprayer frequently, preferably daily.[52] However, the lack of reliability and the necessity for constant care of such automatic sprayers has limited their use.

4. Dust Bags

Dust bags are a further development of the self-application, dustrubber device. The fact that the face fly♦, *Musca autumnalis* De Geer, was difficult to control with conventionally applied body sprays or dusts,[53] led to the development of dust bags that dispensed insecticide dusts when contacted by cattle. Turner[54] suspended dust bags around salt boxes or in aisles used by cattle so that the animals' heads and shoulders would be treated as they touched the bags. Such self-treatment dusting stations were highly effective in applying dusts of a variety of insecticides to cattle for the control of horn flies, but were less effective against face flies.[55-57]

5. Experimental Application Methods
a. Attractant-Toxicant Device
After first determining that horn flies were attracted to ultraviolet (UV) radiation from blacklight blue (BLB) fluorescent lamps,[58] Morgan[59] controlled horn flies on dairy cattle assembled in the dark near attractant-toxicant devices that consisted of a box enclosure that contained a BLB lamp that was covered with a gauze impregnated with stirofos. Flies left the cows, were attracted to the UV radiation, and were killed by the treated gauze.

b. Ultra-Low-Volume Aerial Application
A single ultra-low-volume (ULV) aerial application of technical malathion, sprayed onto cattle, controlled horn flies and face flies for 1 week.[60,61] Trichlorfon was also effective.[62,63] When applied to widely scattered range cattle, aerial ULV applications of malathion, fenthion, and trichlorfon controlled horn flies but were more expensive to apply than conventional sprays.[64] Other ULV treatments included stirofos, trichlorfon, fenthion, and naled,[65,66] a mixture of stirofos plus dichlorvos, and dichlorvos.[67] All treatments afforded short residual activity of less than 1 week. Aerial applications of malathion, stirofos, or a mixture of stirofos plus dichlorvos controlled horn flies for less than 1 week and did not affect most of the arthropods found in the bovine dung.[68]

Kinzer[69] placed a ULV air blast applicator on a pickup truck and applied malathion or fenthion to cattle which were gathered around congregation sites. The treatments controlled horn flies for less than 1 week.

c. Wax Bar Application
Another experimental treatment method used to apply insecticides dermally to cattle to control horn flies was the rubbing of a crotoxyphos-impregnated wax bar on the backs of cattle.[70] The wax bar method was effective because a concentrated amount of toxicant remained on the back where horn flies are found, a situation similar to that which provides for the effectiveness of pouron treatments. Treatment of only 25 to 33% of the cattle in a herd with a crotoxyphos-impregnated wax bar controlled horn flies on the entire herd; treatment of less that 12% of the herd was less satisfactory.[71]

d. Spoton Application
The spoton treatment technique, used to apply concentrated insecticides to a single spot on the back of cattle at a specific volume to weight dosage to control cattle grubs and lice, was also used to apply insecticides to cattle to control horn flies. A single spoton treatment of 2 cm^3 of a chlorpyrifos concentrate per 43 kg of body weight controlled horn flies for 4 to 6 weeks.[72]

D. Pyrethroid Treatments
In the late 1970s, pyrethroid insecticides were found to be highly effective against a variety of arthropods. Permethrin was very effective when applied topically to cattle to control horn flies.[73] The spraying of only 1 animal with permethrin in a herd of 10 to 32 head usually gave >90% reduction of horn flies on all cattle for 1 week.[74] Also, permethrin sprayed onto cattle with ULV ground equipment controlled horn flies for 7 days.[75] Permethrin in marking fluid in a chin-ball on a bull was transferred to cows and controlled horn flies. The treatment

was effective for 3 weeks after the bull was removed from the pasture.[76] *Insecticide and Acaricide Tests* contain many reports on the effectiveness of sprays and dusts of permethrin, fenvalerate, and other pyrethroids for the control of horn flies.

E. Insecticide-Impregnated Ear Tags
1. Organophosphorus Insecticides

A significant advance in the methods used to apply insecticides to cattle to control horn flies was the insecticide-impregnated ear tag. In pioneering research, Harvey and Brethour[77] placed dichlorvos-impregnated plastic strips on ear tags, on neck chains, or as collars around the necks of cattle and controlled horn flies for 1 week to 1 month. In order to determine the extent of transfer of material from devices attached to the bodies of cattle, pads containing a dye were attached to a neckband, halter, tail tag, ear tag, and leg band.[78] There was considerable coverage of the body surfaces of cattle with the dye as a result of movement and self-grooming of the cattle. Dichlorvos-impregnated resin blocks attached to leg bands fastened to the lower rear legs of cattle controlled horn flies for 10 weeks.[79] Dichlorvos-impregnated plastic tags attached to the tails of cattle controlled horn flies despite the loss of ca. 50% of the tags.[80] Stirofos-impregnated ear tags, used principally for the control of the Gulf Coast tick♦, *Amblyomma maculatum* Koch, controlled horn flies for 12 to 14 weeks.[81] Stirofos-impregnated ear tags controlled horn flies for several months, but treatments were less effective when not all cattle were treated with one tag per ear.[82-84]

2. Pyrethroid Insecticides

Control of horn flies for the entire season (>20 weeks in South Texas) was obtained with ear tags impregnated with fenvalerate.[85] Permethrin, decamethrin, and fenvalerate in ear tags also controlled horn flies, but generally were less effective against face flies.[86-91] Issues of *Insecticide and Acaricide Tests* and *Pesticide Research Reports* (Agriculture Canada) in the late 1970s and through the 1980s contain many reports on the effectiveness of pyrethroid-impregnated ear tags applied to cattle at various rates to control horn flies and, to a lesser extent, face flies on cattle.

The application of fenvalerate-impregnated ear tags only to nursing calves[92] was a convenient and highly effective treatment for the control of horn flies on their dams. Organophosphorus- or pyrethroid-impregnated ear tags attached to self-applicating backrubbers or sand-filled dust bags also provided excellent horn fly control.[93] Ear tags impregnated with fenvalerate, permethrin, and flucythrinate were readily accepted by ranchers as an efficient method to control horn flies and were extremely effective for several years. However, their widespread use and the continuous selection pressure that they placed on local populations of horn flies has led to the appearance of resistance in horn flies to pyrethroids. The subject of resistance in horn flies will be covered in detail in Chapter 19.

III. ORAL TREATMENTS

Finally, one other technique used to administer insecticides to cattle for the control of horn flies should be discussed. Because horn flies and face flies breed in fresh, undisturbed bovine manure, and a variety of other filth or nuisance flies breed in diluted manure and other livestock wastes, such as soiled straw and spilled feed, larvicides applied to these breeding materials should control the flies that breed there. In Chapter 18, we discuss control of the house fly♦, *Musca domestica* Linnaeus, stable flies, and other species of flies that breed in manure and other wastes around structures, and Chapter 6 contains a section that discusses control of face flies in undisturbed manure. In this section, we will review the developments in research that led to the technology of the administration of chemicals orally to cattle to control horn fly larvae in manure. Miller[94] briefly reviewed early research on the use of orally administered larvicides to control several species of fly larvae in the manure of cattle. Recently, Miller and Miller[95] presented a concise review of the major developments in the use of chemicals as feed-through treatments to control fly larvae in the manure of livestock.

A. Early Treatment Technology

In early research, specifically with the horn fly, tannic acid, stockholm tar, linseed oil, or a mixture of magnesium sulfate plus sodium chloride or ferrous sulfate added to drinking water of cows did not control horn fly larvae in manure of treated cattle.[96] Oral administration of phenothiazine prevented development of horn fly larvae in manure of treated animals.[97,98] Of 29 chemicals given as single oral treatments to cattle,[99] rotenone killed horn fly larvae at dosages lower than several other effective treatments. Zinc oxide was also effective orally.[100] Arsenic injected intravenously did not kill horn flies feeding on the treated animal, but the animal's manure was toxic to horn fly larvae.[101] In the only reported tests with organochlorine insecticides, manure from cattle given daily oral treatments of lindane, dieldrin, and aldrin was toxic to horn fly larvae.[102]

B. Organophosphorus Treatments

Coumaphos, Dition®, and Bayer 22408 controlled horn fly larvae when added to the feed of cattle.[103] In field tests with a commercially available mineral mixture that contained ronnel, consumption varied considerably. When a sufficient quantity of medicated mixture was consumed, control of horn flies (and cattle grubs) was excellent; however, less than adequate consumption was a continual problem.[104-106] Coumaphos-salt mixtures provided erratic control of horn fly and face fly larvae.[107]

During the late 1960s and 1970s, a variety of organophosphorus insecticides was tested as short-term feed additives to control horn fly larvae and other fly larvae in cattle manure. Effective treatments included coumaphos, Bayer 22408, famphur, fenthion, phosmet, bromophos, stirofos, and dichlofenthion.[108,109] Stirofos[110] was developed as a commercial "feed-thru" mineral block or mineral mix treatment to control horn flies, house flies, stable flies, and face flies. The encapsulation of stirofos, in order to lessen degredation in the gastrointestinal tract of cattle, afforded greater larvicidal (house fly) effectiveness in manure than unencapsulated chemical.[111] The feeding of stirofos to dairy cattle for extended periods did not affect the health or reproductive performance of the cows, and the residues in milk were generally below tolerance levels.[112] Particles of technical stirofos less than 74 μg were less effective against house fly larvae than larger particles.[113] Stirofos and a pelleted formulation of dichlorvos given to cows in feed controlled horn fly larvae.[114]

C. *Bacillus thuringiensis*

Spores and/or crystals of *Bacillus thuringiensis thuringiensis* Berliner (BT), effective as feed additives for control of house fly larvae in bovine manure,[115,116] were also effective against horn fly larvae.[117] The soluble toxins were not as effective as the whole product.[118] The β-exotoxin of BT, found to be the fraction that was active against fly larvae,[119] was formulated into range cubes and, when fed to cows, controlled horn fly larvae in manure of the treated animals.[120] The use of BT as an oral treatment for the control of dipterous larvae in manure has been viewed with renewed interest recently with the finding that crystals and low-density particulate matter (fraction 3) of *B. thuringiensis* subsp. *israelensis* (BTI) were toxic to horn fly larvae.[121]

D. Insect Growth Regulators

The insect growth regulator methoprene prevented the eclosion of horn flies from pupae of larvae that developed in manure of cattle treated orally.[122] Methoprene in mineral blocks for free-choice consumption by cattle reduced the numbers of horn flies that emerged from treated manure, but there was no reduction in populations of horn flies on treated cattle because of the lack of isolation from nearby untreated cattle.[123,124] Mineral blocks or granules containing methoprene not only prevented eclosion of horn flies from treated manure but also reduced populations of adult flies.[125] Methoprene was developed as a commercial feed additive-mineral mixture or free-choice mineral block treatment for the control of horn flies, but not other manure-breeding flies, which were not affected by the dosage provided. Encapsulation or impregnation in plastic did not improve effectiveness of methoprene, and the use of a commercially available, protein-mineral block for free-choice treatment reduced populations of horn flies, but not face flies, on pastured dairy heifers.[126]

Methoprene metered into the drinking water of cattle provided excellent reduction of the horn fly population.[127] A modified water treatment technique[128] was used successfully as part of a pilot sterile insect technique project (see Chapter 20) to suppress populations of horn flies on cattle on Molokai, Hawaii.[129]

Diflubenzuron, a compound that inhibits chitin synthesis in insects, applied topically to cattle as a dust or spray, reduced the hatch of eggs and survival of larvae of horn flies that fed on treated cattle.[130-132] Diflubenzuron as a feed additive controlled house fly and stable fly larvae.[133-135] As a mineral block treatment, diflubenzuron inhibited development of horn fly larvae but did not reduce fly populations on the nonisolated cattle.[136]

E. Sustained-Release Technology

An advance in the oral administration of larvicides to cattle was the development of a sustained-release bolus formulation. Generally, the "free-choice" consumption of orally administered chemicals is subject to both over- or undertreatment. A sustained-release bolus, located in the reticulum or rumen, slowly erodes at a fairly constant rate and provides a measured amount of active ingredient in the manure. A bolus that contained methoprene[137] controlled horn fly larvae in manure for 10 to 12 weeks. Wide-scale testing[138] showed that a methoprene bolus could control horn flies for 28 to 32 weeks and face flies for 10 to 12 weeks.

The sustained release bolus technology could be used to meter a variety of substances into the system or the gastrointestinal tract of cattle. A recently discovered systemic insecticide and anthelmintic is ivermectin, a chemically derived fermentation product of the fungus *Streptomyces avermitilis*.[139] Ivermectin, a very effective animal systemic insecticide,[140] controlled horn fly larvae at extremely low daily dosages administered orally or subcutaneously, and a single subcutaneous injection controlled horn fly larvae in mamure for up to 4 weeks.[141]

IV. OVERVIEW AND CURRENT TECHNOLOGY

There is an extensive history of the development and use of diverse technologies to control the horn fly, the most important arthropod pest of pastured cattle. Early treatments, such as spraying or dipping cattle in a variety of chemicals, usually provided relatively short-term control of horn flies. A revolution in the effectiveness of sprays, dips, and dusts for the control of horn flies occurred when chlorinated hydrocarbon insecticides became available after World War II. A single application of DDT and other insecticides controlled flies for 2 weeks or much longer. Because of residues in milk and meat of treated cattle, most of these insecticides were limited in their use for the control of horn flies, especially on dairy cattle.

The development of backrubbers, dustrubbers, and dust bag treatments so that cattle could treat themselves allowed for the control of horn flies without gathering of cattle for treatment. The forced use of these self-application devices by placing them in locations where they must be used by cattle daily or more frequently provides greater control of flies than when these devices are available for use by cattle on a free-choice basis.

A variety of organophosphorus insecticides controlled horn flies when used as sprays, dips, dusts, and in backrubbers or dust bags. The pouron technique, used to apply systemic insecticides to cattle to control cattle grubs, was also a convenient and easy way to apply insecticides to cattle to control horn flies. Other application techniques, such as automatic sprayers, ULV aerial application, attractant-toxicant devices, wax bar application, and spoton treatments, were used experimentally but generally are not included in current technology for horn fly control.

Pyrethroid insecticides are generally available as practical, long-lasting treatments as sprays and dusts for the control of horn flies.

Undoubtedly, the most significant advance in recent technology for the control of horn flies on cattle has been the development and widespread use of insecticide-impregnated ear tags. This technology provided for the season-long control of horn flies. Unfortunately, the presence of an insecticide in the environment of horn flies for long periods of time and the widespread uses of treated ear tags led to the selection of populations of horn flies that are resistant to pyrethroid and, to a lesser extent, organophosphorus insecticides.

Another technology for the control of horn flies is the oral treatment of cattle to control horn fly larvae in manure. A feed treatment of phenothiazine has been available for years for the control of horn fly larvae. More recently, commercially available oral treatments include stirofos, effective against horn fly, stable fly, house fly, and face fly larvae, and methoprene, effective against horn fly larvae only. Both ronnel and coumaphos are registered but not commercially available.

In the summer of 1986, a sustained-release bolus containing diflubenzuron, became commercially available in the U.S. to control horn fly and face fly larvae in the manure of cattle.

If strategies are not developed to cope with the resistant populations of horn flies, the status of horn fly control will revert to technologies used before the introduction of treated ear tags. To date, suitable alternative chemistries for use in sustained-release matrixes to replace the pyrethroid-impregnated ear tags have not been developed. Strategies to manage resistant populations of horn flies are available but often are not compatible with current cattle management practices. The economic considerations of the producer magnify the problems; their quest for short-term fly control, using products and technologies that enhance the resistance problems, may well lead to a long-term failure of the control technology. Control strategies and pest management plans need to be developed for those producers whose ranching practices will allow for a resistance management program.

REFERENCES

1. **Morgan, C. E. and Thomas, G. D.,** Annotated bibliography of the horn fly, *Haematobia irritans* (L.), including references on the buffalo fly, *H. exigua* (de Meijere), and other species belonging to the genus *Haematobia*, *U.S. Dep. Agric. Misc. Publ.*, 1278, 1974.
2. **Morgan, C. E. and Thomas, G. D.,** Supplement I: annotated bibliography of the horn fly, *Haematobia irritans irritans* (L.), including references on the buffalo fly, *H. irritans exigua* (de Meijere), and other species belonging to the genus *Haematobia*, *U.S. Dep. Agric. Misc. Publ.*, 1278, 1977.
3. **Bruce, W. G.,** The history and biology of the horn fly, *Haematobia irritans* (Linnaeus); with comments on control, *N.C. Agric. Exp. Stn. Tech. Bull.*, 157, 1964.
4. **Riley, C. V.,** The horn fly, *Insect Life*, 2, 93, 1889.
5. **Osborn, H.,** Insects affecting domestic animals: an account of the species of importance in North America, with mention of related forms occurring on other animals, *U.S. Dep. Agric. Entomol. Bull.*, 5, 1896.
6. **Marlatt, C. L.,** The horn fly (*Haematobia serrata* Rob.-Desv.), *U.S. Dep. Agric. Entomol. Bull.*, 115, 1910.
7. **Bishopp, F. C.,** Some important insect enemies of live stock in the United States, *U.S. Dep. Agric. Yearb. Agric.*, 383, 1912.

8. **Cory, E. N.,** The protection of dairy cattle from flies, *J. Econ. Entomol.,* 10, 111, 1917.
9. **Cory, E. N., Harns, H. G., and Anderson, W. H.,** Dusts for control of flies on cattle, *J. Econ. Entomol.,* 29, 331, 1936.
10. **Bruce, W. G.,** The horn fly and its control, *U.S. Dep. Agric.* Leaflet No. 205, 1940.
11. **Bruce, W. G.,** A practical trap for the control of horn flies on cattle, *J. Kans. Entomol. Soc.,* 11, 88, 1938..
12. **Wells, R. W.,** DDT as a flyspray on range cattle, *J. Econ. Entomol.,* 37, 136, 1944.
13. **Laake, E. W.,** DDT for the control of the horn fly in Kansas, *J. Econ. Entomol.,* 39, 65, 1946.
14. **Bruce, W. G. and Blakeslee, E. B.,** DDT to control insect pests affecting livestock, *J. Econ. Entomol.,* 39, 367, 1946.
15. **Bruce, W. G. and Blakeslee, E. B.,** Factors affecting tests with DDT sprays to control horn flies, *J. Econ. Entomol.,* 41, 39, 1948.
16. **Cory, E. N. and Langford, G. S.,** Fly control in dairy barns and on livestock by cooperative spray services, *J. Econ. Entomol.,* 40, 425, 1947.
17. **Eddy, G. W. and Graham, O. H.,** Tests to control horn flies with new insecticides, *J. Econ. Entomol.,* 42, 265, 1949.
18. **Smith, C. L.,** Chlorinated hydrocarbon insecticides for control of the horn fly on dairy cattle in Texas, *J. Econ. Entomol.,* 42, 981, 1949.
19. **Laake, E. W.,** Chlorinated hydrocarbon insecticides for the control of the horn fly on beef cattle in Kansas and Missouri, *J. Econ. Entomol.,* 42, 143, 1949.
20. **McGregor, W. S.,** Field tests of insecticides and spraying methods to control horn flies in dairy herds, *J. Econ. Entomol.,* 42, 641, 1949.
21. **Smith, C. L. and Gates, D. E.,** County-wide control of the horn fly with DDT, *J. Econ. Entomol.,* 42, 847, 1949.
22. **Carter, R. H., Wells, R. W., Radeleff, R. D., Smith, C. L., Hubanks, P. E., and Mann, H. D.,** The chlorinated hydrocarbon content of milk from cattle sprayed for control of horn flies, *J. Econ. Entomol.,* 42, 116, 1949.
23. **Denning, D. G. and Pfadt, R. E.,** Evaluation of certain insecticides in horn fly control, *J. Econ. Entomol.,* 43, 557, 1950.
24. **Laake, E. W., Howell, D. E., Dahm, P. A., Stone, P. C., and Cuff, R. L.,** Relative effectiveness of various insecticides for control of house flies in dairy barns and horn flies on cattle, *J. Econ. Entomol.,* 43, 858, 1950.
25. **Cuff, R. L.,** Fused bentonite sulphur to prolong horn fly protection on beef cattle, *J. Econ. Entomol.,* 43, 111, 1950.
26. **Eddy, G. W.,** Flies on livestock, *U.S. Dep. Agric. Yearb. Agric.,* 657, 1952.
27. **Lindquist, A. W. and Hoffman, R. A.,** Effectiveness of cattle-rubbing devices and hand dusting for horn fly control, *J. Econ. Entomol.,* 47, 79, 1954.
28. **DeFoliart, G. R.,** Dusting for horn fly control on beef herds, *J. Econ. Entomol.,* 49, 393, 1956.
29. **Bruce, W. N.,** Automatic sprayer for control of biting flies on cattle, *Ill. Nat. Hist. Surv. Biol. Notes,* 27, 1952.
30. **Granett, P., Hansens, E. J., and O'Connor, C. T.,** Automatic cattle sprayers for fly control in New Jersey, *J. Econ. Entomol.,* 48, 386, 1955.
31. **Cheng, T. H., Patterson, R. E., Avery, B. W., and Vanderberg, J. P.,** An electric-eye-controlled sprayer for application of insecticides to livestock, *Pa. Agric. Exp. Stn. Bull.,* 626, 1957.
32. **Rogoff, W. M. and Moxon, A. L.,** Cable type back rubbers for horn fly control on cattle, *J. Econ. Entomol.,* 45, 329, 1952.
33. **DeFoliart, G. R.,** Horn fly control with chlorinated insecticides, *J. Econ. Entomol.,* 47, 266, 1954.
34. **Goodwin, W. J.,** Control of horn flies on cattle with treated rubbing devices, *J. Econ. Entomol.,* 49, 407, 1956.
35. **Knipling, E. F. and McDuffie, W. C.,** Controlling flies on dairy cattle and in dairy barns, *Bull. WHO,* 16, 865, 1957.
36. **Hargett, L. T. and Turner, E. C., Jr.,** Horn fly control by the use of insecticidal dusts in self-applicating devices, *J. Econ. Entomol.,* 51, 795, 1958.
37. **Hargett, L. T. and Goulding, R. L.,** Rotenone and methoxychlor dust in backrubbers for horn fly control in dairy herds, *J. Econ. Entomol.,* 52, 762, 1959.
38. **Roberts, R. H.,** Field tests with five insecticides for the control of horn flies, *J. Econ. Entomol.,* 52, 1216, 1959.
39. **Brundrett, H. M., Deer, J. A., and Graham, O. H.,** Control of horn flies in the Rio Grande Valley of Texas with Bayer 21/199 sprays, *J. Econ. Entomol.,* 51, 746, 1958.
40. **Hays, K. L.,** Korlan for control of the hornfly, *Down Earth,* 15, 1, 1959.
41. **Burns, E. C., McCraine, S. E., and Moody, D. W.,** Ronnel and Co-ral for horn fly control on cable type back rubbers, *J. Econ. Entmol.,* 52, 648, 1959.

42. **Turner, E. C., Jr. and Hargett, L. T.**, The effect of residual barn sprays on control of horn flies, *J. Econ. Entomol.*, 51, 559, 1958.

43. **Dorsey, C. K., Heishman, J. O., and Taylor, C. H.**, Horn fly control — using spray, dust, and pour-on formulations, *J. Econ. Entomol.*, 55, 425, 1962.

44. **Hoffman, R. A. and Roberts, R. H.**, Horn fly control studies in Mississippi, 1961, *J. Econ. Entomol.*, 56, 258, 1963.

45. **Witherspoon, B. and Burns, E. C.**, Control implications of a behavioral trait in male horn flies, *J. Econ. Entomol.*, 60, 1280, 1967.

46. **Rogoff, W. M. and Kohler, P. H.**, Horn fly control by the pour-on technique using Ruelene or toxaphene, *J. Econ. Entomol.*, 54, 1101, 1961.

47. **Rogoff, W. M., Kohler, P. H., and Hintz, S. D.**, Pour-on treatments of DDT or toxaphene for horn fly control, *J. Econ. Entomol.*, 56, 82, 1963.

48. **Hoffman, R. A., Berry, I. L., and Graham, O. H.**, Control of flies on cattle by frequent low-volume mist spray applications of Ciodrin, *J. Econ. Entomol.*, 58, 815, 1965.

49. **Berry, I. L. and Hoffman, R. A.**, Use of step-on switches for control of automatic sprayers, *J. Econ. Entomol.*, 56, 888, 1963.

50. **Miller, A. and Eschle, J. L.**, An automatic cattle sprayer for ultra-low-volume applications, *U.S. Dep. Agric. Agric. Res. Serv. 42-125*, 1967.

51. **Miller, A., Eschle, J. L., and Pickens, M.**, Design and performance of an ultralow-volume automatic sprayer for applying insecticide to cattle, *Am. Soc. Agric. Eng.*, 12, 368, 1969.

52. **Eschle, J. L. and Miller, A.**, Ultra-low-volume application of insecticides to cattle for control of the horn fly, *J. Econ. Entomol.*, 61, 1617, 1968.

53. **Wallace, J. B. and Turner, E. C., Jr.**, Experiments for control of the face fly in Virginia, *J. Econ. Entomol.*, 55, 415, 1962.

54. **Turner, E. C., Jr.**, Area control of the face fly using self-applicating devices, *J. Econ. Entomol.*, 58, 103, 1965.

55. **Adkins, T. R., Jr. and Seawright, J. A.**, A simplified dusting station to control face flies and horn flies on cattle, *J. Econ. Entomol.*, 60, 864, 1967.

56. **Kolach, A. J.**, Dust bags for horn fly control on beef cattle, *Manit. Entomol.*, 1, 34, 1967.

57. **Janes, M. J., Hayes, B. W., and Beardsley, D. W.**, Horn fly control with coumaphos, *J. Econ. Entomol.*, 61, 1176, 1968.

58. **Morgan, N. O.**, Ultraviolet radiation as an attractant for adult horn flies, *J. Econ. Entomol.*, 59, 1416, 1966.

59. **Morgan, N. O.**, Control of horn flies by an electrochemical device, *J. Econ. Entomol.*, 60, 750, 1967.

60. **Dobson, R. C. and Sanders, D. P.**, Low-volume, high-concentration spraying for horn fly and face fly control on beef cattle, *J. Econ. Entomol.*, 58, 379, 1965.

61. **Kantack, B. H., Berndt, W. L., and Balsbaugh, E. U., Jr.**, Horn fly and face fly control on range cattle with aerial applications of ultra-low-volume malathion sprays, *J. Econ. Entomol.*, 60, 1766, 1967.

62. **Knapp, F. W.**, Aerial application of trichlorfon for horn fly and face fly control on cattle, *J. Econ. Entomol.*, 59, 468, 1966.

63. **Knapp, F. W.**, Ultra-low-volume aerial application of trichlorfon for control of adult mosquitoes, face flies, and horn flies, *J. Econ. Entomol.*, 60, 1193, 1967.

64. **Kinzer, H. G.**, Aerial applications of ultra-low-volume insecticides to control the horn fly on unrestrained range cattle, *J. Econ. Entomol.*, 62, 1515, 1969.

65. **Balsbaugh, E. U., Jr., Alleman, G. A., Kantack, B. H., and Berndt, W. L.**, Aerial application of ULV organic phosphate insecticides for controlling livestock insect pests, *J. Econ. Entomol.*, 63, 548, 1970.

66. **Campbell, J. B. and Raun, E. S.**, Aerial ULV and LV applications of insecticides for control of the stable fly and the horn fly, *J. Econ. Entomol.*, 64, 1170, 1971.

67. **Balsbaugh, E. U., Jr. and Kessler, H.**, Further tests of aerial applications of ULV organic phosphate insecticdes for controlling the horn fly in South Dakota, *J. Econ. Entomol.*, 63, 1915, 1970.

68. **Del Fosse, E. S. and Balsbaugh, E. U., Jr.**, Effects of ULV organophosphates on horn flies and face flies of cattle, and on the bovine coprocoenosis, *Environ. Entomol.*, 3, 919, 1974.

69. **Kinzer, H. G.**, Ground application of ultra-low-volume malathion and fenthion for horn fly control in New Mexico, *J. Econ. Entomol.*, 63, 736, 1970.

70. **Harvey, T. L. and Ely, D. G.**, Wax-bar applications of Ciodrin for horn fly control, *J. Econ. Entomol.*, 62, 1386, 1969.

71. **Harvey, T. L. and Ely, D. G.**, Partial herd treatment with crotoxyphos in wax-bars to control horn flies, *J. Econ. Entomol.*, 63, 671, 1970.

72. **Deutscher, G. H. and MacLean, G. J.**, South Dakota hornfly control trial in pasture cattle with topical insecticide (Dursban 44 Insecticide), *Down Earth*, 36, 18, 1980.

73. **Schmidt, C. D., Matter, J. J., Meurer, J. H., Reeves, R. E., and Shelley, B. K.,** Evaluation of a synthetic pyrethroid for control of stable flies and horn flies on cattle, *J. Econ. Entomol.,* 69, 484, 1976.

74. **Harvey, T. L. and Brethour, J. R.,** Treatment of one beef animal per herd with permethrin for horn fly control, *J. Econ. Entomol.,* 72, 532, 1979.

75. **Walker, T. W., Lancaster, J. L., Jr., Eberhardt, W. L., Turner, R. W., Williams, D. C., and Meisch, M. V.,** Efficacy of ULV insecticides applied by truck mounted cold aerosol generator against horn flies *(Haematobia irritans)* on cattle, *Mosq. News,* 42, 436, 1982.

76. **Harvey, T. L. and Brethour, J. R.,** Chin-ball application of permethrin to cows for horn fly (Diptera: Muscidae) control, *J. Econ. Entomol.,* 77, 655, 1984.

77. **Harvey, T. L. and Brethour, J. R.,** Horn fly control with dichlorvos-impregnated strips, *J. Econ. Entomol.,* 63, 1688, 1970.

78. **Beadles, M. L., Gingrich, A. R., and Miller, J. A.,** Slow-release devices for livestock insect control: cattle body surfaces contacted by five types of devices, *J. Econ. Entomol.,* 70, 72, 1977.

79. **Beadles, M. L., Miller, J. A., Shelley, B. K., and Reeves, R. E.,** Horn flies: control with dichlorvos-impregnated resin blocks attached to bands on the rear legs of cattle, *J. Econ. Entomol.,* 71, 287, 1978.

80. **Beadles, M. L., Miller, J. A., Shelley, B. K., and Ingenhuett, D. P.,** Comparison of the efficacy of ear tags, leg bands, and tail tags for control of the horn fly on range cattle, *Southwest. Entomol.,* 4, 70, 1979.

81. **Ahrens, E. H.,** Horn fly control with an insecticide-impregnated ear tag, *Southwest. Entomol.,* 2, 8, 1977.

82. **Wilson, N. L., Huston, J. E., and Davis, D. I.,** Effectiveness of stirofos impregnated ear tags for control of horn flies and horse flies on cattle in Central Texas, *Southwest. Vet.,* 31, 197, 1978.

83. **Sheppard, C.,** Stirofos impregnated cattle ear tags at four rates for horn fly control, *J. Econ. Entomol.,* 73, 276, 1980.

84. **Lewis, D. J. and Block, E.,** Efficacy of tetrachlorvinphos-impregnated cattle ear tags against livestock Diptera in southern Quebec, *Can. J. Anim. Sci.,* 62, 1249, 1982.

85. **Ahrens, E. H. and Cocke, J.,** Season long horn fly control with an insecticide-impregnated ear tag, *J. Econ. Entomol.,* 72, 215, 1979.

86. **Williams, R. E. and Westby, E. J.,** Evaluation of pyrethroids impregnated in cattle ear tags for control of face flies and horn flies, *J. Econ. Entomol.,* 73, 791, 1980.

87. **Harvey, T. L. and Brethour, J. R.,** Control of horn fly, *Haematobia irritans* (L.) (Diptera: Muscidae) on cattle by partial herd treatment with fenvalerate-impregnated ear tags, *Prot. Ecol.,* 2, 313, 1981.

88. **Schmidt, C. D. and Kunz, S. E.,** Fenvalerate and stirofos ear tags for control of horn flies on range cattle, *Southwest. Entomol.,* 5, 202, 1980.

89. **Knapp, F. W. and Herald, F.,** Face fly and horn fly reduction on cattle with fenvalerate ear tags, *J. Econ. Entomol.,* 74, 295, 1981.

90. **Williams, R. E., Westby, E. J., Hendrix, K. S., and Lemenager, R. P.,** Use of insecticide-impregnated ear tags for the control of face flies and horn flies on pastured cattle, *J. Anim. Sci.,* 53, 1159, 1981.

91. **Williams, R. E. and Westby, E. J.,** Comparison of three insecticide-impregnated cattle ear tags for face fly and horn fly control (Diptera: Muscidae), *J. Kans. Entomol. Soc.,* 55, 335, 1982.

92. **Harvey, T. L. and Brethour, J. R.,** Controlling horn fly (Diptera: Muscidae) in cow-calf herds with insecticide-impregnated ear tag treatments of nursing calves, *J. Econ. Entomol.,* 76, 117, 1983.

93. **Harvey, T. L., Brethour, J. R., and Broce, A. B.,** Horn fly (Diptera: Muscidae) control of cattle with insecticide ear tags attached to backrubbers and dust bags, *J. Econ. Entomol.,* 76, 96, 1983.

94. **Miller, R. W.,** Larvicides for fly control — a review, *Bull. Entomol. Soc. Am.,* 16, 154, 1970.

95. **Miller, R. W. and Miller, J. A.,** Feed-through chemicals for insect control in animals, in *Agricultural Chemicals of the Future,* (BARC Symp. 8), Hilton, J. L., Ed., Rowman & Allanheld, Totowa, N.J., 1984, 355.

96. **Gallagher, B. A.,** Special report on horn fly experiment, *Hawaii Forest. Agric.,* 25, 144, 1928.

97. **Knipling, E. F.,** Internal treatment of animals with phenothiazine to prevent development of horn fly larvae in the manure, *J. Econ. Entomol.,* 31, 315, 1938.

98. **Bruce, W. G.,** The use of phenothiazine in the medication of cattle for the control of horn flies, *J. Econ. Entomol.,* 32, 704, 1939.

99. **Bruce, W. G.,** The medication of cattle for the control of horn flies, *J. Kans. Entomol. Soc.,* 13, 41, 1940.

100. **Bruce, W. G.,** Zinc oxide: a new larvicide for use in the medication of cattle for the control of horn flies, *J. Kans. Entomol. Soc.,* 15, 105, 1942.

101. **Bruce, W. G.,** Intravenous injections of arsenic ineffective in controlling horn flies on cattle, *J. Kans. Entomol. Soc.,* 13, 128, 1940.

102. **Eddy, G. W., McGregor, W. S., Hopkins, D. E., and Dreiss, J. M.,** Effects on some insects of the blood and manure of cattle fed certain chlorinated hydrocarbon insecticides, *J. Econ. Entomol.,* 47, 35, 1954.

103. **Eddy, G. W. and Roth, A. R.,** Toxicity to fly larvae of the feces of insecticide-fed cattle, *J. Econ. Entomol.,* 54, 408, 1961.

104. **Medley, J. G., Drummond, R. O., and Graham, O. H.,** Field tests with low-level feeding of ronnel for control of cattle grubs and horn flies, *J. Econ. Entomol.,* 56, 500, 1963.

105. **Simco, J. and Lancaster, J. L., Jr.,** Low-level feeding of ronnel for controlling hornflies and cattle grubs, *Arkansas Farm Res.,* 13, 16, 1964.

106. **Kinzer, H. G. and Bullard, R. G.,** Animal systemic insecticides for control of the horn fly, *N. M. State Univ. Agric. Exp. Stn. Res. Rep.,* 129, 1967.

107. **Knapp, F. W.,** The effect of free-choice coumaphos salt mixtures on cattle and cattle parasites, *J. Econ. Entomol.,* 58, 197, 1965.

108. **Drummond, R. O.,** Toxicity to house flies and horn flies of manure from insecticide-fed cattle, *J. Econ. Entomol.,* 56, 344, 1963.

109. **Drummond, R. O., Whetstone, T. M., and Ernst, S. E.,** Control of larvae of the house fly and the horn fly of manure of insecticide-fed cattle, *J. Econ. Entomol.,* 60, 1306, 1967.

110. **Miller, R. W., Gordon, C. H., Bowman, M. C., Beroza, M., and Morgan, N. O.,** Gardona as a feed additive for control of fly larvae in cow manure, *J. Econ. Entomol.,* 63, 1420, 1970.

111. **Miller, R. W. and Gordon, C. H.,** Encapsulated rabon for larval house fly control in cow manure, *J. Econ. Entomol.,* 65, 455, 1972.

112. **Miller, R. W. and Gordon, C. H.,** Effect of feeding rabon to dairy cows over extended periods, *J. Econ. Entomol.,* 66, 135, 1973.

113. **Miller, R. W. and Gordon, C. H.,** Technical rabon for larval house fly control in cow manure, *J. Econ. Entomol.,* 65, 1064, 1972.

114. **Butler, J. F. and Greer, N. I.,** Toxicity of SD 8447 and dichlorvos to larvae of the horn fly, *Haematobia irritans* (Diptera: Muscidae), in manure of insecticide-fed cattle, *Fla. Entomol.,* 56, 103, 1973.

115. **Harvey, T. L. and Brethour, J. R.,** Feed additives for control of house fly larvae in livestock feces, *J. Econ. Entomol.,* 53, 774, 1960.

116. **Dunn, P. H.,** Control of house flies in bovine feces by a feed additive containing *Bacillus thuringiensis* var. *thuringiensis* Berliner, *J. Insect. Pathol.,* 2, 13, 1960.

117. **Gingrich, R. E.,** *Bacillus thuringiensis* as a feed additive to control dipterous pests of cattle, *J. Econ. Entomol.,* 58, 363, 1965.

118. **Gingrich, R. E. and Eschle, J. L.,** Preliminary report on the larval development of the horn fly, *Haematobia irritans,* in feces from cattle given fractions of a commercial preparation of *Bacillus thuringiensis, J. Invert. Pathol.,* 8, 285, 1966.

119. **Gringrich, R. E. and Eschle, J. L.,** Susceptibility of immature horn flies to toxins of *Bacillus thuringiensis, J. Econ. Entomol.,* 64, 1183, 1971.

120. **Gingrich, R. E.,** Control of the horn fly, *Haematobia irritans,* with *Bacillus thuringiensis, Comp. Pathobiol.,* 7, 47, 1984.

121. **Temeyer, K. B.,** Larvicidal activity of *Bacillus thuringiensis* subsp. *israelensis* in the dipteran *Haematobia irritans, Appl. Environ. Microbiol.,* 47, 952, 1984.

122. **Harris, R. L., Frazar, E. D., and Younger, R. L.,** Horn flies, stable flies, and house flies: development in feces of bovines treated orally with juvenile hormone analogues, *J. Econ. Entomol.,* 66, 1099, 1973.

123. **Harris, R. L., Chamberlain, W. F., and Frazar, E. D.,** Horn flies and stable flies: free-choice feeding of methoprene mineral blocks to cattle for control, *J. Econ. Entomol.,* 67, 384, 1974.

124. **Bay, D. E. and Scofield, M. L.,** Evaluation of methoprene impregnated mineral blocks for horn fly control, *Tex. Agric. Exp. Stn. Misc. Publ.,* 1278, 1976.

125. **Paysinger, J. T. and Adkins, T. R., Jr.,** Efficacy of methoprene (Altoside® IGR), against the horn fly, when fed to cattle in mineral supplements, *J. Ga. Entomol. Soc.,* 12, 255, 1977.

126. **Miller, R. W. and Pickens, L. G.,** Evaluation of methoprene formulations for fly control, *J. Econ. Entomol.,* 68, 810, 1975.

127. **Beadles, M. L., Miller, J. A., Chamberlain, W. F., Eschle, J. L., and Harris, R. L.,** The horn fly: methoprene in drinking water of cattle for control, *J. Econ. Entomol.,* 68, 781, 1975.

128. **Miller, J. A., Chamberlain, W. F., Beadles, M. L., Pickens, M. O., and Gingrich, A. R.,** Methoprene for control of horn flies: application to drinking water of cattle via a tablet formulation, *J. Econ. Entomol.,* 69, 330, 1976.

129. **Miller, J. A., Eschle, J. L., Hopkins, D. E., Wright, F. C., and Matter, J. J.,** Methoprene for control of horn flies: a suppression program on the island of Molokai, Hawaii, *J. Econ. Entomol.,* 70, 417, 1977.

130. **Kunz, S. E., Schmidt, C. D., and Harris, R. L.,** Effectiveness of diflubenzuron applied as dust to inhibit reproduction in horn flies, *Southwest. Entomol.,* 1, 190, 1976.

131. **Kunz, S. E., Harris, R. L., Hogan, B. F., and Wright, J. E.,** Inhibition of development in a field population of horn flies treated with diflubenzuron, *J. Econ. Entomol.,* 70, 298, 1977.

132. **Wright, J. E. and Harris, R. L.,** Ovicidal activity of Thompson-Hayward TH 6040 in the stable fly and horn fly after surface contact by adults, *J. Econ. Entomol.,* 69, 728, 1976.

133. **Miller, R. W.,** TH 6040 as a feed additive for control of the face fly and house fly, *J. Econ. Entomol.,* 67, 697, 1974.

134. **Wright, J. E.,** Insect growth regulators: development of house flies in feces of bovines fed TH 6040 in mineral blocks and reduction in field populations by surface treatments with TH 6040 or a mixture of stirofos and dichlorvos at larval breeding areas, *J. Econ. Entomol.,* 68, 322, 1975.

135. **Barker, R. W. and Newton, G. L.,** Dimilin: evaluation as a livestock dietary feed additive for control of *Musca domestica* larvae in cattle waste, *J. Ga. Entomol. Soc.,* 11, 71, 1976.

136. **Barker, R. W. and Jones, R. L.,** Inhibition of larval horn fly development in the manure of bovines fed Dimilin® mineral blocks, *J. Econ. Entomol.,* 69, 441, 1976.

137. **Miller, J. A., Beadles, M. L., Palmer, J. S., and Pickens, M. O.,** Methoprene for control of the horn fly: a sustained-release bolus formulation for cattle, *J. Econ. Entomol.,* 70, 589, 1977.

138. **Miller, J. A., Knapp, F. W., Miller, R. W., and Pitts, C. W.,** Sustained-release boluses containing methoprene for control of the horn fly and face fly, *Southwest. Entomol.,* 4, 195, 1979.

139. **Campbell, W. C., Fisher, M. H., Stapley, E. O., Alberts-Schonberg, G., and Jacob, T. A.,** Ivermectin: a potent new antiparasitic agent, *Science,* 221, 823, 1983.

140. **Drummond, R. O.,** Effectiveness of Ivermectin for control of arthropod pests of livestock, *Southwest. Entomol., Suppl.* 7, 34, 1985.

141. **Miller, J. A., Kunz, S. E., Oehler, D. D., and Miller, R. W.,** Larvicidal activity of Merck MK-933, an avermectin, against the horn fly, stable fly, face fly, and house fly, *J. Econ. Entomol.,* 74, 608, 1981.

Chapter 3

CONTROL OF STABLE FLIES AND THE USE OF REPELLENTS ON CATTLE*

I. INTRODUCTION

The stable fly*, *Stomoxys calcitrans* (Linnaeus), is an important pest of cattle, horses, and other livestock held in or near barns or stables, or confined in feedlots and other enclosures. The adults, which feed by sucking blood from the extremities of livestock, can be very annoying to animals. Stable flies breed in all types of decaying vegetable matter or in manure mixed with hay, feed, silage, and other materials often found in abundance near structures that house animals. An annotated bibliography of stable flies and other *Stomoxys* species was presented by Morgan et al.[1]

Stable flies can also be an important pest of man. From late summer until frost, beaches along the western Gulf Coast of Florida often become infested with stable flies. These flies, called "dog flies", attack bathers, fishermen, and others who frequent the beaches and cause pain and annoyance. Although stable flies were believed to breed extensively in seashore wastes, it has been recently demonstrated that many of the stable flies at the beach have migrated there from inland breeding sites with the aid of weather systems.[2]

Control of stable flies depends primarily upon the elimination of breeding sites. Sanitation around structures or where breeding materials accumulate is absolutely essential to any stable fly control program. Removing and spreading of manure and other breeding materials to allow them to dry makes them unsuitable as a larval breeding medium. Chemical technologies to control larvae include topical application of insecticides to breeding materials or by feeding insecticides and insect growth regulators to cattle in order to treat manure. Technologies to control adult stable flies include applying insecticides with extended residual activity to barns, sheds, fences, stables, and other structures where stable flies rest before and after they have fed or applying insecticides as mists or fogs to livestock and the structures that house them. Usually these "space" treatments are intended to provide a quick kill of flies and generally have short residual activity. Control of stable flies and other flies in manure and in structures is discussed in Chapter 18.

Stable flies may be killed by insecticides applied directly to cattle as dips, sprays, pourons, spotons, dusts, etc. Because of the fact that stable flies visit cattle for only short periods of time in order to feed, insecticides applied directly to cattle do little to eliminate populations of flies, although some temporary control may be obtained.

Finally, repellents may be applied to cattle to repel stable flies and other biting flies, especially horse and deer flies. Repellents should prevent flies from feeding, but their residual activity, if any, is very short lived.

Because the control of stable flies has involved and continues to involve the use of a variety of control technologies, this chapter will focus on the development and use of toxicants, repellents, and traps.

In his classic work in 1896, Osborn[3] devoted only two paragraphs to the stable fly, and the only control technique listed was "prompt disposal of dung". *U.S. Dep. Agric. Farmers' Bulletin* No. 540 in 1913[4] described the life history, hosts, habits, and distribution of the stable fly and emphasized that control of the species was found only by attacking the immature stages. Larvae were controlled by heat and drying of the larval medium, by predation by

---

* Common names of insects and acarines, as listed in *Common Names of Insects and Related Organisms* (published by the Entomological Society of America), are marked with a * the first time they are cited preceding the scientific name.

hogs, poultry, and certain insects, and by parasitic wasps. The proper stacking of straw and other breeding materials and their protection from rain was helpful, but the most effective measure was the proper disposal and care of manure. He stated "there are far more manure piles than straw stacks". Repellents were not very effective and livestock were protected by blankets or nets. Bishopp[5] described severe stable fly outbreaks in several states, reported on research on the life history and biology of the pest, and listed control measures of destruction of breeding places, such as straw stacks and manure piles, and protection of livestock with cloth coverings or by treatment with repellents.

U.S. Dep. Agric. Farmers' Bulletin No. 1097,[6] which superseded Bulletin No. 540 in 1920, updated biological information on the species and listed all of the earlier-described control measures. The 1931 revision of Bulletin No. 1097[7] listed all of the previously listed control techniques and added that treating manure with hellebore or borax killed larvae of the house fly*, *Musca domestica* Linnaeus, and the stable fly. A special mention was made that cattle that consumed sulfur added to common salt were not protected from flies. The 1939 revision[8] again presented no changes in control technology.

II. TOXICANTS

An emulsion of pine tar and creosote sprayed daily onto dairy cows freed the animals of stable flies and the horn fly*, *Haematobia irritans* (Linnaeus).[9]

A thorough spraying of cattle, especially their legs and lower body areas, with DDT or moving cattle through a wading vat charged with DDT, and spraying all of the nearby structures with DDT provided excellent control of a very large population of stable flies for 2 weeks.[10] DDT, its bromine analogues, and methoxychlor applied to screen wire cages controlled stable flies in excess of 100 days.[11] Stable flies were controlled by light, daily applications of sprays of methoxychlor or synergized pyrethrins.[12]

Backrubber treatments of DDT or methoxychlor, with or without the addition of butoxy polypropylene glycol, controlled horn flies but were not effective against stable flies.[13] Methoxychlor, with or without butoxy polypropylene glycol, Lethane 384®, or synergized pyrethrins in backrubbers controlled horn flies but not stable flies.[14]

During the 1950s, several automatic sprayers were developed to apply small amounts of toxicants, repellents, or their mixtures to cattle daily to control a variety of biting fly pests of cattle. An initial version[12] was activated when cattle stepped on a treadle and applied synergized pyrethrins which controlled stable flies, horn flies, and horse flies. A similar sprayer that applied pyrethrins plus a variety of repellents for two to four times per day controlled a mixed population of stable flies, horn flies, and horse flies.[14] Combinations of methoxychlor, synergized pyrethrins, deet, dimethoate, Thanite®, Lethane 384®, and R-1207 applied daily or more often, with an electric-eye-controlled automatic sprayer, controlled horn flies, but were less effective against stable flies and horse flies.[15-18] A mist spray of crotoxyphos applied with an automatic sprayer activated by a step-on switch controlled horn flies but was not effective against stable flies.[19] Generally, the maintenance requirements to keep the automatic sprayers working satisfactorily are more than most stock raisers are willing to provide.

Dichlorvos, naled, fenthion, and a mixture of dichlorvos and stirofos, applied with fixed-wing aircraft or helicopter at the rate of 47 ℓ/ha low volume (LV) or 0.73 ℓ/ha ultra low volume (ULV) to cattle in dairy farms or feedlots, afforded partial reduction in numbers of stable flies feeding on treated cattle for only 1 day posttreatment.[20] Of nine insecticides evaluated as residual sprays for the control of stable flies, only stirofos, Mobam®, and propoxur gave 50% control of flies feeding on cattle for 2 weeks or longer; crotoxyphos or methoxychlor sprayed onto cattle controlled stable flies for 4 days and space sprays of mists of dichlorvos or naled afforded only partial control for 1 day.[21]

Chlorfenvinphos sprayed onto cattle did not reduce the numbers of stable flies per leg, but large numbers of dead stable flies were collected from the floor of the barn that held treated cattle for 8 days posttreatment.[22]

In large-cage tests in which sprayed cattle were held in large screened cages and infested periodically with stable flies, permethrin spray controlled stable flies for 7 to 10 days.[23] Deltamethrin applied to a spot on cattle not only repelled stable flies, but remained active as a toxicant when it no longer repelled flies and they fed on the treated area.[24]

Ear tags impregnated with flucythrinate and tag tapes containing permethrin placed around existing ear tags controlled stable flies for 10 weeks.[25] A period of 2 to 3 weeks was necessary to lower fly populations to zero to one fly per animal.

Articles of *Insecticide and Acaricide Tests* since 1977 have reported on the effectiveness of naled and dichlorvos aerial sprays to cattle to reduce feeding of stable flies, effectiveness of sprays of permethrin and fenvalerate applied to cattle, short residual activity (1 day only) of permethrin pouron, and variable control of stable flies on cattle treated with ear tags impregnated with permethrin and deltamethrin.

III. REPELLENTS

A. Treatment Technology

The only repellent listed in *U.S. Dep. Agric. Farmers' Bulletins* from 1913 to 1939 was a mixture of fish oil, pine tar oil, pennyroyal oil, and kerosene. Graybill[26] reviewed the literature on repellents, listed pyrethrins or tobacco powders and Beaumont crude oil, fish oil, tar oil, and cottonseed oil as popular repellents, and, of a number of repellents tested, only carbolic acid in cottonseed oil, pine tar oil, and tar oil repelled flies for 1 day or less. He stated that oral administration of repellents to animals "seems to be an extremely unpromising means of repelling flies".

Of a variety of commercial and home-mixed repellents sprayed daily onto milk cows[27] to repel stable flies and horn flies, the most satisfactory in terms of effectiveness, cost, and practicality was a home-mixed spray of used crankcase oil and oil of tar.

Sprays of pyrethrins and/or pine oil in a petroleum oil base repelled stable flies and house flies for only 5 to 8 hr.[28] Cattle dusted with pyrethrins and rotenone were freed of flies, but the apparent repellent activity was actually the result of rapid knockdown and kill of flies.[29] Sprays of Thanite® and pyrethrins repelled stable flies for up to 84 hr.[30]

Butoxy polypropylene glycol, in oil or water, repelled stable flies and house flies,[31] and, when combined with pyrethrins, allethrin, or Thanite® was highly effective against stable flies and horn flies for at least 1 day.[32] Cyclethrin, a pyrethroid, synergized with piperonyl butoxide or sulfoxide, as a whole body aqueous spray, repelled stable flies and horn flies for 3 to 5 days.[33]

MGK Repellent 11® and 326® repelled stable flies, house flies, and horn flies for several days and had much longer residual effectiveness on animals held in the shade than on those in the sun.[34] Sprays of Tabutrex® and MGK Repellent 326® repelled stable flies for 1 to 6 days and were more effective than synergized pyrethrins.[35]

B. Testing Techniques

A new technique for evaluating repellents[36] took into consideration the relative susceptibility of individual cows to stable flies and was modified later[37] to include the spraying of the untreated cows with the base oil. A "one-half cow" technique, in which half of a cow was sprayed with a repellent and the other half unprotected, was described[38] as an efficient method to evaluate repellents. The nature of and need for fly repellents were explained and only oil sprays of pyrethrins extract of Lethane 384® were identified as effective repellents.[39]

During the early 1940s, there was an emphasis on the need for the standardization of the testing of repellents. The details of several methods used to test repellents on cattle in the field and to test repellents and toxicants in the laboratory were presented by Nelson.[40] Balanced trials, statistical analysis, and mathematically transformed observed data on fly counts were needed to accurately define repellency.[41,42]

A treated cheese cloth/rabbit test was used[43] to screen repellents, but little relationship was found between repellent activity in screening tests and effectiveness when applied to cattle in the field. Candidate toxicants and repellents were sprayed onto white mice which were exposed to stable flies periodically after treatment.[44] Materials found effective in the screening test were sprayed onto cattle and also killed or repelled stable flies. A sandwich-bait method was used to screen hundreds of chemicals.[45] An animal-derived membrane was used[46] to evaluate repellents, and the activity of repellents in field tests with horn flies and stable flies on cattle showed some relationship to their activity in the membrane test. A sandwich-bait screening tests, and a secondary test in which the skin of a mouse was treated and exposed to starved stable flies was used to evaluate repellents.[47]

Repellents or toxicants were sprayed onto small test areas, called "spots", on cattle,[48] and stable flies were confined onto the treated spots. This test could discriminate between toxicants and repellents in that repellents prevented flies from feeding and toxicants killed flies during or after feeding. Results of this "spot test" technique compared favorably with results of subsequent "large-cage"tests in which repellents or toxicants were applied as whole body sprays onto cattle which were then confined in large screened cages and subjected to attack by stable flies. In a series of large-cage tests,[49] the effectiveness of repellents for stable flies was related to the amount of pyrethrins they contained rather than to additives, such as Tabutrex®, butoxy polypropylene glycol, piperonyl butoxide, and other repellents. In large-cage tests, deet repelled stable flies for only 4 hr even when applied at rates to cattle that caused adverse toxicological symptoms, such as excessive salivation and nasal discharge.[50] Of 639 compounds screened by the spot test technique from 1967 through 1973, 53 repelled stable flies for 4 days or longer and 149 were toxic for 8 days or longer.[51]

A review of literature on the testing of repellents[52] focused on protecting humans, but is of value to those interested in the protection of cattle.

IV. TRAPS

A. Early Traps

As described in early *U.S. Dep. Agric. Farmers' Bulletins,* Hodge fly traps placed in the windows of buildings trapped stable flies as they were attracted from the insides of buildings to the light. Manure boxes could be fitted with fly traps, and manure could be placed on maggot traps, similar to those (see Chapter 18) used for larvae of the house fly.

B. Attractant Traps

Early traps were "passive" traps in that they only trapped stable flies and other flies as the flies left darkened places. More recent traps were "active" traps in that flies actively sought them out as a response to CO_2, light, color, or an attractant aspect of the trap. The design and use of a variety of traps with or without CO_2 to attract and collect horse and deer flies are discussed in detail in Chapter 5. With respect to stable flies, Malaise traps baited with CO_2 caught about three times more flies than did nonbaited traps or traps baited with CO.[53] Stable flies and house flies inside a barn were attracted to and killed by a trap that combined BLB fluorescent lamps and an electrocutor grid.[54] Plywood panels painted with a sticky adhesive captured marked stable flies.[55] The combination of an electrocutor grid plus release of CO_2 attracted and killed thousands of stable flies and was more effective than the combination of the grid plus ultraviolet light or the grid plus clear plexiglass.[56]

A new type of trap, constructed of translucent white Alsynite® fiberglass panels and coated with an adhesive, was more effective than previously used box traps to capture stable flies.[57] When the toxicant, permethrin, replaced the sticky material, the traps attracted and killed enough stable flies to reduce local populations by 84 to 90%.[58] These "Williams" traps, coated with an adhesive, reduced numbers of stable flies by about 80% in a zoo, but required a high level of maintenance.[59] They have also been used to measure migration[2] and population levels[60] of the stable fly.

V. OVERVIEW AND CURRENT TECHNOLOGY

The primary technology for the control of stable flies is the elimination of the breeding of larvae that takes place in manure, wastes, feed, and other media found around structures that hold livestock. Sanitation is absolutely essential to any stable fly control program.

The application of toxicants and/or repellents to cattle provided variable control or repelling of stable flies. Toxicants or repellents applied to cattle by automatic sprayers or by air provided some control or repelling of stable flies but were not suitable for practical application. In general, the pyrethroid insecticides appear to provide more control of stable flies than has been achieved with previous treatments applied to cattle.

Traps have been designed that attract and capture or kill large numbers of stable flies. Their use as a practical technology to reduce populations of stable flies has yet to be determined.

With stable flies or other pest flies, in which only a small portion of the total local population is found around cattle and other livestock at any time, the killing or repelling of these individuals has little effect on the population as a whole.

REFERENCES

1. **Morgan, C. E., Thomas, G. D., and Hall, R. D.,** Annotated bibliography of the stable fly, *Stomoxys calcitrans* (L.), including references on other species belonging to the genus *Stomoxys, Univ. Mo. Agric. Exp. Stn. Res. Bull.,* 1049, 1983.
2. **Hogsette, J. A. and Ruff, J. P.,** Stable fly (Diptera: Muscidae) migration in northwest Florida, *Environ. Entomol.,* 14, 170, 1985.
3. **Osborn, H.,** Insects affecting domestic animals: an account of the species of importance in North America, with mention of related forms occurring on other animals, *U.S. Dep. Agric. Bull.,* 5, 1896.
4. **Bishopp, F. C.,** The stable fly, *U.S. Dep. Agric. Farmers' Bull.,* 540, 1913.
5. **Bishopp, F. C.,** The stable fly, (*Stomoxys calcitrans* L.), an important livestock pest, *J. Econ. Entomol.,* 6, 112, 1913.
6. **Bishopp, F. C.,** The stable fly: how to prevent its annoyance and its losses to livestock, *U.S. Dep. Agric. Farmers' Bull.,* 1097, 1920.
7. **Bishopp, F. C.,** The stable fly: how to prevent its annoyance and its losses to livestock, *U.S. Dep. Agric. Farmers' Bull.,* 1097, 1931.
8. **Bishopp, F. C.,** The stable fly: how to prevent its annoyance and its losses to livestock, *U.S. Dep. Agric. Farmers' Bull.,* 1097, 1939.
9. **Cory, E. N.,** The protection of dairy cattle from flies, *J. Econ. Entomol.,* 10, 111, 1917.
10. **Bruce, W. G. and Blakeslee, E. B.,** DDT to control insect pests affecting livestock, *J. Econ. Entomol.,* 39, 367, 1946.
11. **Eddy, G. W. and McGregor, W. S.,** Residual action of organic insecticides against stable flies, *J. Econ. Entomol.,* 42, 547, 1949.
12. **Bruce, W. N.,** Automatic sprayer for control of biting flies on cattle, *Ill. Nat. Hist. Surv. Biol. Notes,* 27, 1952.
13. **Raun, E. S. and Casey, D. J.,** A comparison of back rubber formulations for controlling horn and stable flies in Iowa, *J. Econ. Entomol.,* 49, 395, 1956.
14. **Cheng, T. H. and Vanderberg, J. P.,** The treadle sprayer and the cable-type back rubber for control of biting flies on cattle in Pennsylvania, *J. Econ. Entomol.,* 51, 149, 1958.

15. **Granett, P., Hansens, E. J., and O'Connor, C. T.,** Automatic cattle sprayers for fly control in New Jersey, *J. Econ. Entomol.,* 48, 386, 1955.
16. **Cheng, T. H., Frear, D. E. H., and Enos, H. F., Jr.,** The use of treatments containing methoxychlor against biting flies on cattle and the determination of methoxychlor residues in milk, *J. Econ. Entomol.,* 51, 618, 1958.
17. **Cheng, T. H., Frear, D. E. H., and Enos, H. F., Jr.,** Effectiveness of aerosol formulations containing methoxychlor and other insecticide-repellents against biting flies on cattle, and analyses of milk from treated animals, *J. Econ. Entomol.,* 52, 866, 1959.
18. **Cheng, T. H., Frear, D. E. H., and Enos, H. F., Jr.,** The use of spray and aerosol formulations containing R-1207 and dimethoate for fly control on cattle and the determination of dimethoate residues in milk, *J. Econ. Entomol.,* 55, 39, 1962.
19. **Hoffman, R. A., Berry, I. L., and Graham, O. H.,** Control of flies on cattle by frequent, low-volume mist spray applications of Ciodrin, *J. Econ. Entomol.,* 58, 815, 1965.
20. **Campbell, J. B. and Raun, E. S.,** Aerial ULV and LV applications of insecticides for control of the stable fly and horn fly, *J. Econ. Entomol.,* 64, 1170, 1971.
21. **Campbell, J. B. and Hermanussen, J. F.,** Efficacy of insecticides and methods of insecticidal application for control of stable flies in Nebraska, *J. Econ. Entomol.,* 64, 1188, 1971.
22. **Roberts, R. H., Wrich, M. J., Hoffman, R. A., and Jones, C. M.,** Control of horn flies and stable flies with three General Chemical compounds, *J. Econ. Entomol.,* 54, 1047, 1961.
23. **Schmidt, C. D., Matter, J. J., Meurer, J. H., Reeves, R. E., and Shelley, B. K.,** Evaluation of a synthetic pyrethroid for control of stable flies and horn flies on cattle, *J. Econ. Entomol.,* 69, 484, 1976.
24. **Schmidt, C. D. and Matter, J. J.,** Systemic activity of the pyrethroid NRDC 161 against stable flies on cattle, *Southwest. Entomol.,* 3, 133, 1978.
25. **Hogsette, J. A. and Ruff, J. P.,** Evaluation of flucythrinate- and fenvalerate-impregnated ear tags and permethrin ear tapes for fly (Diptera: Muscidae) control on beef and dairy cattle in northwest Florida, *J. Econ. Entomol.,* 79, 152, 1986.
26. **Graybill, H. W.,** Repellents for protecting animals from the attacks of flies, U.S. Dep. Agric. Bull., 131, 1914.
27. **Cleveland, C. R.,** Repellent sprays for flies attacking dairy cattle, *J. Econ. Entomol.,* 19, 529, 1926.
28. **Freeborn, S. B. and Regan, W. M.,** Fly sprays for dairy cows — a progress report, *J. Econ. Entomol.,* 25, 167, 1932.
29. **Cory, E. N., Harns, H. G., and Anderson, W. H.,** Dusts for control of flies on cattle, *J. Econ. Entomol.,* 29, 331, 1936.
30. **Shaw, A. O., Smith, R. C., Atkeson, F. W., Fryer, H. C., Borgmann, A. R., and Holmes, F. J.,** Tests of fly repellents of known ingredients and of selected commercial sprays on dairy cattle, *J. Econ. Entomol.,* 36, 23, 1943.
31. **Granett, P., Haynes, H. L., Connola, D. P., Bowery, T. G., and Barber, G. W.,** Two butoxypoly-propylene glycol compounds as fly repellents for livestock, *J. Econ. Entomol.,* 42, 281, 1949.
32. **Granett, P., Haynes, H. L., and Helm, R. W.,** Further evaluation of butoxypolypropylene glycol as a fly repellent for dairy cattle, *J. Econ. Entomol.,* 44, 97, 1951.
33. **Granett, P. and Haynes, H. L.,** Use of cyclethrin in livestock sprays for control of flies, *J. Econ. Entomol.,* 48, 409, 1955.
34. **Howell, D. E. and Goodhue, L. D.,** Fly repellents, *Soap Chem. Spec.,* 31, 181, 1955.
35. **Bruce, W. N. and Decker, G. C.,** Experiments with several repellent formulations applied to cattle for the control of stable flies, *J. Econ. Entomol.,* 50, 709, 1957.
36. **Pearson, A. M., Wilson, J. L., and Richardson, C. H.,** Some methods used in testing cattle fly sprays, *J. Econ. Entomol.,* 26, 269, 1933.
37. **Pearson, A. M.,** An improved method for the determination of cattle fly spray repellence, *J. Econ. Entomol.,* 28, 160, 1935.
38. **MacCreary, D. and Goddin, A. H.,** Tests of cattle fly sprays by the "one-half cow" method, *J. Econ. Entomol.,* 30, 478, 1937.
39. **Searls, E. M. and Synder, F. M.,** Cattle sprays their composition and application, *Soap Chem. Spec.,* 14, 103, 1938.
40. **Nelson, F. C.,** Cattle spray testing, *Soap Sanit. Chem.,* 17, 92, 1941.
41. **Fryer, H. C., Shaw, A. O., Atkeson, F. W., Smith, R. C., and Borgmann, A. R.,** Techniques for conducting fly-repellency tests on cattle, *J. Econ. Entomol.,* 36, 33, 1943.
42. **Fryer, H. C., Atkeson, F. W., and Smith, R. C.,** Comparison of methods for testing repellent-type fly sprays, *J. Econ. Entomol.,* 41, 80, 1948.
43. **Starnes, E. B. and Granett, P.,** A laboratory method for testing repellents against biting flies, *J. Econ. Entomol.,* 46, 420, 1953.
44. **Eddy, G. W. and McGregor, W. S.,** Use of white mice for testing materials used as repellents and toxicants for stable flies, *J. Econ. Entomol.,* 42, 461, 1949.

45. **Goodhue, L. D. and Stansbury, R. E.,** Some new fly repellents from laboratory screening tests, *J. Econ. Entomol., 46,* 982, 1953.
46. **Granett, P.,** Use of an animal membrane in the evaluation of chemical repellents against the stable fly, *J. Econ. Entomol., 53,* 432, 1960.
47. **Yeoman, G. H. and Warren, B. C.,** Repellents for *Stomoxys calcitrans* (L.), the stable fly: techniques and a comparative laboratory assessment of butyl methylcinchoninate, *Bull. Entomol. Res., 59,* 563, 1970.
48. **Roberts, R. H., Jones, C. M., and Gless, E. E.,** Methods for the evaluation of stable fly toxicants and repellents, *J. Econ. Entomol., 53,* 301, 1960.
49. **Roberts, R. H., Harris, R. L., and Graham, O. H.,** Effects of additives on the toxicity of pyrethrins to stable flies and horn flies, *J. Econ. Entomol., 56,* 699, 1963.
50. **Blume, R. R., Roberts, R. H., Eschle, J. L., and Matter, J. J.,** Tests of aerosols of deet for protection of livestock from biting flies, *J. Econ. Entomol., 64,* 1193, 1971.
51. **Matter, J. J., Schmidt, C. D., and Blume, R. R.,** Compounds screened as animal protectant sprays at Kerrville, Texas, 1967-1973, *U.S. Dep. Agric. Agric. Res. Serv. S-125,* 1976.
52. **Schreck, C. E.,** Techniques for the evaluation of insect repellents: A critical review, *Annu. Rev. Entomol., 22,* 101, 1977.
53. **Hoy, J. B.,** Trapping the stable fly by using CO_2 or CO as attractants, *J. Econ. Entomol., 63,* 792, 1970.
54. **Morgan, N. O., Pickens, L. G., and Thimijan, R. W.,** House flies and stable flies captured by two types of traps, *J. Econ. Entomol., 63,* 672, 1970.
55. **Bailey, D. L., Whitfield, T. L., and Smittle, B. J.,** Flight and dispersal of the stable fly, *J. Econ. Entomol., 66,* 410, 1973.
56. **Schreck, C. E., Posey, K., and Gouck, H. K.,** Evaluation of the electrocutor grid trap baited with carbon dioxide against the stable fly, *Stomoxys calcitrans* (L.) (Diptera: Muscidae), *J. Med. Entomol., 12,* 338, 1975.
57. **Williams, D. F.,** Sticky traps for sampling populations of *Stomoxys calcitrans, J. Econ. Entomol., 66,* 1279, 1973.
58. **Meifert, D. W., Patterson, R. S., Whitfield, T., LaBrecque, G. C., and Weidhaas, D. E.,** Unique attractant-toxicant system to control stable fly populations, *J. Econ. Entomol., 71,* 290, 1978.
59. **Rugg, D.,** Effectiveness of Williams traps in reducing the numbers of stable flies (Diptera: Muscidae), *J. Econ. Entomol., 75,* 857, 1982.
60. **Scholl, P. J., Lowry, S. R., and Rabe, G. G.,** Modified Williams' sticky traps used to measure activity of adult stable flies, *Stomoxys calcitrans* (L.) in eastern Nebraska, *Southwest. Entomol., 10,* 32, 1985.

Chapter 4

CONTROL OF "SMALL" BITING AND NUISANCE FLIES ON CATTLE*

I. INTRODUCTION

"Small" biting and nuisance flies are defined as those flies smaller than mosquitoes that are pests of cattle, other livestock, and, often, humans. Many species are pests because they suck blood from cattle and other livestock. Other species do not "bite" animals, but their constant presence around livestock is a nuisance to the animals. There is a considerable body of literature on the biology and control of these flies in relation to humans. We will limit ourselves to a review of the technology used to control small biting and nuisance flies in the families of Simuliidae, Chloropidae, and Ceratopogonidae, as they relate to cattle and other livestock.

The interested reader is referred to the reviews on northern biting flies by Hocking,[1] bionomics and control of *Culicoides* and *Leptoconops* by Kettle,[2] biting flies in temperate regions by Service,[3] black flies by Jamnback,[4] black flies in Canada by Fredeen,[5] and blood-sucking ceratopogonids by Kettle.[6] The book, *Blackflies, The Future for Biological Methods in Integrated Control,* edited by Laird,[7] presents a broad summary of the status of a variety of control measures for black flies. A bibliography and keyword index of the Ceratopogonidae contains 3527 references.[8]

There are two facets to the technologies used to control these flies: (1) "personal" protection or the application of toxicants, repellents, or devices to livestock to kill, repel, or prevent the flies from biting or being a nuisance, and (2) area control of adults or larvae by adulticiding with residual sprays or space sprays or by larviciding with insecticides applied to breeding sites.

II. CONTROLLING OR REPELLING ADULTS ON LIVESTOCK

In 1896, Osborn[9] described losses in animal production due to buffalo gnats, *Simulium* spp., and listed the following remedies for protecting animals: smudges (smoke-producing fires), coating animals with a layer of mud or syrup, keeping animals, especially horses, in darkened buildings, and applying sprays or washes of kerosene emulsion, pyrethrins, dilute carbon bisulfide or dissolved tobacco soap, which were effective for only 2 hr. The most effective treatments were greases — cottonseed oil, "stinking" oils, fish oil, and gnat oil — which repelled flies and often injured the animals as well. He strongly recommended a wash of water-based oil of tar and speculated that future control should be directed toward the destruction of immature forms in breeding sites and noted that some chemical treatments killed larvae, but their use on a large scale was not considered practical.

Little has been reported on the use of repellents or toxicants applied to animals to repel or control adults. An emulsion of potash, fish oil, or used crankcase oil plus soap diluted with water applied to cattle repelled the southern buffalo gnat♦, *Cnephia pecuarum* (Riley), for 3 to 8 hr.[10] *C. pecuarum* was repelled by smudges, oils, or a "new" repellent of pine-tar oil plus soap in water applied to animals.[11] Cloth sleeves were used to cover the ears of livestock to prevent feeding of black flies, and heavy applications of grease to ears repelled black flies.[12]

---

* Common names of insects and acarines, as listed in *Common Names of Insects and Related Organisms* (published by the Entomological Society of America), are marked with a ♦ the first time they are cited preceding the scientific name.

Several organophosphorus and pyrethroid insecticides were tested against black flies. A pouron treatment of cattle with phosmet had an immediate repellent effect and a long-term insecticidal effect that reduced the number of black flies, mostly *Simulium arcticum* Malloch, feeding on cattle for several weeks.[13] Additional studies showed that phosmet pouron[14] controlled black flies and also reduced black fly toxicosis in cattle.

Ethanolic solutions or aqueous emulsions of permethrin sprayed onto cattle repelled black flies for 8 to 11 days depending on dosage. Sprays of cypermethrin and resmethrin were effective for 5 and 2 days, respectively, and a permethrin dust repelled black flies for up to 8 days.[15] Deet repelled black flies for up to 4 days; older repellents, such as citronella, camphor, cedar oil, tar oil, castor oil, ammonia, and pine tar, were effective for a very short time, but pyrethroids were very effective.[16]

In Australia, mortality of adult *Culicoides brevitarsis* Kieffer was as high as 99% for 10 days posttreatment when the flies fed on cattle treated with a single subcutaneous injection of ivermectin.[17]

III. AREA CONTROL OF ADULTS AND LARVAE

The area control of small biting flies with residual or space sprays or control of their larvae with larvicides was not a practical possibility until the advent of chlorinated hydrocarbon insecticides during World War II.

A. Adults

A thermal aerosol fog generator was used to apply DDT and benzene hexachloride (BHC) to land areas, including pastures and stables, and the treatment controlled black flies and a variety of other biting flies.[18] Fogging or misting of small areas (1200 ha) with lindane, DDT, or malathion afforded relief from black fly biting (of humans) for only a few hours.[19]

Adult *Hippelates pusio* Loew, an eye gnat, held in cages, were treated with thermal fogs of insecticides. Propoxur and naled were most toxic, DDT was least toxic, and fenthion, dichlorvos, chlorpyrifos, stirofos, iodofenphos, and a mixture of malathion and Lethane 384® had intermediate toxicity.[20] Ultra-low-volume (ULV) (7 to 14 mℓ/ha) aerial sprays of stirofos and naled controlled caged *Hippelates* spp., fenthion was partially effective, and propoxur was ineffective.[21] Only about 50% control of *H. pusio* was obtained on treatment day by ULV applications of stirofos, naled, and malathion.[22] Area control of *H. consullor* (Townsend) was obtained by twice-weekly applications of an attractant plus sugar plus a toxicant, such as dichlorvos or trichlorfon.[23,24]

Residual sprays or thermal aerosols of DDT killed adult *Leptoconops kerteszi* Kieffer.[25] Adulticiding with fogs of fenthion or naled was of doubtful value for the control of *Culicoides variipennis* (Coquillett).[26]

B. Larvae
1. Simuliidae

An oil emulsion of pyrethrins extract applied to a stream eliminated a heavy population of black fly larvae for as far as 200 m downstream without apparent harm to fishes and frogs, but the treatment eliminated nontarget insects as well.[27] Black fly larvae in streams were controlled by treating water with DDT,[28,29] lindane, chlordane, and toxaphene.[30] Treating rivers in Canada with DDT controlled larvae of a black fly, *S. arcticum*, for 27 km downstream, and some effects were noted for as far as 145 km.[31] Heptachlor suspensions were more effective than DDT, while TDE, malathion, schradan, endrin, isodrin, and dieldrin were less effective,[32] DDT treatment of streams practically eliminated the feeding of black flies on cattle in nearby pastures.[33]

The accumulation of DDT in fish and other aquatic life and its effect on fish reproduction called for research to find substitute larvicides for black flies. Temephos was more effective than fenthion and was not as hazardous to nontarget arthropods.[34] Chlorpyrifos was more effective than temephos, methoxycholor, or ronnel.[35] Resistance of black fly larvae to DDT was detected in 1970.[36] Larviciding with DDT for 19 years and methoxychlor for the following 10 years prevented damaging outbreaks of black flies in Western Canada.[37] The larviciding of streams with temephos yearly for 5 years substantially reduced populations of black flies.[38]

Black fly larvae were also controlled when streams were treated with *Bacillus thuringiensis* var. *israelensis* (BTI).[39-41] The effectiveness of BTI as a biological control agent for black fly larvae was reviewed by Gaugler and Finney.[42] BTI readily controlled black fly larvae[43] with little effect on other aquatic insects. BTI treatment, however, did not control the anthropophilic *Prosimulium* species.[44]

Temephos, FMC-45497, and diflubenzuron were evaluated for the control of *Simulium* larvae. Temephos was most specific for *Simulium* larvae, FMC-45497 affected nontarget organisms, and the effectiveness of diflubenzuron, because of its slow-acting activity, was difficult to assess.[45]

2. Chloropidae

Treating soil with sprays or granules of DDT, aldrin, chlordane, BHC, and heptachlor gave moderate to good initial control and some residual control of larvae of *Hippelates* spp.[46,47] Treatments with Shell SD-4402 were effective for 12 months.[48] Populations of *Hippelates* larvae were reduced by herbiciding of weeds, frequent tillage, and nonincorporation of weeds into soil.[49,50] Plowing increased numbers of eye gnats emerging from the soil.[51] Control of larvae of *H. collusor* was obtained by treating breeding areas with granular formulations of sprays of urea.[52]

3. Ceratopogonidae

Outbreaks of *L. kerteszi* were controlled by applying DDT to the ground to kill larvae and pupae.[25] Larvae of *L. kerteszi* were controlled by treating breeding areas in the soil with granular formulations or sprays of urea.[52]

Control of *C. variipennis* larvae was obtained with aerial applications of dieldrin and shoreline treatments of fenthion and diesel oil.[26] Strategies for the control of *Culicoides* have emphasized the use of larvicides plus alteration of larval breeding sites by the implementation of improved methods of waste disposal at sewage plants and feedlots.[53] A series of laboratory tests determined the relative toxicity of fenthion, chlorpyrifos, and temephos to larvae of *C. variipennis*.[54] In field trials, granular formulations of chlorpyrifos, fention, and temephos controlled larvae of *C. variipennis*.[55]

Recently, Holbrook[56] presented an overview of technologies that can be used for control of *Culicoides*. Experimental control strategies for *Culicoides* larvae included water management to decrease breeding of larvae.[57] The management of water and the use of temephos as a larvicide in a 10,000-ha area reduced populations of adult *C. variipennis*.[58] A late fall application of temephos to known overwintering larval sites reduced and delayed spring peaks of adult activity. The treatment of an alkaline lake with permethrin controlled *C. variipennis* larvae, and four treatments over a 2-month period greatly reduced populations of adults.[59]

IV. OVERVIEW AND CURRENT TECHNOLOGY

It is obvious that little technology exists for the control of small biting and nuisance flies of cattle and other livestock. Sprays of pyrethorids or pourons of phosmet applied to cattle have been shown to provide some control of black flies for several days, but such control was only temporary.

Injections of Ivermectin controlled *Culicoides* that fed on treated cattle for several days after treatment. Even if the period of effectiveness of the treatment could be extended considerably by sustained release technology, it is unlikely that such a treatment would affect the total population of flies. Those flies which fed on the treated cattle, even if they were all killed by the treatment, would be only a small segment of the total population. Thus, little control, if any, of the total population would result from such a treatment or any toxicant that killed only a portion of the population.

Control of adults of small biting flies by residual or space sprays has been of little value. However, control of larvae of black flies in certain streams and rivers in Canada has been accomplished by the selective use of water treatments of DDT, methoxychlor, and temephos. Recently, BTI has been shown to be an effective larvicide. Soil treatments, as well as soil management practices, controlled *Hippelates* larvae.

Recent studies have shown that water management and selective use of larvicides control *Culicoides* larvae. Such treatments, if applied on an area-wide basis, may also reduce populations of adults.

REFERENCES

1. **Hocking, B.,** Northern biting flies, *Annu. Rev. Entomol.,* 5, 135, 1960.
2. **Kettle, D. S.,** The bionomics and control of *Culicoides* and *Leptoconops* (Diptera, Ceratopogonidae-Heleidae), *Annu. Rev. Entomol.,* 7, 401, 1962.
3. **Service, M. W.,** Conservation and the control of biting flies in temperate regions, *Biol. Conserv.,* 3, 113, 1971.
4. **Jamnback, H.,** Recent developments in control of blackflies, *Annu. Rev. Entomol.,* 18, 281, 1973.
5. **Fredeen, F. J. H.,** A review of the economic importance of black flies *(Simuliidae)* in Canada, *Quaest. Entomol.,* 13, 219, 1977.
6. **Kettle, D. S.,** Biology and bionomics of bloodsucking ceratopogonids, *Annu. Rev. Entomol.,* 22, 33, 1977.
7. **Laird, M., Ed.,** *Blackflies: The Future for Biological Methods in Integrated Control,* Academic Press, New York, 1981.
8. **Atchley, W. R., Wirth, W. W., Gaskins, C. T., and Strauss, S. L.,** A bibliography and keyword index of the biting midges (Diptera: Ceratopogonidae), *U.S. Dep. Agric. Bibliogr. Lit. Agric.,* 13, 1981.
9. **Osborn, H.,** Insects affecting domestic animals: an account of the species of importance in North America with mention of related forms occurring on other animals, *U.S. Dep. Agric. Bull.,* 5, 1896.
10. **Schwardt, H. H.,** Lubricating oil emulsion as a buffalo gnat repellent, *J. Kans. Entomol. Soc.,* 8, 141, 1935.
11. **Bishopp, F. C.,** The southern buffalo gnat, *U.S. Dep. Agric. Bull.,* E-401, 1941.
12. **Snow, W. E., Pickard, E., and Moore, J. B.,** Observations on blackflies *(Simuliidae)* in the Tennessee river basin, *J. Tenn. Acad. Sci.,* 33, 5, 1958.
13. **Khan, M. A.,** Protection of pastured cattle from black flies (Diptera: Simuliidae): improved weight gains following a dermal application of phosmet, *Vet. Parasitol.,* 8, 327, 1981.
14. **Khan, M. A. and Kosub, G. C.,** Response of Angus, Charolais, and Hereford bulls to black flies *(Simulium* spp.), with and without phosmet treatment, *Can. J. Anim. Sci.,* 65, 269, 1985.
15. **Shemanchuk, J. A.,** Repellent action of permethrin, cypermethrin and resmethrin against black flies *(Simulium* spp.) attacking cattle, *Pestic. Sci.,* 12, 412, 1981.
16. **Shemanchuk, J. A. and Taylor, W. G.,** Repellents protect cattle from black flies, *Can. Agric.,* 29, 14, 1983.
17. **Standfast, H. A., Muller, M. J., and Wilson, D. D.,** Mortality of *Culicoides brevitarsis* (Diptera: Ceratopogonidae) fed on cattle treated with Ivermectin, *J. Econ. Entomol.,* 77, 419, 1984.
18. **Glasgow, R. D. and Collins, D. L.,** The thermal aerosol fog generator for large scale application of DDT and other insecticides, *J. Econ. Entomol.,* 39, 227, 1946.
19. **McComb, C. W. and Bickley, W. E.,** Observations on black flies in two Maryland counties, *J. Econ. Entomol.,* 52, 629, 1959.
20. **Axtell, R. C. and Edwards, T. D.,** Susceptibility of adult *Hippelates pusio* to insecticidal fogs, *J. Econ. Entomol.,* 63, 1184, 1970.

21. **Axtell, R. C.,** Ultralow volume aerial sprays for the control of *Hippelates* gnats and other flies, *J. Ga. Entomol. Soc.,* 6, 101, 1971.

22. **Axtell, R. C.,** *Hippelates pusio* eye gnat control by ultralow volume aerial sprays, *J. Ga. Entomol. Soc.,* 7, 119, 1972.

23. **Mulla, M. S., Axelrod, H., and Ikeshoji, T.,** Attractants for synanthropic flies: area-wide control of *Hippelates collusor* with attractive baits, *J. Econ. Entomol.,* 67, 631, 1974.

24. **Mulla, M. S. and Axelrod, H.,** Attractants for synanthropic flies: longevity of attractant and toxicant formulations evaluated against *Hippelates collusor, J. Econ. Entomol.,* 67, 641, 1974.

25. **Rees, D. M. and Smith, J. V.,** Effective control methods used on biting gnats in Utah during 1949 (Diptera: Ceratopogonidae), *Mosq. News,* 10, 9, 1950.

26. **Apperson, C. S.,** Biological activity of insecticides against *Culicoides variipennis* (Coquillett) (Diptera: Ceratopogonidae), *Proc. Annu. Conf. Calif. Mosq. Cont. Assoc.,* 43, 118, 1975.

27. **Glasgow, R. D.,** Control of blackflies *(Simuliidae), J. Econ. Entomol.,* 32, 882, 1939.

28. **Fairchild, G. B. and Barreda, E. A.,** DDT as a larvicide against *Simulium, J. Econ. Entomol.,* 38, 694, 1945.

29. **Gjullin, C. M., Sleeper, D. A., and Husman, C. N.,** Control of black fly larvae in Alaskan streams by aerial applications of DDT, *J. Econ. Entomol.,* 42, 392, 1949.

30. **Gjullin, C. M., Cope, O. B., Quisenberry, B. F., and DuChanois, F. R.,** The effect of some insecticides on black fly larvae in Alaskan streams, *J. Econ. Entomol.,* 42, 100, 1949.

31. **Arnason, A. P., Brown, A. W. A., Fredeen, F. J. H., Hopewell, W. W., and Rempel, J. G.,** Experiments in the control of *Simulium arcticum* Malloch by means of DDT in the Saskatchewan River, *Sci. Agric.,* 29, 527, 1949.

32. **Hocking, B.,** Developments in the chemical control of black flies (Diptera: Simuliidae), *Can. J. Agric. Sci.,* 33, 572, 1953.

33. **Curtis, L. C.,** Observations on a black fly pest of cattle in British Columbia (Diptera: Simuliidae), *Proc. Entomol. Soc. B.C.,* 51, 3, 1954.

34. **Swabey, Y. H., Schenk, C. F., and Parker, G. L.,** Evaluation of two organophosphorus compounds as blackfly larvicides, *Mosq. News,* 27, 149, 1967.

35. **Travis, B. V. and Schuchman, S. M.,** Tests (1967) with black fly larvicides, *J. Econ. Entomol.,* 61, 843, 1968.

36. **Jamnback, H. and West, A. S.,** Decreased susceptibility of blackfly larvae to p,p'-DDT in New York State and Eastern Canada, *J. Econ. Entomol.,* 63, 218, 1970.

37. **Fredeen, F. J. H.,** Black fly control and environmental quality with reference to chemical larviciding in Western Canada, *Quaest. Entomol.,* 13, 321, 1977.

38. **Baldwin, W. F., Gross, H. P., Wilson, M. L., Keill, D. J., Stuart, R. J., Sebastien, R. J., Knight, A. G., Chant, G. D., Knight, P. A., and West, A. S.,** Suppression of black fly populations in Deep River, Ontario, *Can. Entomol.,* 109, 249, 1977.

39. **Undeen, A. H.,** Control of black flies *(Simuliidae)* using *Bacillus thuringiensis* var. *israelensis, Proc. 51st Meet. Fla. Anti-Mosq. Assoc.,* 55, 1980.

40. **Molloy, D. and Jamnback, H.,** Field evaluation of *Bacillus thuringiensis* var. *israelensis* as a black fly biocontrol agent and its effect on nontarget stream insects, *J. Econ. Entomol.* 74, 314, 1981.

41. **Molloy, D., Gaugler, R., and Jamnback, H.,** Factors influencing efficacy of *Bacillus thuringiensis* var. *israelensis* as a biological control agent of black fly larvae, *J. Econ. Entomol.,* 74, 61, 1981.

42. **Gaugler, R. and Finney, J. R.,** A review of *Bacillus thuringiensis* var. *israelensis* (Serotype 14) as a biological control agent of black flies *(Simuliidae), Misc. Publ. Entomol. Soc. Am.,* 12, 1, 1982.

43. **Lacey, L. A. and Undeen, A. H.,** Effect of formulation, concentration, and application time on the efficacy of *Bacillus thuringiensis* (H-14) against black fly (Diptera: Simuliidae) larvae under natural conditions, *J. Econ. Entomol.,* 77, 412, 1984.

44. **White, D. J. and Morris, C. D.,** Seasonal abundance of anthropophilic Simuliidae from the Adirondack mountains of New York State and effectiveness of an experimental treatment program using *Bacillus thuringiensis* var. *israeliensis, Environ. Entomol.,* 14, 464, 1985.

45. **Mohsen, Z. H. and Mulla, M. S.,** Field evaluation of *Simulium* larvicides: effects on target and nontarget insects, *Environ. Entomol.,* 11, 390, 1982.

46. **Dow, R. P. and Willis, M. J.,** Evaluation of insecticides for the control of *Hippelates pusio* in soil, *J. Econ. Entomol.,* 52, 68, 1959.

47. **Mulla, M. S., Barnes, M. M., and Garber, M. J.,** Soil treatments with insecticides for control of the eye gnats *Hippelates collusor* and *H. hermsi, J. Econ. Entomol.,* 53, 362, 1960.

48. **Mulla, M. S.,** Control of *Hippelates* gnats with soil treatments using organochlorine insecticides, *J. Econ. Entomol.,* 54, 636, 1961.

49. **Mulla, M. S.,** An ecological basis for the suppression of *Hippelates* eye gnats, *J. Econ. Entomol.,* 56, 768, 1963.

50. **Mulla, M. S., Garber, M. J., Axelrod, H., and Andrews, F. G.,** Control of *Hippelates* eye gnats with herbicidal oils, *J. Econ. Entomol.,* 59, 552, 1966.
51. **Gaydon, D. M. and Adkins, T. R., Jr.,** Effect of cultivation on emergence of eye gnats (*Hippelates* spp.) in South Carolina, *J. Econ. Entomol.,* 62, 312, 1969.
52. **Legner, E. F., Sjogren, R. D., Olton, G. S., and Moore, L.,** Control of biting and annoying gnats with fertiziler, *Calif. Agric.,* 30, 14, 1976.
53. **Jones, R. H., Luedke, A. J., Walton, T. E., and Metcalf, H. E.,** Bluetongue in the United States an entomological perspective toward control, *World Anim. Rev.,* 38, 2, 1981.
54. **Holbrook, F. R.,** Evaluations of three insecticides against colonized and field-collected larvae of *Culicoides variipennis* (Diptera: Ceratopogonidae), *J. Econ. Entomol.,* 75, 736, 1982.
55. **Holbrook, F. R. and Agun, S. K.,** Field trials of pesticides to control larval *Culicoides variipennis* (Ceratopogonidae), *Mosq. News,* 44, 233, 1984.
56. **Holbrook, F. R.,** An overview of *Culicoides* control, in *Bluetongue and Related Orbiviruses,* Barber, T. L. and Jochim, M. M., Eds., Alan R. Liss, New York, 1985, 607.
57. **Mullens, B. A., Loomis, E. C., and Anderson, J. R.,** Clues to control of bluetongue virus: control strategy aimed at early life stages of vector gnats is one possibility, *Calif. Agric.,* 40, 23, 1986.
58. **Holbrook, F. R.,** Research on the control of bluetongue in livestock by vector suppression, in *Bluetongue and Related Orbiviruses,* Barber, T. L. and Jochim, M. M., Eds., Alan R. Liss, New York, 1985, 617.
59. **Woodward, D. L., Colwell, A. E., and Anderson, N. L.,** Use of pyrethrin larvicide to control *Culicoides variipennis* (Diptera: Ceratopogonidae) in an alkaline lake, *J. Am. Mosq. Cont. Assoc.,* 1, 363, 1985.

Chapter 5

CONTROL OF HORSE FLIES AND DEER FLIES ON CATTLE*

I. INTRODUCTION

Biting flies in the family Tabanidae, horse flies and deer flies, can affect the productiveness and well-being of cattle, horses, and large wildlife. Their blood-feeding activities can cause considerable blood loss in livestock, and tabanids transmit organisms that cause diseases, including anthrax, equine infectious anemia, tularemia, and anaplasmosis. In the U.S. and Canada there are over 300 species of tabanids, and the most important pests of livestock are found in the genera *Tabanus, Chrysops,* and *Hybomitra.* Horse and deer flies are very difficult to control with chemicals, for the female flies are found on livestock for only short periods of time as they imbibe blood and are only briefly in contact with repellents or toxicants applied to the animals. Eggs are generally laid on vegetation in moist or wet areas, and the free-living larvae are generally found in moist soil or in water. Most larvae are predaceous or cannibalistic, but some are herbivorous. We know very little about the biology, life history, and habitats of adult or larval tabanids.

Controlling or repelling horse and deer flies has been attempted by treating animals with toxicants or repellents and by the use of space sprays to kill flies in the air or on vegetation. Traps have attracted adults and provided limited control of tabanids. Also, insecticides have been applied to the soil to kill horse fly larvae. Use of repellents on cattle is addressed in Chapter 3. Biocontrol of horse flies is briefly discussed in Chapter 21.

II. TOXICANTS OR REPELLENTS APPLIED TO CATTLE

A. Early Treatment Technology

In 1896, Osborn[1] described several species of horse and deer flies and listed the draping of cloth nets over cattle and horses to protect them from fly attack. Nothing available had sufficient repellency to keep horse flies away from cattle, but oil and other substances used to repel bot flies may be of value. Control remedies consisted of fly nets to cover livestock or a kerosene emulsion applied with an atomizer or hand sprayer.[2] *U.S. Dep. Agric. Bulletin* No. 1218 in 1924[3] reported that hoods of burlap or canvas protected the heads and necks of horses from horse flies; none of the materials tested repelled flies and the traps tested did not trap flies.

B. Organochlorine Insecticides and Repellents

DDT sprayed onto dairy cattle did not cause a noticeable reduction in the numbers of *Chrysops discalis* Williston.[4] Although DDT sprays controlled the horn fly*, *Haematobia irritans* (Linnaeus), stable flies, and a variety of other pests of cattle, they had no effect on numbers of tabanids on the cattle.[5] Because of sprays of DDT, benzene hexachloride (BHC), chlordane, and toxaphene controlled several species of horse flies for 1 to 2 days after spraying, but afforded little repellency, cattle were sprayed with pyrethrins plus piperonyl butoxide, piperonyl cyclonene, or rotenone. Only pyrethrins plus piperonyl butoxide provided fair protection for 2 to 3 days.[6] Spraying of dairy cows with pyrethrins plus piperonyl butoxide reduced numbers of *T. sulcifrons* Macquart feeding on cattle. Sprays of pyrethrins plus piperonyl butoxide were more effective repellents than sprays of butoxy polypropylene

---

* Common names of insects and acarines, as listed in *Common Names of Insects and Related Organisms* (published by the Entomological Society of America), are marked with a * the first time they are cited preceding the scientific name.

glycol, lindane plus bentonite sulfur, or a dust of allethrin for *T. quinquevittatus* Wiedemann.[7] The 1952 *U.S. Dep. Agric. Yearbook of Agriculture*[8] listed that sprays of pyrethrins plus piperonyl butoxide repelled horse flies for about 1 day and that results of tests with chlorinated hydrocarbon insecticides as toxicants were extremely inconsistent, although DDT and methoxychlor often provided high mortality of flies for 5 days. Further tests with pyrethrins plus piperonyl butoxide indicated that a single treatment repelled several species of horse flies for 5 to 7 days.[9] Some 250 chemicals were tested as repellents against *C. discalis* when applied topically to white mice, and, of five selected repellents sprayed onto calves, only pyrethrins repelled deer flies for a short time without some deleterious effect to the skin or hair of the calves.[10]

C. Automatic Sprayers

Treatment of beef cattle with a mixture of pyrethrins plus piperonyl butoxide applied with a treadle-activated automatic sprayer reduced numbers of *T. sulcifrons* feeding on cattle.[11] In further tests with the sprayer, pyrethrins plus piperonyl butoxide, butoxy polypropylene glycol, Thanite®, allethrin, and MGK 264® repelled *T. sulcifrons* satisfactorily, but application technology and proper knowledge of animal routine were more important factors in the determination of relative effectiveness of the repellents than the repellents themselves.[12] A mixture of synergized pyrethrins and butoxy polypropylene glycol applied daily with an electric-eye-controlled automatic sprayer controlled *T. sulcifrons* and *T. giganteus* (De-Geer).[13] Pyrethrins plus piperonyl butoxide applied to cattle with an electric-eye or self-activated automatic sprayer reduced populations of horse flies and also reduced transmission of anaplasmosis.[14,15]

D. Other Treatment Technologies

BW-11Z70 sprays controlled horse flies for 1 to 3 weeks.[16] Weekly spraying of steers with a combination of methoxychlor, carbaryl, and pyrethrins plus piperonyl butoxide provided good to excellent control of horse flies on the day after treatment, and there was still some control evident on the day before the next treatment.[17] A spray of dust of permethrin controlled *T. subsimilis* Bellardi, *T. sulcifrons,* and *T. proximus* Walker confined in cages on the cattle for up to 2 weeks for posttreatment.[18,19]

Stirofos-impregnated ear tags did not control horse flies.[20] In contrast, ear tags impregnated with fenvalerate or treated with tapes of permethrin reduced numbers of horse flies similar to the reduction that was obtained from permethrin pouron or spray.[21]

Lindane, aldrin, and dieldrin injected into mice controlled *C. discalis.*[22] Only lindane injections gave partial control of deer flies and horse flies that fed on treated cattle.

III. AREA CONTROL OF FLIES

DDT in oil sprayed onto a shoreline afforded season-long control of adult salt marsh greenhead flies, *T. nigrovittatus* Macquart.[23] Methoxychlor, toxaphene, chlordane, or DDT dissolved in oil and cyclohexanone applied by aircraft to wooded areas did not decrease numbers of *T. abactor* Philip, *T. sulcifrons,* and other species of horse flies attacking draft horses.[24] The aerial application of lindane controlled horse flies and deer flies in open areas but not in dense forest, and DDT and dieldrin were generally ineffective.[25] Aerial applications of naled afforded excellent control of tabanids at 1 day and 1 week posttreatment,[26] and naled applied to a tree- and shrub-lined river bank reduced numbers of horse flies, especially *T. lineola,* collected from cattle in the area.[27] Mist sprays of resmethrin and permethrin, applied to woods near fields by large- or low-volume mist blowers or by ULV sprayer, reduced catches of a deer fly, *C. atlanticus* Pechuman, for less than 24 hr.[28]

IV. TRAPS

Female *C. discalis* were attracted to boards as sites for oviposition, and stakes coated with two nondrying butylene polymer adhesives placed at oviposition locations captured hundreds of flies.[29] Horse flies and other biting flies were captured in a steer-baited trap.[30] A sticky trap, constructed as a cylinder to simulate the shape of a cow[31] and baited with dry ice as a source of CO_2, caught significantly more female horse flies than an unbaited trap.[32] These traps captured thousands of horse flies, and numbers of flies observed feeding on cattle were decreased during the trapping periods.[33] A CO_2-baited cylinder trap caught more specimens and more species of tabanids than a standard animal-baited trap.[34] A conical trap, baited with dry ice, collected a variety of tabanids and other blood-sucking flies.[35]

A Manitoba fly trap, which consisted of a cone located over a black decoy target, attracted and captured a number of species of horse flies.[36] This trap captured more tabanids than either an animal silhouette trap or use of a hand-held aerial sweep net.[37] Malaise traps, described in detail by Townes,[38] baited with CO_2, collected more horse and deer flies than unbaited traps.[39] A Malaise trap baited with CO_2 or a steer captured more horse flies, stable flies, and mosquitoes than an unbaited Malaise trap.[40] A canopy trap, which combined features of several previous traps, baited with dry ice, collected as many as 1000 tabanids per hour during peak seasons.[41] The Manning trap,[42] superior to the Manitoba fly trap in capturing *T. nigrovittatus,* caught thousands of flies when placed in a salt marsh.[43] A modified canopy trap captured horse flies and other species of blood-sucking flies on golf courses.[44] Studies with several trap designs, use of CO_2 baits, and types of black decoys[45,46] indicated that traps varied considerably in their ability to trap tabanids, CO_2 increased catches of tabanids, and that the black decoys and CO_2 were sampling the same population of flies. The Assateague trap, which contained a blacklight ultraviolet fluorescent lamp, was unique in that from midnight until dawn it captured large numbers of male *T. lineola* Fabricius not collected by other types of traps.[47] Drum traps, made from the halves of a 55-gal drum, were more successful than Manning traps in collecting *T. nigrovittatus* and were also more durable.[48] The use of traps to collect tabanids was reviewed by Roberts.[49]

A modifed cattle-baited trap that used a movable, collapsible cloth suspended over an arch-shaped frame to cover a bait animal collected horse flies and a variety of other blood-sucking flies.[50]

V. AREA CONTROL OF LARVAE

Plots of marsh land were treated topically with granular formulations of dieldrin, aldrin, DDT, or lindane, and only the highest dieldrin treatment reduced numbers of larvae of *T. nigrovittatus,* but also seriously damaged other animal life.[51] Dieldrin granules were more effective than granules of aldrin, chlordane, heptachlor, and DDT for the control of *Tabanus* larvae. Treatment of an isolated area with dieldrin reduced populations of adult horse flies, especially *T. nigrovittatus,* but did not reduce populations in a nonisolated area.[52] Although a number of organophosphorus insecticides were toxic to larvae of *C. flavidus* Wiedemann in laboratory tests, none was used in field tests.[53]

VI. OVERVIEW AND CURRENT TECHNOLOGY

It is obvious that there are limited technologies available to control horse and deer flies. Frequent application of chlorinated hydrocarbon insecticides and repellents to cattle provided some control of tabanids. Tests with permethrin indicated that sprays of this pyrethroid (and possibly other pyrethroids as well) could control tabanids for limited periods.

Applying insecticides to vegetation to control adults or to the ground to control larvae appears to hold little promise as a practical control technology. This technology not only fails to provide effective control, but also generally requires environmentally unsound uses of insecticide.

The use of traps, which can attract and capture large numbers of tabanids, appears to be limited because of constraints on numbers of traps needed and costs to purchase and maintain them. Traps appear to be more of a survey tool than a control technology.

A major problem in the development of control technologies for tabanids is our inadequate knowledge of their biology and life history. There is yet to be established a reproducing laboratory colony of any species. An in vitro colony could supply adequate numbers of larvae and flies for testing chemicals and other control technologies. Such colonies would also allow for the accumulation of knowledge about the biology and life history of pest species. There is also a need for broad based research on the field biology and ecology of tabanids before much progress can be made in the development of control technologies.

We await a practical control technology for horse and deer flies.

REFERENCES

1. **Osborn, H.,** Insects affecting domestic animals: an account of the species of importance in North America with mention of related forms occurring on other animals, *U.S. Dep. Agric. Bull.,* 5, 1896.
2. **Hine, J. S.,** A preliminary report on the horseflies of Louisiana with a discussion of remedies and natural enemies, *La. State Crop Pest Comm. Circ.,* 6, 1906.
3. **Webb, J. L. and Wells, R. W.,** Horse-flies: biologies and relation to western agriculture, *U.S. Dep. Agric. Bull.,* 1218, 1924.
4. **Gjullin, C. M. and Mote, D. C.,** Notes on the biology and control of *Chrysops discalis* Williston (Diptera, Tabanidae), *Proc. Entomol. Soc. Wash.,* 47, 236, 1945.
5. **Bruce, W. G. and Blakeslee, E. B.,** DDT to control insect pests affecting livestock, *J. Econ. Entomol.,* 39, 367, 1946.
6. **Howell, D. E.,** Piperonyl formulations as horse fly repellents, *J. Econ. Entomol.,* 42, 401, 1949.
7. **Goodwin, W. J., Sloan, M. J., and Schwardt, H. H.,** Repellency test for horse flies and horn flies in New York State, *J. Econ. Entomol.,* 45, 121, 1952.
8. **Eddy, G. W.,** Flies on livestock, *U.S. Dep. Agric. Yearb. Agric.,* 657, 1952.
9. **Goodwin, W. J., Moore, S., III, and Schwardt, H. H.,** Horse fly and horn fly repellent tests on cattle in New York, *J. Econ. Entomol.,* 46, 1088, 1953.
10. **Roth, A. R., Mote, D. C., and Lindquist, D. A.,** Tests of repellents against tabanids, *U.S. Dep. Agric. Agric. Res. Serv. 33-2,* 1954.
11. **Bruce, W. N. and Decker, G. C.,** Tabanid control on dairy and beef cattle with synergized pyrethrins, *J. Econ. Entomol.,* 44, 154, 1951.
12. **Bruce, W. N. and Decker, G. C.,** Factors affecting the performance of treadle sprayers, *J. Econ. Entomol.,* 48, 167, 1955.
13. **Cheng, T. H., Patterson, R. E., Avery, B. W., and Vanderberg, J. P.,** An electric-eye-controlled sprayer for application of insecticides to livestock, *Pa. Agric. Exp. Stn. Bull.,* 626, 1957.
14. **Hoffman, R. A., Smith, K. O., Collins, J. C., Mott, L. O., and Scales, J. W.,** Summary of 1959 and 1960 Mississippi experiments relative to the influence of insect control on transmission of bovine anaplasmosis, *Miss. State Univ. Agric. Exp. Stn. Inform. Sheet,* 699, 1961.
15. **Wilson, B. H., Burns, E. C., Oglesby, W. T., Myers, R. B., Rogers, T. E., and Wimblery, J.,** The effect of horse fly control on rate of infection of bovine anaplasmosis under field conditions in Louisiana, *J. Econ. Entomol.,* 56, 578, 1963.
16. **Brown, L. and Lancaster, J. L., Jr.,** Controlling horse flies on cattle, *Arkansas Farm Res.,* 22, 6, 1973.
17. **Roberts, R. H. and Pund, W. A.,** Control of biting flies on beef steers: effect on performance in pasture and feedlot, *J. Econ. Entomol.,* 67, 232, 1974.
18. **Bay, D. E., Ronald, N. C., and Harris, R. L.,** Evaluation of a synthetic pyrethroid for tabanid control on horses and cattle, *Southwest. Entomol.,* 1, 198, 1976.
19. **Bay, D. E. and Carroll, S. C.,** Control of horse flies on cattle with a synthetic pyrethroid, *Tex. Agric. Exp. Stn. Prog. Rep.,* 3644, 105, 1976.

20. **Wilson, N. L., Huston, J. E., and Davis, D. I.,** Effectiveness of stirofos impregnated ear tags for control of horn flies and horse flies on cattle in central Texas, *Southwest. Vet.,* 31, 197, 1978.

21. **Huston, J. E., Fuchs, T. W., DeBord, J., and Bales, K.,** Control of horn flies and horseflies in beef cattle with synthetic pyrethroid insecticides, *Tex. Agric. Exp. Stn. Prog. Rep.,* 4111, 105, 1983.

22. **Linquist, A. W., Roth, A. R., Hoffman, R. A., Yates, W. W., and Ritcher, P. O.,** Chemotherapeutic use of insecticides for control of bloodsucking insects, *J. Econ. Entomol.,* 46, 610, 1953.

23. **Gerry, B. I.,** Control of a salt marsh tabanid by means of residual DDT-oil spray, *J. Econ. Entomol.,* 42, 888, 1949.

24. **Howell, D. E., Eddy, G. W., and Cuff, R. L.,** Effect on horse fly populations of aerial spray applications to wooded areas, *J. Econ. Entomol.,* 42, 644, 1949.

25. **Brown, A. W. A. and Morrison, P. E.,** Control of adult tabanids by aerial spraying, *J. Econ. Entomol.,* 48, 125, 1955.

26. **Hagen, A. F.,** Area control of tabanids with naled, 1976, *Insectic. Acaric. Tests,* 2, 146, 1977.

27. **Campbell, J. B.,** ULV aerial applications of naled for control of a complex of livestock insects on Platte River pastures in Nebraska, 1975-1976, *Insectic. Acaric. Tests,* 2, 138, 1977.

28. **Hansens, E. J.,** Resmethrin and permethrin sprays to reduce annoyance from a deer fly, *Chrysops atlanticus, J. Econ. Entomol.,* 74, 3, 1981.

29. **Roth, A. R. and Lindquist, A. W.,** Ecological notes on the deer fly at Summer Lake, Oregon, *J. Econ. Entomol.,* 41, 473, 1948.

30. **Roberts, R. H.,** A steer-baited trap for sampling insects affecting cattle, *Mosq. News,* 25, 281, 1965.

31. **Tugwell, P., Burns, E. C., and Witherspoon, B.,** Notes on the flight behavior of the horn fly *Haematobia irritans* (L.) (Diptera: Muscidae), *J. Kans. Entomol. Soc.,* 39, 561, 1966.

32. **Wilson, B. H., Tugwell, N. P., and Burns, E. C.,** Attraction of tabanids to traps baited with dry ice under field conditions in Louisiana, *J. Med. Entomol.,* 3, 148, 1966.

33. **Wilson, B. H.,** Reduction of tabanid populations on cattle with sticky traps baited with dry ice, *J. Econ. Entomol.,* 61, 827, 1968.

34. **Everett, R. and Lancaster, J. L., Jr.,** A comparison of animal- and dry-ice-baited traps for the collection of tabanids, *J. Econ. Entomol.,* 61, 863, 1968.

35. **DeFoliart, G. R. and Morris, C. D.,** A dry ice-baited trap for the collection and field storage of hematophagous Diptera, *J. Med. Entomol.,* 4, 360, 1967.

36. **Thorsteinson, A. J., Braken, G. K., and Hanec, W.,** The orientation behaviour of horse flies and deer flies (Tabanidae, Diptera). III. The use of traps in the study of orientation of tabanids in the field, *Entomol. Exp. Appl.,* 8, 189, 1965.

37. **Thompson, P. H.,** Collecting methods for Tabanidae (Diptera), *Ann. Entomol. Soc. Am.,* 62, 50, 1969.

38. **Townes, H.,** Design for a Malaise trap, *Proc. Entomol. Soc. Wash.,* 64, 253, 1962.

39. **Roberts, R. H.,** Tabanidae collected in a Malaise trap baited with CO_2, *Mosq. News,* 30, 52, 1970.

40. **Roberts, R. H.,** Relative attractiveness of CO_2 and a steer to Tabanidae, Culicidae, and *Stomoxys calcitrans* (L.), *Mosq. News,* 32, 208, 1972.

41. **Catts, E. P.,** A canopy trap for collecting Tabanidae, *Mosq. News,* 30, 472, 1970.

42. **Granger, C. A.,** Trap design and color as factors in trapping the salt marsh greenhead fly, *J. Econ. Entomol.,* 63, 1670, 1970.

43. **Hansens, E. J., Bosler, E. M., and Robinson, J. W.,** Use of traps for study and control of saltmarsh greenhead flies, *J. Econ. Entomol.,* 64, 1481, 1971.

44. **Adkins, T. R., Jr., Ezell, W. B., Jr., Sheppard, D. C., and Askey, M. M., Jr.,** A modified canopy trap for collecting Tabanidae (Diptera), *J. Med. Entomol.,* 9, 183, 1972.

45. **Roberts, R. H.,** The comparative efficiency of six trap types for the collection of Tabanidae (Diptera), *Mosq. News,* 36, 530, 1976.

46. **Roberts, R. H.,** Attractancy of two black decoys and CO_2 to tabanids (Diptera: Tabanidae), *Mosq. News,* 37, 169, 1977.

47. **Morgan, N. O. and Uebel, E. C.,** Efficacy of the Assateague insect trap in collecting mosquitoes and biting flies in a Maryland salt marsh, *Mosq. News,* 34, 196, 1974.

48. **Morgan, N. O.,** Drum trap captures saltmarsh greenheads, *Southwest. Entomol.,* 6, 331, 1981.

49. **Roberts, R. H.,** Horse flies and Deer flies (family Tabanidae). in Surveillance and Collection of Arthropods of Veterinary Importance, Bram, R. A., Ed., *U.S. Dep. Agric. Agric. Handb.,* 518, 1978, 46.

50. **McCreadie, J. W., Colbo, M. H., and Bennett, G. F.,** A trap design for the collection of haematophagous Diptera from cattle, *Mosq. News,* 44, 212, 1984.

51. **Hansens, E. J.,** Granulated insecticides against greenhead *(Tabanus)* larvae in the salt marsh, *J. Econ. Entomol.,* 49, 401, 1956.

52. **Jamnback, H. and Wall, W.,** Control of salt marsh *Tabanus* larvae with granulated insecticides, *J. Econ. Entomol.,* 50, 379, 1957.

53. **Hoffman, R. A.,** Laboratory evaluation of several insecticides against *Chrysops* larvae, *J. Econ. Entomol.,* 53, 262, 1960.

Chapter 6

CONTROL OF FACE FLIES ON CATTLE*

I. INTRODUCTION

The appearance of the face fly*, *Musca autumnalis* DeGeer, in North America in the early 1950s[1] and its subsequent spread throughout most of Canada and the U.S. has been documented by Sabrosky.[2] It moved across southern Canada and the northern U.S., and it also rapidly spread southward in the U.S. until it is now found in every state except Arizona, New Mexico, Texas, and Florida.

When face flies are first found in the area, beef and dairy cattle herdsmen become quickly aware of these "new" flies that feed around the eyes and nostrils of their cattle. Affected cattle cluster and do not feed, and often eye disorders, such as infectious bovine kerato-conjunctivitis (pinkeye) and excessive lacrimation, become common. The habits and ecology of face flies make them difficult to control with conventional insecticidal treatments. Some treatments may provide partial control for limited periods of time. After several years of experiencing face flies on their cattle, the herdsmen usually accept face flies as part of the general complex of arthropod pests found on their animals. Also, populations of face flies tend to become somewhat regulated by parasites, predators, and other natural mechanisms, so that populations increase and decrease through the years, but seldom seem to reach the levels that occurred when face flies first infested an area.

Nevertheless, the presence of the face fly in North America has called for research on the biology and control of this pest in the last 30 years. Smith et al.[3] presented an annotated bibliography of articles published from 1952 through 1965 on the face fly. Pickens and Miller[4] reviewed the literature on face fly biology and control not only from North America since 1953, but also from Europe and other places where face flies had previously been studied. Morgan et al.[5] presented an annotated bibliography of the face fly which contained 844 citations.

Control of the face fly has been attempted by the application of insecticides topically to cattle to kill the adults and orally to cattle to kill or prevent the development of larvae in manure. This chapter is divided into three sections, two on the control technologies described above and a third on integrated pest management schemes to control the face fly.

II. DERMAL TREATMENTS

A. Face and Body Treatments
Spraying barns, trees, sheds, fences, and other sites where adults rest, spraying the bodies of cattle with insecticides commonly used to control biting flies, and applying repellents to the animals' heads were generally ineffective.[6] Dichlorvos or dimethoate in corn syrup bait applied with a paint brush (the "brush-on" treatment) to heads of cattle provided some control of face flies for 1 to 5 days. Daily treatments for the 1st week and at 2- to 5-day intervals after that reduced face fly populations through 3 weeks.

Repellents and insecticides with or without attractive baits applied as wipes, paints, streaks, or sprays to the faces of cattle gave only a few hours control or were relatively ineffective,[7] and the baits caused the hair to become matted and sticky — a problem in itself. Insecticidal

* Common names of insects and acarines, as listed in *Common Names of Insects and Related Organisms* (published by the Entomological Society of America), are marked with a * the first time they are cited preceding the scientific name.

baits were not effective, and less than 1 day of control was obtained from low-volume sprays or wipe-on or brush-on applications of repellents and trichlorfon or dichlorvos.[8] A variety of insecticides combined with repellents was applied to dairy cattle as aerosols, oil-based wipe-ons, or low-pressure sprays, and only the treatments that contained dichlorvos controlled face flies for 1 day.[9] Face sprays of diazinon and dimethoate, face smears of diazinon, trichlorfon, dimethoate, coumaphos, and ronnel, or dusts of diazinon, carbaryl, and coumaphos gave fair to good protection for 7 to 14 days.[10] Body sprays or face and head dusting with coumaphos, diazinon, naled, trichlorfon, crufomate, and carbaryl were ineffective.[11] Of a variety of liquids and dusts, only trichlorfon and naled controlled face flies for 6 to 9 hr (naled irritated cattle and appliers as well). Body treatments of crotoxyphos and chlorfenvinphos controlled horse flies and the stable fly♦, *Stomoxys calcitrans* (Linnaeus), but afforded little protection against face flies.[12] Dichlorvos in syrup, if applied to the face daily, but not if applied irregularly, controlled face flies.[13] Crotoxyphos as a body spray or face treatment (with sugar added) was superior to other materials tested, and chlorfenvinphos, pyramat, and dimetilan gave promising results.[14]

Dimethoate in honey bait applied to the face controlled face flies, and some control was obtained with a body spray of a DDT-lindane mixture.[15] DeFoliart[16] recognized the need to start control measures early in the spring and reapply them regularly in order to control face flies and other fly pests. Only brush-on applications of syrup baits containing dichlorvos or naled controlled face flies for 1 day. Dusts of malathion, methoxychlor, and ronnel and sprays of coumaphos failed to control face flies, and face wipes of dimethoate gave inconsistent control.[17]

B. Ultra-Low-Volume Aerial Application

The application of ultra-low-volumes (ULV) of high concentrations of malathion by airplane to grazing cattle controlled face flies for several days.[18] Aerially applied ULV trichlorfon controlled face flies for 24 hr,[19] but, in a second test, control was much less, presumably due to immigrating flies.[20] Malathion ULV sprays applied by airplane four times during the summer lowered face fly populations.[21] ULV aerial sprays of malathion, stirofos, and a mixture of stirofos plus dichlorvos controlled face flies for 1 day, but provided no residual control.[22]

C. Self-Application Devices

Research on automatic mechanical sprayers that were activated by photoelectric cells or other devices showed that such sprayers could apply small amounts of insecticides when activated by cattle. Sprays or aerosols of Stauffer® R-1207 and dimethoate applied daily with an automatic sprayer or aerosol applicator controlled the horn fly♦, *Haematobia irritans* (Linnaeus), and stable flies, but were less effective against face flies.[23] Sprays of crotoxyphos applied through a four-nozzle manually activated spraying system thoroughly treated the face and body and afforded excellent control of face flies, stable flies, and horn flies for 3 days or longer.[24] The need for constant maintenance and care has limited the practical use of these systems.

Because there was still a need to apply insecticides frequently to cattle in order to control face flies, considerable research centered around the use of maintenance-free, nonautomatic self-application devices so that cattle could treat themselves as needed. Methoxychlor, ronnel, DDT, and toxaphene in self-application cable-type backrubbers reduced face fly populations, but dichlorvos, butoxy polypropylene glycol, and dimethoate in backrubbers were ineffective.[25] DDT, methoxychlor, dioxathion, and toxaphene in backrubbers were ineffective.[15] The use of self-application dust bags containing a variety of dusts or wettable powders (used as dusts) in dusting stations[26,27] reduced numbers of face flies, were more effective than backrubbers, but did not give complete control. Better control of face flies was obtained when cattle were forced to use the devices daily (or more frequently) than when cattle used the devices free choice. Usually self-application devices provided high levels of horn fly control and generally only moderate control of face flies.[28] Dusts of dimetilan, stirofos, coumaphos, and malathion dispensed from dust bags at a simplified dusting station[29] reduced the number of face flies on cattle that had daily access to the bags. Coumaphos, methoxychlor, crotoxyphos, and a mixture of toxaphene-DDT-lindane in self-application dust bags gave generally good to excellent control of face flies.[30] Coumaphos or fenthion in dust bags or tank- or cable-type backrubbers controlled face flies if cattle used them more than twice daily.[32] In other studies,[32] neither dust bags charged with crotoxyphos nor backrubbers charged with toxaphene effectively controlled face flies. Starting in 1976, each issue of *Insecticide and Acaricide Tests* has contained short reports on the testing of insecticides and other materials applied to cattle topically as sprays, pourons, dusts, by backrubbers, face-rubbers, dust bags, or walk-through sprayers to control face flies and other flies, especially horn flies, on cattle.

D. Insecticide-Impregnated Ear Tags

Insecticide-impregnated ear tags that control horn flies on cattle have also been very extensively evaluated for control of face flies. Fenvalerate, deltamethrin, permethrin, or stirofos in ear tags[33-40] generally gave excellent, season-long horn fly control. Control of face flies was fair to good with populations reduced from 50 to 75% of those on untreated cattle. In recent studies, age structure of face flies captured from cattle was used to evaluate the effectiveness of treatments.[41] Because ear tag treatments did not cause a significant change in proportions of parous and nonparous face flies, data suggested that the treatments did not control flies. *Insecticide and Acaricide Tests* since 1969 contains many reports on use of a number of insecticide-impregnated ear tags for the control of horn flies and face flies.

III. ORAL TREATMENTS

Because face flies breed in fresh, undisturbed cow manure, another method to control this species is treating cattle orally to control larvae in the manure. Miller[42] reviewed the early use of this treatment methodology.

A. Organophosphorus Treatments

Anthony et al.[43] reviewed the very limited early research on oral treatments of cattle to control manure-breeding flies and found that coumaphos, ronnel, and Bayer 22408 in the daily feed of cattle completely inhibited the development of larvae of the face fly and the house fly♦, *Musca domestica* Linnaeus, in manure. In laboratory tests, coumaphos, fenthion, crotoxyphos, ronnel, and Zytron® in the feed of cattle controlled face fly larvae. In field tests, free-choice consumption by cattle of mineral blocks containing ronnel provided variable control of face fly larvae in manure and some reduction of face fly populations on the animals.[44] A ronnel salt-mineral mixture, available free choice for cattle, afforded 95% control of face fly larvae provided the consumption was adequate; however, the numbers of flies on cattle remained high in small-[45] and large-scale tests[46] as a result of immigrating flies.

Coumaphos in the feed of cattle or sprayed onto grass that was eaten by cattle eliminated face fly breeding in manure, but there was no decrease in the number of flies on treated cattle.[47] In other feed additive tests,[48] zinc oxide, fenthion, barthrin, dimethrin, coumaphos, ronnel, and Bayer 22408 were effective, while *Bacillus thuringiensis,* carbaryl, methoxychlor, malathion, diazinon and others did not control face fly larvae. Feed treatments of coumaphos, stirofos, chlorfenvinphos, and phosmet were also effective.[49]

A polyvinyl chloride resin formulation of dichlorvos, previously ineffective as a face fly larvicide because cattle refused to eat the treated ration,[44] was highly effective when eaten by cattle. The treatment, which was protected from degradation while passing through cattle, did not adversely affect the animals.[50] Polyvinyl chloride pellets containing diazinon, dichlorvos, dimethoate, and dimetilan were more effective than technical material given orally to cows, but in subsequent field tests, a dichlorvos pellet formulation did not control face fly larvae.[51]

In field tests, a coumaphos salt mixture afforded only partial reduction of the population of face flies, and a famphur salt mixture was ineffective.[28] Coumaphos salt mixture available free choice to cattle controlled face fly larvae in manure, but effects on numbers of adults were very erratic.[52] Ronnel mineral blocks or granules were not completely effective against face fly larvae and numbers of flies on cattle were not decreased.[53] Stirofos in feed controlled horn fly larvae in manure but did not have any marked effect on face fly populations.[54] Stirofos in salt caused a significant decrease in numbers of face fly larvae in manure and only slightly affected the rate of decomposition of manure pats and the tunneling of beetles.[55]

B. Other Materials

Materials other than organic chemical toxicants have been given orally to cattle to control face fly and other fly larvae in manure. *Bacillus thuringiensis* was toxic to face fly larvae when fed to dairy cattle.[56,57]

Methoprene, an insect growth regulator which prevents the emergence of adults, highly effective as an oral treatment for horn flies, was found to be effective against face flies as well.[58] However, the dosage needed to prevent emergence of face flies was about six times higher than the dosage needed for horn flies.[59] Mineral blocks or loose mineral containing methoprene at levels higher than those registered for use for horn fly control prevented emergence of face flies, but numbers of adults on cattle were only slightly reduced.[60] Of six arylterpenoid juvenile hormone mimics evaluated, three fed to cattle were highly effective against face fly and other fly larvae.[61]

Diflubenzuron, a compound that inhibits chitin synthesis in insects, was effective as a feed additive for the control of face fly and house fly larvae in manure.[62] Diflubenzuron in salt controlled face fly larvae in manure, and the treatment slightly affected the rate of decomposition of the manure pats and tunneling of a beetle, *Sphaeridium scarabaeoides* (Linnaeus).[55]

Monensin, a biologically active compound that alters rumen fermentation, caused a decrease in pupal weights, and highest dosages prevented pupation and eclosion of adult face flies.[63] The feeding of a dye, erthrosin B, to cattle caused not only a decrease in survival and pupation of face fly larvae, but many of the adults that emerged from treated pupae were not morphologically normal.[64] A triazine insect growth regulator, Larvadex®, was active against face fly larvae when given orally to cattle.[65]

Ivermectin, a chemical modification of a fermentation product of a fungus, *Streptomyces avermitilis,* is a unique, highly effective animal parasiticide. The systemic activity of ivermectin against arthropod pests of livestock was reviewed by Drummond.[66] A single subcutaneous treatment of cattle with ivermectin controlled face fly larvae in manure of treated cattle for ca. 2 weeks.[67] Daily subcutaneous injections were also effective.[68] Face fly larvae, as well as larvae of other species of pest flies that breed in manure, were controlled by ivermectin given to cattle orally, as a subcutaneous injection, or as a sustained-release bolus.[69]

C. Sustained-Release Bolus

A problem associated with free-choice consumption of "feed-thru" products in feed, mineral, or salt mixes has been one of over- and underconsumption of the treatment. Since both methoprene and diflubenzuron are active at very low dosages, researchers became interested in incorporating these materials in sustained-release boluses, which, when given to cattle, erode at a fairly constant rate that provides sufficient active ingredient in manure to control fly larvae for many weeks. A bolus containing methoprene gave 80 to 90% inhibition of emergence of face flies from manure for 10 to 12 weeks.[70] A single bolus containing diflubenzuron controlled face fly larvae for at least 20 weeks and two boluses controlled larvae for excess of 30 weeks.[71] A minimum of four boluses containing stirofos was needed to control face fly larvae.[72]

Recently, Miller and Miller[73] summarized the development of "feed-thru" chemicals to control flies that develop in manure of cattle. They reported that phenothiazine, ronnel, coumaphos, stirofos, and methoprene were registered for that use, ten chemicals had been tested but not registered, and eight chemicals have been tested as sustained-release boluses.

IV. INTEGRATED PEST MANAGEMENT TECHNOLOGY

Pioneering studies by Pickens et al.[74] showed that panels of various materials painted white and coated with a sticky substance attracted and collected face flies and could be used to reduce numbers of face flies on cattle. Screen wire disks painted white also trapped male face flies.[75] White, pyramidal, sticky traps trapped face flies in proportion to numbers of traps per site, sites per area, and cattle per trap.[76]

In a 4-year study, neither sticky, white tetrahedral traps nor stirofos as an oral larvicide used separately reduced face fly populations, but when these two control techniques were combined, the combination suppressed populations of face flies on cattle in an area of Howard County, Maryland.[77] The combination of fenvalerate-impregnated ear tags with stirofos oral larvicide[78] provided good control of face flies during the summer and prevented the late-season buildup of face fly populations.

V. OVERVIEW AND CURRENT TECHNOLOGY

The face fly has been found in the U.S. and Canada for only slightly over 30 years, but its habit of feeding around the faces of cattle and its ability to transmit pinkeye have made it an arthropod pest of considerable importance.

Only limited control of the face fly is obtained with insecticides and repellents applied to the faces of cattle. Aerial ULV spraying of cattle with insecticides is not used for face fly control. Some control has been obtained with the use of nonautomatic self-application dust bags that are available free choice for use by cattle or are positioned so that cattle are forced to use them daily or more frequently. Forced use of these systems usually provides greater control than free choice use. Insecticide-impregnated ear tags have provided some control of face flies for extended periods of time.

Oral treatment of cattle with insecticides and other materials has been shown to be highly effective against face fly larvae in the manure of treated animals. However, in many instances the populations of face flies on cattle have not been affected as the result of immigration of flies from untreated cattle.

Stirofos, commercially available as a feed-through treatment for beef and lactating dairy cattle, is effective against horn fly, face fly, house fly, and stable fly larvae. The commercially available treatments of methoprene and phenothiazine are effective against horn fly larvae only. Certainly, the effectiveness of Ivermectin at very low dosages against a variety of fly larvae in manure makes this compound an excellent candidate for a feed-through treatment or incorporation into a sustained-release implant or bolus. The development of sustained-release bolus technology has proceeded to the point that, in the summer of 1986, a bolus containing diflubenzuron became commercially available in the U.S. for the control of horn flies and face flies.

Because of the immigration of flies, the oral treatments will be most effective when used on a large scale or when used as part of integrated pest mangement (IPM) technologies. The limited data on the effectiveness of IPM technology for face flies indicates that the combination of several treatment technologies, such as attractant traps, oral treatment, and ear tags may provide sustained control of the face fly.

REFERENCES

1. **Vockeroth, J. R.,** *Musca autumnalis* Deg. in North America (Diptera: Muscidae), *Can. Entomol.,* 85, 422, 1953.
2. **Sabrosky, C. W.,** Our first decade with the face fly, *Musca autumnalis, J. Econ. Entomol.,* 54, 761, 1961.
3. **Smith, T. A., Linsdale, D. D., and Burdick, D. J.,** An annotated bibliography of the face fly, *Musca autumnalis* DeGeer, in North America, *Calif. Vector Views,* 13, 43, 1966.
4. **Pickens, L. G. and Miller, R. W.,** Biology and control of the face fly, *Musca autumnalis* (Diptera: Muscidae), *J. Med. Entomol.,* 17, 195, 1980.
5. **Morgan, C. E., Thomas, G. D., and Hall, R. D.,** Annotated bibliography of the face fly, *Musca autumnalis* (Diptera: Muscidae), *J. Med. Entomol.,* Suppl. 4, 1, 1983.
6. **Bruce, W. N., Moore, S., III, and Decker, G. C.,** Face fly control, *J. Econ. Entomol.,* 53, 450, 1960.
7. **Granett, P. and Hansens, E. J.,** Tests against face flies on cattle in New Jersey during 1960, *J. Econ. Entomol.,* 54, 562, 1961.
8. **Fales, J. H., Keller, J. C., and Bodenstein, O. F.,** Experiments on control of the face fly, *J. Econ. Entomol.,* 54, 1147, 1961.
9. **Matthysse, J. G.,** Controlling the face fly on dairy cattle, *Stn. Stn. Res. News,* 7, 1, 1961.
10. **Dorsey, C. K., Kidder, H. E., and Cunningham, C. J.,** Face fly control studies in West Virginia in 1960 and 1961, *J. Econ. Entomol.,* 55, 369, 1962.
11. **Wallace, J. B. and Turner, E. C., Jr.,** Experiments for control of the face fly in Virginia, *J. Econ. Entomol.,* 55, 415, 1962.
12. **Granett, P., Hansens, E. J., and Forgash, A. J.,** Tests against face flies on cattle in New Jersey during 1961, *J. Econ. Entomol.,* 55, 655, 1962.
13. **Holdsworth, R. P.,** Control of face flies attacking commercial dairy herds, *J. Econ. Entomol.,* 55, 146, 1962.
14. **Hansens, E. J. and Granett, P.,** Tests of Ciodrin and other materials against face fly, *Musca autumnalis, J. Econ. Entomol.,* 56, 24, 1963.
15. **Benson, O. L. and Wingo, C. W.,** Investigations of the face fly in Missouri, *J. Econ. Entomol.,* 56, 251, 1963.
16. **DeFoliart, G. R.,** Preventive spraying schedules for dairy farm fly control, *J. Econ. Entomol.,* 56, 649, 1963.
17. **Ode, P. E. and Matthysse, J. G.,** Face fly control experiments, *J. Econ. Entomol.,* 57, 631, 1964.
18. **Dobson, R. C. and Sanders, D. P.,** Low-volume, high-concentration spraying for horn fly and face fly control on beef cattle, *J. Econ. Entomol.,* 58, 379, 1965.
19. **Knapp, F. W.,** Aerial application of trichlorfon for horn fly and face fly control on cattle, *J. Econ. Entomol.,* 59, 468, 1966.
20. **Knapp, F. W.,** Ultra-low-volume aerial application of trichlorfon for control of adult mosquitoes, face flies and horn flies, *J. Econ. Entomol.,* 60, 1193, 1967.
21. **Kantack, B. H., Berndt, W. L., and Balsbaugh, E. U., Jr.,** Horn fly and face fly control on range cattle with aerial applications of ultra-low-volume malathion sprays, *J. Econ. Entomol.,* 60, 1766, 1967.
22. **Del Fosse, E. S. and Balsbaugh, E. U., Jr.,** Effects of ULV organophosphates on horn flies and face flies of cattle, and on the bovine coprocoenosis, *Environ. Entomol.,* 3, 919, 1974.
23. **Cheng, T. H., Frear, D. E. H., and Enos, H. F., Jr.,** The use of spray and aerosol formulations containing R-1207 and dimethoate for fly control on cattle and the determination of dimethoate residues in milk, *J. Econ. Entomol.,* 55, 39, 1962.
24. **Cheng, T. H., Hower, A. A., and Sprenkel, R. K.,** Oil-based and water-based Ciodrin sprays for fly control on dairy cattle, *J. Econ. Entomol.,* 58, 910, 1965.
25. **Dobson, R. C. and Huber, D. A.,** Control of face flies *(Musca autumnalis)* on beef cattle in Indiana, *J. Econ. Entomol.,* 54, 434, 1961.

26. **Hair, J. A. and Adkins, T. R., Jr.,** Dusting stations and cable backrubbers as self-applicatory devices for control of the face fly, *J. Econ. Entomol.,* 58, 39, 1965.

27. **Turner, E. C., Jr.,** Area control of the face fly using self-applicating devices, *J. Econ. Entomol.,* 58, 103, 1965.

28. **Dorsey, C. K., Heishmann, J. O., and Cunningham, C. J.,** Face fly and horn fly control on cattle — 1962—64, *J. Econ. Entomol.,* 59, 726, 1966.

29. **Seawright, J. A. and Adkins, T. R., Jr.,** Dust stations for control of the face fly in South Carolina, *J. Econ. Entomol.,* 61, 504, 1968.

30. **Poindexter, C. E. and Adkins, T. R., Jr.,** Control of the face fly and the horn fly with self-applicatory dust bags, *J. Econ. Entomol.,* 63, 946, 1970.

31. **Wrich, M. J.,** Horn fly and face fly control on beef cattle using back rubbers and dust bags containing coumaphos or fenthion, *J. Econ. Entomol.,* 63, 1123, 1970.

32. **Kessler, H. and Berndt, W. L.,** Comparison of dust bags to backrubbers for control of horn flies and face flies on beef cattle in east-central South Dakota, *J. Econ. Entomol.,* 64, 1465, 1971.

33. **Knapp, F. W. and Herald, F.,** Efficacy of permethrin ear tags against face flies and horn flies on pastured cattle, *Southwest. Entomol.,* 5, 183, 1980.

34. **Williams, R. E. and Westby, E. J.,** Evaluation of pyrethroids impregnated in cattle ear tags for control of face flies and horn flies, *J. Econ. Entomol.,* 73, 791, 1980.

35. **Knapp, F. W. and Herald, F.,** Face fly and horn fly reduction on cattle with fenvalerate ear tags, *J. Econ. Entomol.,* 74, 295, 1981.

36. **Williams, R. E., Westby, E. J., Hendrix, K. S., and Lemenager, R. P.,** Use of insecticide-impregnated ear tags for the control of face flies and horn flies on pastured cattle, *J. Anim. Sci.,* 53, 1159, 1981.

37. **Williams, R. E. and Westby, E. J.,** Comparison of three insecticide-impregnated cattle ear tags for face fly and horn fly control (Diptera: Muscidae), *J. Kan. Entomol. Soc.,* 55, 335, 1982.

38. **Hall, R. D. and Fischer, F. J.,** Cattle ear tags containing amitraz and permethrin for the control of face flies and horn flies on pastured herds, *J. Agric. Entomol.,* 1, 282, 1984.

39. **Knapp, F. W. and Herald, F.,** Effects of application date and selective tagging of cows and calves with fenvalerate ear tags for the control of the horn fly and face fly, *J. Agric. Entomol.,* 1, 58, 1984.

40. **Miller, R. W., Hall, R. D., Knapp, F. W., Williams, R. W., Doisy, K. E., Herald, F., and Towell, C. A.,** Permethrin ear tags evaluated in four states for control of the horn fly and face fly, *J. Agric. Entomol.,* 1, 264, 1984.

41. **Krafsur, E. S.,** Use of age structure to assess insecticidal treatments of face fly populations, *Musca autumnalis* DeGeer (Diptera: Muscidae), *J. Econ. Entomol.,* 77, 1364, 1984.

42. **Miller, R. W.,** Larvicides for fly control — a review, *Bull. Entomol. Soc. Am.,* 16, 154, 1970.

43. **Anthony, D. W., Hooven, N. W., and Bodenstein, O.,** Toxicity to face fly and house fly larvae of feces from insecticide-fed cattle, *J. Econ. Entomol.,* 54, 406, 1961.

44. **Treece, R. E.,** Feed additives for control of face fly larvae in cattle dung, *J. Econ. Entomol.,* 55, 765, 1962.

45. **Wallace, J. B. and Turner, E. C., Jr.,** Experiments for control of the face fly in Virginia, *J. Econ. Entomol.,* 55, 415, 1962.

46. **Wallace, J. B. and Turner, E. C., Jr.,** Low-level feeding of ronnel in a mineral salt mixture for area control of the face fly, *Musca autumnalis, J. Econ. Entomol.,* 57, 264, 1964.

47. **Jones, C. M. and Medley, J. G.,** Control of the face fly on cattle with Co-ral in grain and on pasture, *J. Econ. Entomol.,* 56, 214, 1963.

48. **Ode, P. E. and Matthysse, J. G.,** Feed additive larviciding to control face fly, *J. Econ. Entomol.,* 57, 637, 1964.

49. **Treece, R. E.,** Evaluation of some chemicals as feed additives to control face fly larvae, *J. Econ. Entomol.,* 57, 962, 1964.

50. **Pitts, C. W. and Hopkins, T. L.,** Toxicological studies on dichlorvos feed-additive formulations to control house flies and face flies in cattle feces, *J. Econ. Entomol.,* 57, 881, 1964.

51. **Lloyd, J. E. and Matthysse, J. G.,** Polyvinyl chloride-insecticide pellets fed to cattle to control face fly larvae in manure, *J. Econ. Entomol.,* 63, 1271, 1970.

52. **Knapp, F. W.,** The effect of free-choice coumaphos salt mixtures on cattle and cattle parasites, *J. Econ. Entomol.,* 58, 197, 1965.

53. **Knapp, F. W.,** Free choice feeding of ronnel mineral block and granules for face fly, horn fly, and cattle grub control, *J. Econ. Entomol.,* 58, 836, 1965.

54. **Miller, R. W. and Pickens, L. G.,** Feed additives for control of flies on dairy farms, *J. Med. Entomol.,* 12, 141, 1975.

55. **Cook, C. W. and Gerhardt, R. R.,** Selective mortality of insects in manure from cattle fed Rabon® and Dimilin®, *Environ. Entomol.,* 6, 589, 1977.

56. **Yendol, W. G. and Miller, E. M.,** Susceptibility of the face fly to commercial preparations of *Bacillus thuringiensis, J. Econ. Entomol.,* 60, 860, 1967.

57. **Hower, A. A., Jr. and Cheng, T. H.,** Inhibitive effect of *Bacillus thuringiensis* on the development of the face fly in cow manure, *J. Econ. Entomol.,* 61, 26, 1968.

58. **Miller, R. W. and Uebel, E. C.,** Juvenile hormone mimics as feed additives for control of the face fly and house fly, *J. Econ. Entomol.,* 67, 69, 1974.

59. **Miller, R. W. and Pickens, L. G.,** Evaluation of methoprene formulations for fly control, *J. Econ. Entomol.,* 68, 810, 1975.

60. **Miller, R. W., Pickens, L. G., and Hunt, L. M.,** Methoprene: field tested as a feed additive for control of face flies, *J. Econ. Entomol.,* 71, 274, 1978.

61. **Schwarz, M., Miller, R. W., Wright, J. E., Chamberlain, W. F., and Hopkins, D. E.,** Compounds related to juvenile hormone. Exceptional activity of arylterpenoid compounds in four species of flies, *J. Econ. Entomol.,* 67, 598, 1974.

62. **Miller, R. W.,** TH 6040 as a feed additive for control of the face fly and house fly, *J. Econ. Entomol.,* 67, 697, 1974.

63. **Herald, F. and Knapp, F. W.,** Effects of monensin on development of the face fly and the horn fly, *J. Econ. Entomol.,* 73, 762, 1980.

64. **Fairbrother, T. E., Essig, H. W., Combs, R. L., and Heitz, J. R.,** Toxic effects of rose bengal and erythrosin B on three life stages of the face fly, *Musca autumnalis, Environ. Entomol.,* 10, 506, 1981.

65. **Miller, R. W., Corley, C., Cohen, C. F., Robbins, W. E., and Marks, E. P.,** CGA-19255 and CGA-72662: efficacy against flies and possible mode of action and metabolism, *Southwest. Entomol.,* 6, 272, 1981.

66. **Drummond, R. O.,** Effectiveness of Ivermectin for control of arthropod pests of livestock, *Southwest. Entomol.,* Suppl. 7, 34, 1985.

67. **Meyer, J. A., Simco, J. S., and Lancaster, J. L., Jr.,** Control of face fly larval development with the Ivermectin, MK-933, *Southwest. Entomol.,* 5, 207, 1980.

68. **Meyer, J. A., Simco, J. S., and Lancaster, J. L., Jr.,** Control of face fly larval development in bovine feces with daily injections of the Ivermectin, MK-933, *Southwest. Entomol.,* 6, 269, 1981.

69. **Miller, J. A., Kunz, S. E., Oehler, D. D., and Miller, R. W.,** Larvicidal activity of Merck MK-933, an avermectin, against the horn fly, stable fly, face fly, and house fly, *J. Econ. Entomol.,* 74, 608, 1981.

70. **Miller, J. A., Knapp, F. W., Miller, R. W., and Pitts, C. W.,** Sustained-release boluses containing methoprene for control of the horn fly and face fly, *Southwest. Entomol.,* 4, 195, 1979.

71. **Miller, J. A. and Miller, R. W.,** Sustained-release bolus formulations containing insect growth regulators for control of livestock pests, in Proc. 5th Int. Symp. Controlled Release Bioactive Material, 1978, 52.

72. **Riner, J. L., Byford, R. L., and Hair, J. A.,** Sustained-release rabon bolus for face fly control in cattle feces, *J. Econ. Entomol.,* 74, 359, 1981.

73. **Miller, R. W. and Miller, J. A.** Feed-through chemicals for insect control in animals, in *Agricultural Chemicals of the Future (BARC Symposium),* Hilton, J. L., Ed., Rowman & Allanheld, Totowa, N.J., 1985, 355.

74. **Pickens, L. G., Miller, R. W., and Grasela, J. J.,** Sticky panels as traps for *Musca autumnalis, J. Econ. Entomol.,* 70, 549, 1977.

75. **Peterson, R. D., II and Meyer, H. J.,** Trapping technique for male face flies, *J. Econ. Entomol.,* 71, 40, 1978.

76. **Pickens, L. G.,** Relationship between the capture of marked face flies and the number of sticky traps used, *Southwest. Entomol.,* 6, 326, 1981.

77. **Miller, R. W., Pickens, L. G., and Nafus, D. M.,** Use of white tetrahedral traps and stirofos oral larvicide for area-wide control of the face fly, *J. Agric. Entomol.,* 1, 126, 1984.

78. **Miller, R. W., Pickens, L. G., Schmidtmann, E. T., and Kunkle, W. E.,** Fenvalerate ear tags with and without stirofos oral larvicide for control of horn flies and face flies, *Southwest. Entomol.,* 9, 79, 1984.

Chapter 7

CONTROL OF SCREWWORMS ON CATTLE AND OTHER LIVESTOCK*

I. INTRODUCTION

The screwworm◆, *Cochliomyia hominivorax* (Coquerel), was described in 1896 by Osborn[1] as "unquestionably one of the most important of all the insects that affect domestic animals". This species is limited in its distribution to the Western Hemisphere and is an obligate, myiasis-producing parasite of warm-blooded animals. Cattle and other livestock, especially sheep, are also infested with larvae of other myiasis-producing flies, including the black blow fly◆, *Phormia regina* (Meigen); the secondary screwworm◆, *Cochliomyia macellaria* (Fabricius); *Lucilia sericata* (Meigen); *Protophormia terrae-novae* (Robineau-Desvoidy); and other species. Control of these "secondary" species, usually called "fleece worms" or "wool maggots", is discussed in detail in Chapter 13. Information on the development of the sterile male technique that has been used to eradicate the screwworm from the U.S. and most of Mexico will be presented in some detail in Chapter 19. In this chapter we shall confine our discussion to the technologies used to control screwworms on cattle and other livestock. Because screwworms parasitize a wide variety of hosts, our discussion encompasses all livestock.

Because of its importance as a parasite and as the object of the pioneering use of the sterile insect technique, the screwworm has been the subject of a number of publications. Snow et al.[2] listed 621 references in their annotated bibliography. A concise review of the chemicals applied to livestock to control screwworms was presented by Graham.[3]

II. EARLY TREATMENT TECHNOLOGY

Osborn[1] described in detail a number of larval infestations in domestic animals and man and stated that control of the species, then called *Compsomyia macellaria* Fabricius, consisted of treating infested wounds with carbolic acid to kill larvae and the coating of treated wounds with pine tar to repel flies.

In the early literature, myiasis caused by the "true" or "primary" screwworm was not differentiated from that caused by the more numerous secondary screwworm. This fact is illustrated by Bishopp,[4] who stated "The screwworm, *C. macellaria*, has developed a very marked tendency to attack living animals, although it breeds in greatest numbers in carcasses." He cited the need for the scheduling of ranching operations so that wounds would be created in the wintertime when flies were absent or populations were low. He recommended treatment of wounds with chloroform and creosote products to control larvae and with pine tar to repel flies. The original issue of *U.S. Dep. Agric. Farmers' Bulletin* No. 734 in 1915[5] recommended the use of conical hoop traps baited with "gut slime" (the mucous membrane from the lining of intestines of hogs), blood tankage, and other malodorous substances to trap screwworm flies and other blow flies. The original issue of *U.S. Dep. Agric. Farmers' Bulletin* No. 857 in 1917[6] listed control measures as burning or burying carcasses ("by far the best method of control"), avoiding infestations by the timing of ranching operations, avoiding injury to livestock, destroying ticks, poisoning or trapping flies, and treating wounds with chloroform to kill larvae and with pine tar to repel flies.

---

* Common names of insects and acarines, as listed in *Common Names of Insects and Related Organisms* (published by the Entomological Society of America), are marked with a ◆ the first time they are cited preceding the scientific name.

Other wound treatments, such as turpentine, kerosene, gasoline, cobalt solution, and ether, were less effective. The 1922 revision of Bulletin No. 857[7] contained no changes in control measures.

In tests with *C. macellaria* and other species of flies, benzol was more effective as a larvicide than chloroform; pine tar oils and other oils were repellent, and dried egg was the most satisfactory bait for use in traps.[8] Benzol applied to a wound with cotton or cloth was an effective, practical larvicide.[9] Of a large variety of repellents tested, chloropicrin, a tear gas, was the most effective but was difficult to use.[10] The 1926 revision of Bulletin No. 857[11] listed all of the previous control measures but stated that nothing better than benzol had been found for controlling larvae in wounds and that a coating of pine tar protected wounds from reinfestation. Continuing studies on baits and repellents[12-15] identified beef or hog liver or rabbit meat as the best baits. Although pine tar oil was an effective repellent, the search for future repellents may lie in the use of chemicals that prevent the formation and emission of volatile attractant compounds from wounds rather than repel flies.

The 1930 revision of Bulletin No. 734[16] had an enlarged section on trapping of the screwworm fly and recommended the use of conical hoop traps baited with carcasses of rabbits or other wild animals, dried "gut slime", or dried whole egg mixed with water. Size of the bait pans and number and location of traps were critical aspects of successful trapping. Extensive trapping over ca. 63,000 ha in Texas reduced the incidence of infestation of screwworms in animals. Millions of flies were trapped, but the expense of trapping was too great for the program to be recommended for general use.[17]

An important addition to our knowledge about screwworms and blow flies occurred in 1933 when Cushing and Patton[18] determined that the true primary screwworm, which they named *C. americana,* was an obligate parasite that was morphologically different from the more numerous facultative parasite, *C. macellaria.* Studies on the biology of these two species[19] revealed many differences, especially in their relationships to hosts and in numbers found in nature. Also in 1933, screwworms became established in the southeastern U.S. and immediately became an important problem for livestock owners.[20]

Screwworm larvae in wounds were killed with benzol or soluble pine oils combined with nicotine or methyl thiocyanate.[21] U.S. Department of Agriculture Leaflet No. 162 in 1938[22] presented a variety of measures to prevent screwworm infestations and recommended treating wounds with benzol to kill larvae followed by coating the wounds with pine tar oil to repel flies.

III. EFFECTIVE WOUND TREATMENTS

Most early wound treatments were effective for a very brief period, and wounds had to be treated often to kill larvae as a result of reinfestation before the wounds healed sufficiently so that they were no longer attractive to ovipositing females. In laboratory tests to find longer-lasting treatments, 551 chemicals were tested against screwworm larvae,[23,24] and several, especially phenothiazine, were found to be highly toxic. In field tests with animals, the most effective larvicide and wound protectant was diphenylamine.[25] A revised U.S. Department of Agriculture Leaflet No. 162 in 1943[26] listed Smear 62, a mixture of diphenylamine, benzol, turkey red oil, and lamp black, as a new, effective treatment for screwworm larvae in wounds.

A series of laboratory tests to determine the toxicity of newer organic insecticides to screwworm larvae[27,28] led to the development of Smear EQ-335. This smear contained lindane, pine oil, mineral oil, and other ingredients[29] and killed larvae in wounds and the flies that visited wounds. This smear usually provided protection from reinfestation until the wounds healed and were no longer attractive to ovipositing females. The 1952 *U.S. Dep. Agric. Yearbook of Agriculture*[30] presented an informative summary of the biology and control of screwworms and mentions the use of the sterile insect technique to eliminate screwworms.

IV. SYSTEMIC INSECTICIDES

To determine if chlorinated hydrocarbon insecticides would be effective systemically against screwworm larvae, Eddy et al.[31] placed larvae in larval medium that contained blood obtained from a lindane-treated animal. However, the treatment did not affect larval development, pupation, or eclosion of adults. Subcutaneous injections of dieldrin, aldrin, and lindane killed screwworm larvae in cattle for up to 1 month posttreatment,[32] but extensive residues of these insecticides in tissues of treated animals precluded their use as practical treatments for control of screwworm larvae. Screwworm larvae were used as a test arthropod to screen thousands of potential systemic insecticides when given orally or subcutaneously to guinea pigs.

V. ORGANOPHOSPHORUS LARVICIDES

Ronnel was found to be a highly effective screwworm larvicide when applied to sheep as a spray, smear, or orally.[33] Sprays of coumaphos killed larvae in wounds and protected wounds from infestation for 2 to 3 weeks.[34] Body sprays of ronnel and coumaphos prevented infestation of screwworm larvae without specific treatment of cuts and wounds as was necessary with Smear EQ-335. Sprays of coumaphos were generally more effective than those of ronnel, but both provided greater residual protection from reinfestation than Smear EQ-335.[35] Other organophosphorus insecticides that were effective screwworm larvicides were Bayer 22408,[36] crufomate,[37] and chlorfenvinphos.[38,39] Of 19 candidate insecticides sprayed onto cattle, several, including bromophos, fenthion, and stirofos, killed 1- and 2-day-old screwworm larvae.[40]

Two insect juvenile hormone analogues, methoprene and Stauffer® R-20458, applied topically to fully grown larvae and pupae or placed in the larval diet, prevented emergence of adults. When sprayed onto cattle, these chemicals did not prevent emergence of adults from larvae in wounds on treated cattle.[41]

Because of the success of the screwworm eradication program, there has been little need in the U.S. for research on new screwworm larvicides or other techniques to control screwworms.

VI. OVERVIEW AND CURRENT TECHNOLOGY

The screwworm was an important arthropod pest of livestock and other warm-blooded animals in the U.S. Early measures to control this species consisted of timing of ranch operations so as to avoid wounding of animals when flies were present, the treatment of wounds to kill larvae, and trapping of flies. Wound treatment technology continued to improve with the advent of smears and spray treatments that killed larvae in wounds and protected the wounds from reinfestation until they were healed.

The highly successful sterile insect program has eradicated screwworms from the U.S. and most of Mexico and has eliminated the need for further research on the use of chemicals to control screwworms in cattle and other livestock.

In the absence of screwworms, livestock management practices in many areas of the U.S. have changed drastically. If screwworms should return to these areas, reversion to pre-eradication management practices would be costly in terms of both facilities and labor needs.

REFERENCES

1. **Osborn, H.,** Insects affecting domestic animals: an account of the species of importance in North America, with mention of related forms occurring on other animals, *U.S. Dep. Agric. Bull.,* 5, 1896.
2. **Snow, J. W., Siebenaler, A., and Newell, F. G.,** Annotated bibliography of the screwworm, *Cochliomyia hominivorax* (Coquerel), ARM-S-14, U.S. Department of Agriculture, Washington, D.C., 1981.
3. **Graham, O. H.,** The chemical control of screwworms: a review, *Southwest. Entomol.,* 4, 258, 1979.
4. **Bishopp, F. C.,** Flies which cause myiasis in man and animals — some aspects of the problem, *J. Econ. Entomol.,* 8, 317, 1915.
5. **Bishopp, F. C.,** Flytraps and their operation, *U.S. Dep. Agric. Farmers' Bull.,* 734, 1915.
6. **Bishopp, F. C., Mitchell, J. D., and Parman, D. C.,** Screw-worms and other maggots affecting animals, *U.S. Dep. Agric. Farmers' Bull.,* 857, 1917.
7. **Bishopp, F. C., Mitchell, J. D., and Parman, D. C.,** Screw-worms and other maggots affecting animals, *U.S. Dep. Agric. Farmers' Bull.,* 857, 1922.
8. **Bishopp, F. C., Cook, F. C., Parman, D. C., and Laake, E. W.,** Progress report of investigations relating to repellents, attractants and larvicides for the screw-worm and other flies, *J. Econ. Entomol.,* 16, 222, 1923.
9. **Parman, D. C.,** Benzene as a larvicide for screw worms, *J. Agric. Res.,* 31, 885, 1925.
10. **Bishopp, F. C., Roark, R. C., Parman, D. C., and Laake, E. W.,** Repellents and larvicides for the screw worm and other flies, *J. Econ. Entomol.,* 18, 776, 1925.
11. **Bishopp, F. C., Laake, E. W., and Parman, D. C.,** Screw worms and other maggots affecting animals, *U.S. Dep. Agric. Farmers' Bull.,* 857, 1926.
12. **Laake, E. W., Parman, D. C., Bishopp, F. C., and Roark, R. C.,** Field tests with repellents for the screw worm fly, *Cochliomyia macellaria* Fab., upon domestic animals, *J. Econ. Entomol.,* 19, 536, 1926.
13. **Roark, R. C., Parman, D. C., Bishopp, F. C., and Laake, E. W.,** Repellents for blowflies, *Ind. Eng. Chem.,* 19, 942, 1927.
14. **Parman, D. C., Bishopp, F. C., Laake, E. W., Cook, F. C., and Roark, R. C.,** Chemotropic tests with the screw-worm fly, *U.S. Dep. Agric. Bull.,* 1472, 1927.
15. **Parman, D. C., Laake, E. W., Bishopp, F. C., and Roark, R. C.,** Tests of blowfly baits and repellents during 1926, *U.S. Dep. Agric. Tech. Bull.,* 80, 1928.
16. **Bishopp, F. C.,** Flytraps and their operation, *U.S. Dep. Agric. Farmers' Bull.,* 734, 1930.
17. **Laake, E. W.,** Economic studies of screw worm flies, *Cochliomyia* species (Diptera, Calliphorinae), with special reference to the prevention of myiasis of domestic animals, *Iowa State Coll. J. Sci.,* 10, 345, 1936.
18. **Cushing, E. C. and Patton, W.,** Studies on the higher Diptera of medical and veterinary importance. *Cochliomyia americana* sp. nov., the screw-worm fly of the new world, *Ann. Trop. Med. Parasitol.,* 27, 539, 1933.
19. **Laake, E. W., Cushing, E. C., and Parish, H. E.,** Biology of the primary screw worm fly, *Cochliomyia americana,* and a comparison of its stages with those of *C. macellaria, U.S. Dep. Agric. Tech. Bull.,* 500, 1936.
20. **Dove, W. E. and Parman, D. C.,** Screw worms in the Southeastern states, *J. Econ. Entomol.,* 28, 765, 1935.
21. **McGovran, E. R.,** Insecticides to control blowfly larvae in wounds, *J. Econ. Entomol.,* 30, 876, 1937.
22. **Dove, W. E.,** Screwworm control, *U.S. Dep. Agric. Leaflet,* 162, 1938.
23. **Bushland, R. C.,** The toxicity of phenothiazine and certain related compounds to young screwworms, *J. Econ. Entomol.,* 33, 666, 1940.
24. **Bushland, R. C.,** The toxicity of some organic compounds to young screwworms, *J. Econ. Entomol.,* 33, 669, 1940.
25. **Parish, H. E. and Knipling, E. F.,** Field studies of certain benzene derivatives as larvicides and wound protectors against the screwworm, *J. Econ. Entomol.,* 35, 70, 1942.
26. **Dove, W. E.,** Screwworm control, *U.S. Dep. Agric. Leaflet,* 162, 1943.
27. **Eddy, G. W. and Graham, O. H.,** An improved laboratory method for testing materials as screw-worm larvicides, *J. Econ. Entomol.,* 43, 558, 1950.
28. **Eddy, G. W.,** Toxicity of some organic insecticides to screw-worm larvae, *J. Econ. Entomol.,* 44, 254, 1951.
29. **Eddy, G. W., McGregor, W. S., Hopkins, D. E., Dreiss, J. M., and Cairnes, J.,** EQ-335 and other wound treatments for screw-worm control, U.S. Department of Agriculture Agricultural Research Administration Bureau of Entomology and Plant Quarantine, E-813, U.S. Department of Agriculture, Washington, D.C., 1951.
30. **Bruce, W. G.,** Screw-worms, *U.S. Dep. Agric., Yearb. Agric.,* 666, 1952.
31. **Eddy, G. W., McGregor, W. S., Hopkins, D. E., and Dreiss, J. M.,** Effects on some insects of the blood and manure of cattle fed certain chlorinated hydrocarbon insecticides, *J. Econ. Entomol.,* 47, 35, 1954.

32. **McGregor, W. S., Radeleff, R. D., Claborn, H. V., and Bushland, R. C.,** Dieldrin, aldrin & lindane systemic insecticides against livestock pests, *Agric. Chem.,* 10, 34, 1955.

33. **McGregor, W. S. and Miller, W. O.,** Trolene and korlan show promise for parasite control in sheep, *Down Earth,* 14, 7, 1958.

34. **Brundrett, H. M. and Graham, O. H.,** Bayer 21/199 as a deterrent to screw-worm attack in sheep, *J. Econ. Entomol.,* 51, 407, 1958.

35. **Graham, O. H., Moore, B., Wrich, M. J., Kunz, S., Warren, J. W., and Drummond, R. O.,** A comparison on ronnel and Co-Ral sprays for screw-worm control, *J. Econ. Entomol.,* 52, 1217, 1959.

36. **Wrich, M. J. and Bushland, R. C.,** Screw-worm control with insecticide sprays, *J. Econ. Entomol.,* 53, 1058, 1960.

37. **Wrich, M. J.,** A comparison of Co-Ral, ronnel, and Ruelene dusts for screw-worm control, *J. Econ. Entomol.,* 54, 941, 1961.

38. **Wrich, M. J., Chamberlain, W. F., and Smith, C. L.,** Toxicity of General Chemical compounds 3582, 3583, and 4072 to screw-worms in laboratory and field tests, *J. Econ. Entomol.,* 54, 1049, 1961.

39. **Drummond, R. O., Ernst, S. E., Barrett, C. C., and Graham, O. H.,** Sprays and dips of Shell compound 4072 to control *Boophilus* ticks and larvae of the screw-worm on cattle, *J. Econ. Entomol.,* 59, 395, 1966.

40. **Drummond, R. O., Ernst, S. E., Trevino, J. L., and Graham, O. H.,** Control of larvae of the screw-worm in cattle with insecticidal sprays, *J. Econ. Entomol.,* 60, 199, 1967.

41. **Wright, J. E., Smalley, H. E., Younger, R. L., and Crookshank, H. R.,** Hormones for the control of livestock arthropods. Effects of 2 juvenile hormone analogues against the screwworm *Cochliomyia hominivorax* (Coquerel), *in vitro* and in infested bovine hosts, *J. Med. Entomol.,* 2, 385, 1974.

Chapter 8

CONTROL OF CATTLE GRUBS IN CATTLE*

I. INTRODUCTION

In the U.S. and Canada, cattle are commonly infested with the common cattle grub♦, *Hypoderma lineatum* (Villers), which is found from Canada into Mexico, and the northern cattle grub♦, *H. bovis* (Linnaeus), found from Canada south to about the 35° latitude. When trying to oviposit on cattle, the nonfeeding females of these species, called "heel flies", "gad flies", or "warble flies", cause the cattle to run, stampede, and stand in water in order to escape from the flies. This "gadding" response is well documented as one that calves "learn" from the herd and has a very characteristic pattern. Gadding may cause cattle to injure themselves, graze less, or abort. Eggs are attached to hair on the bodies of cattle. Penetration of the newly hatched larvae through the skin apparently irritates cattle as they are often seen licking the area of penetration. Because of this licking action, many early observers reasoned incorrectly that the eggs or newly hatched larvae were taken into cattle through the mouth. Cattle grub larvae migrate from site of penetration of the skin through the host's body. *H. lineatum* larvae travel to the submucosal tissues of the esophagus where they stay for a period of time before they move to the back. *H. bovis* larvae move to the tissue surrounding the spinal cord inside the spinal column and stay there for a period of time before they move to the back. Between 6 and 8 months after penetration, larvae appear under the skin of the host's back where they make a hole in the hide. The greatest economic damage to cattle is caused by the cattle grub larvae in dermal capsules, called "warbles" or "wolves", in the backs of cattle. In addition to the creation of holes in the hide, larvae damage the underlying flesh, called "licked beef" or "jellied beef", which is the result of reaction of the animal's body to the presence of these hypodermal larvae. Fully grown larvae exit from the warbles and fall to the ground to pupate. Length of the pupal period depends upon temperature. Heel flies and their larvae have been recognized for many years as being of considerable economic importance to the cattle industry. They have been the subject of a number of studies in order to determine their complex, year-long life cycle and to find technologies for their control.

II. EARLY TREATMENT TECHNOLOGY

A. Turn-of-the-Century Technology

Before Osborn's[1] publication in 1896, there already existed an extensive literature on heel flies/cattle grubs (e.g., see Riley[2]). In *U.S. Dep. Agric. Circular* No. 25 in 1897,[3] control of cattle grubs involved preventing oviposition of flies or killing eggs or newly hatched larvae by application of tar, train oil, or other oils, with or without carbolic acid or sulfur, to the body areas where eggs were laid. Larvae in the backs of cattle were controlled by applying kerosene or mercurial ointment into warbles or pressing out the larvae by hand. Because new cattle grub larvae appear in the backs of cattle over a period of several months, it is necessary to treat cattle several times during the warble season in order to make sure that all larvae in newly formed warbles are treated, and thereby reducing the numbers of heel flies the next heel fly season.

---

* Common names of insects and acarines, as listed in *Common Names of Insects and Related Organisms* (published by the Entomological Society of America), are marked with a ♦ the first time they are cited preceding the scientific name.

Spraying legs of cattle only or the use of a wading tank to apply used cylinder oil or coal-tar creosote to the legs and lower body areas of cattle in order to prevent oviposition of heel flies or hatching of eggs prevented larvae from appearing in the backs of laboratory-held cattle, but, in the field, range cattle would not pass through wading tanks voluntarily.[4] The dipping of cattle in arsenic for the fever tick eradication program did not eliminate cattle grub infestations, but the wading tank technique to apply crude petroleum or coal-tar creosote dips to legs of cattle reduced numbers of warbles in backs of cattle.[5]

The first major U.S. compilation of information on the control of cattle grubs was *U.S. Dep. Agric. Bulletin* No. 1369 in 1926,[6] which listed 112 references. Natural control factors included destruction of larvae and pupae by birds, mammals, insects, fungi, submergence in water, soil conditions, and host resistance. Artificial control measures included burying larvae and pupae by plowing or covering them with manure; confining cattle during heel fly season; applying creosol, acetic acid, petroleum, fish oil, or pine tar oil to repel heel flies (none was effective); and treating legs and lower body regions with arsenicals in wading vats or with sprays of oil or coal-tar creosote to kill eggs or newly hatched larvae (none was very effective). The most practical artificial control measures, those directed against larvae in warbles, included extraction of larvae by hand or by suction pump or forceps, injecting benzol or carbon tetrachloride into warbles, or treating warbles with a powder, ointment, or water suspension of rotenone, ointments of iodoform and pyrethrins, or powders of nicotine.

B. Rotenone Treatments of Larvae in Warbles

In the first tests with rotenone, an ointment applied to warbles or a wash applied with a stiff brush to the backs of cattle killed most larvae.[7]

The first issue of *U.S. Dep. Agric. Farmers' Bulletin* No. 1596 in 1929[8] listed most of the control measures presented in Bulletin No. 1369 and recommended the use of nicotine dust as an inexpensive and effective treatment for larvae in warbles. Rotenone, nicotine, and nicotine sulfate applied as dusts to warbles were highly effective in killing larvae.[9] Application of a saturated salt solution into warbles or as a backwash failed to kill cattle grub larvae.[10]

The 1936 revision of Bulletin No. 1596[11] was very similar to the original issue but added that the most effective treatment for control of larvae in warbles was the dusting of the backs of cattle with rotenone and thoroughly rubbing the dust into the warbles. Extensive studies in Canada showed that the application of a rotenone-soap wash onto backs of cattle during the warble season for several years reduced both the extensity and intensity of the infestation.[12] Washes of crude rotenone were more effective than those of pure rotenone.[13] The use of a power sprayer to apply rotenone as a spray at a high pressure was as effective as the wash and was less time consuming because hand scrubbing was not needed to assure treatment of the larvae in warbles.[14] A mixture of rotenone and wettable sulfur powder gave excellent control of larvae in warbles without the need for massaging of the powder into the hair.[15] Rotenone plus wettable sulfur applied to the backs of cattle as a dust, wash, or spray to control larvae in warbles was listed in the 1942 *U.S. Dep. Agric. Yearbook of Agriculture* as the preferred technology to control cattle grubs.[16] In extensive tests with range cattle, the spraying of rotenone was not as effective as a wash applied with a stiff brush, and rotenone dusts were effective only against fully grown larvae.[17] In further testing of rotenone, higher spray pressures were more effective than lower pressures, an increase in rotenone percentage increased effectiveness, increased volume of spray or amount of dust increased effectiveness, as did the addition of wetting agents to the spray.[18-23]

The 1949 revision of Bulletin No. 1596[24] presented few changes but added that power spraying of rotenone at high pressure was effective against larvae in warbles. An excellent review of the literature on earlier research on the biology and control of cattle grubs with data on the effectiveness of rotenone treatments against cattle grub larvae was presented by Scharff.[25] The 1952 *U.S. Dep. Agric. Yearbook of Agriculture*[26] emphasized the need for accurate timing of treatments with rotenone every 30 to 45 days during the warble season to kill newly arrived larvae and the need for cattle grub control programs to be based on a community or area basis. Some 9 years of rotenone treatment resulted in a decrease of warbles and gadding of cattle, but lack of control in 1 year resulted in an increase in gadding and warbles the next year.[27]

C. Organochlorine and Organophosphorus Treatments

1. Control of Larvae in Warbles

In tests to find a substitute for rotenone, which was not available as a result of World War II, DDT was injected into warbles but none of the cattle grub larvae was killed.[17] Treatment of warbles with ointments of toxaphene, benzene hexachloride (BHC), and chlordane afforded some kill of cattle grub larvae, but dusts of BHC and methoxychlor were ineffective.[28] *U.S. Dep. Agric. Bulletin* No. 1596 in 1949[24] reported that none of the new chlorinated hydrocarbon insecticides tested controlled larvae in warbles.

New organophosphorus insecticides were evaluated as backwashes to determine their effectiveness against cattle grub larvae in warbles. Trichlorfon, coumaphos, and diazinon caused larval mortalities equal to those expected from rotenone wash, while malathion, EPN, and dieldrin were ineffective.[29] Washes of coumaphos, Bayer 21/200, trichlorfon, but not chlorthion, and a spray of coumaphos controlled larvae in warbles.[30]

2. Control of Eggs or Heel Flies

DDT sprayed onto the undersides and legs of cattle once before heel fly season did not prevent infestation of cattle.[31] DDT, TDE, methoxychlor, chlordane, toxaphene, and lindane sprayed onto the cattle every other week during heel fly season failed to reduce the number of cattle grub larvae in the backs of treated cattle.[32] The daily application of synergized pyrethrins by an automatic treadle sprayer prevented oviposition by *H. lineatum* females, but was not effective against *H. bovis* females.[33] In order to prevent the appearance of cattle grub larvae in the backs of lactating dairy cows, cows were sprayed twice daily with crotoxyphos in oil for 8 weeks during heel fly season and the treatments caused a 74 to 96% reduction in numbers of larvae.[34]

The 1956 *U.S. Dep. Agric. Yearbook of Agriculture*[35] presents an overview of the cattle grub problem, lists the use of rotenone to destroy larvae in warbles as the only practical treatment, and again emphasized that large-scale area control programs are needed to make an impact on populations of cattle grubs.

III. SYSTEMIC INSECTICIDES

The possibility of using systemic insecticides to control cattle grub larvae and other pests of cattle has intrigued researchers for generations. Systemics, if used after the end of the heel fly season and before the appearance of larvae in the backs of cattle, would control cattle grub larvae before they would cause major losses in cattle production. Also, only a single treatment would control all or most of the larvae. We shall concentrate in this section only on those reports that deal with control of *Hypoderma* larvae with systemics. Early research on the development of systemics for use on animals was reviewed by Bushland et al.[36] and a number of other authors.

A. Early Ineffective Treatments

Preliminary trials indicated that phenothiazine was systemically active against cattle grub larvae. Single oral treatments of cattle with a mixture of phenothiazine, hexachloroethane, and di-*n*-butyltin dilaurate prevented the appearance of warbles in the backs of treated cattle.[37] A small number of cattle given free-choice access to phenothiazine in mineral mixture had significantly fewer larvae in their backs than untreated cattle.[38] In subsequent trials, when phenothiazine was given daily in feed for 1 year to a larger number of cattle, the treated cattle had 2.5 times more larvae in their backs than the untreated animals.[39] Monthly drenching of cattle with a mixture of phenothiazine, hexachloroethane, and di-*n*-butyltin dilaurate during heel fly season or daily feed treatments of phenothiazine during heel fly and warble season did not significantly reduce numbers of cattle infested or numbers of cattle grub larvae per animal.[40] Daily feed treatment of cattle with phenothiazine, alone or in combination with diethylstilbestrol, initiated 45 days before the appearance of first cattle grub larvae in the backs of cattle and continued throughout the warble period, had no effect on numbers of larvae in the backs of treated cattle.[41] Additional large-scale tests with phenothiazine and a combination of phenothiazine, hexachloroethane, and di-*n*-butyltin dilaurate as drenches or phenothiazine in salt confirmed that the treatments had no effect on the number of cattle grub larvae in the backs of cattle.[42]

Several injections of lithium antimony thiomalate for treatment of warts reduced numbers of warbles in the back of a treated heifer.[43] In large-scale tests, injections of lithium antimony thiomalate failed to control larvae in warbles or to prevent the appearance of new larvae in the backs of cattle.[44]

B. Treatment of Larvae in Warbles

Cattle were injected with aldrin, dieldrin, or lindane subcutaneously at 4-week intervals either before larvae were to appear in their backs or during the warble season. The early treatments did not prevent cattle grub larvae from appearing in the animals' backs, but the treatments given later killed most of the larvae in the warbles; however, high residues of all materials were found in the animals' tissues.[45] Dieldrin injections killed many larvae in warbles and prevented adults from emerging from pupae.[46]

A single subcutaneous injection of diazinon gave complete kill of larvae in warbles and those that appeared in the backs during the following 2 weeks. Oral treatments of trichlorfon, chlorthion, and diazinon, but not coumaphos, killed larvae in warbles, but none of these treatments prevented larvae from reaching the animals' backs.[47]

C. Practical Systemic Insecticides

The first practical systemic insecticide to control cattle grub larvae before they reached the backs of cattle was ronnel (Dow ET-57). Oral dosing of cattle with ronnel killed all larvae in warbles and/or prevented new larvae from appearing in the backs of cattle.[48,49] In 1957, a number of tests provided additional evidence that the single oral treatment with ronnel was highly active systemically against first instar cattle grub larvae before they reached the backs of cattle.[50-54] A spray of ronnel was not effective.[55] The efficacy of a single spray of coumaphos to prevent the appearance of cattle grub larvae in backs of cattle was first reported in 1957 by Brundrett et al.[55] Subsequently, large-scale tests confirmed the effectiveness of coumaphos sprays.[56]

The literature from 1957 through 1973 contains a large number of papers on tests on the effectiveness of ''established'' systemics and on preliminary field tests with newly discovered systemics for the control of cattle grubs. Many of these papers are listed in Table 1.

Publications during 1957 to 1973 presented data on effectiveness of new systemics, of treatments applied at different times during the interval after heel fly season and before appearance of cattle grub larvae in cattle's backs, or of systemics administered by different methods of treatment, such as oral drench or bolus, short- or long-term feeding, free-choice treated salt or mineral mix, injection, spray, dip, pouron, dust bag, backrubber, treated drinking water, and spoton. Some of the systemics in Table 1 were developed into com-

Table 1
TESTS WITH SYSTEMICS FOR CONTROL OF
CATTLE GRUBS, *HYPODERMA* SPP.

Systemic	Treatment method	Ref.
1957		
Ronnel	Oral, dermal, s.c.	48
	Oral	49-51, 53, 54
	Spray	55
Coumaphos	Spray	55
1958		
Coumaphos	Spray	56, 59-61, 63
Ronnel	Oral, feed	57, 63
	Oral	59-62
Dowco® 109	Spray, oral	60
	Oral, feed, spray	63
Dimethoate	Oral	60, 63
	Oral, i.m.	58, 61
1959		
Coumaphos	Spray	67, 68, 73
	Oral	68, 77
Ronnel	Oral	65, 70, 78
	Mineral	69
	Feed, oral, mineral	71
	Feed	66
	Oral, feed	72
	Spray	75
Dowco® 109	Oral, spray	64
	Oral, feed	72
	Oral, i.m., spray	74
Crufomate	Oral, feed, spray	76
Dimethoate	Oral, i.m., spray	79
1960		
Dimethoate	i.m.	80
	Oral, i.m.	81
	Oral	88
Ronnel	Oral	81, 87
	Feed, oral	85, 88
	Feed	86
Dowco® 109	Spray	81
	Oral, spray, feed	88
Coumaphos	Spray	81, 83, 84, 86, 88, 89
Crufomate	Pouron, spray	82
1961		
Chlorfenvinphos	Spray	90
Dimethoate	i.m., feed	96
Ronnel	Oral, feed	91
	Oral	93
	Feed	97
	Spray, spray-dip, backrubber	95

Table 1 (continued)
TESTS WITH SYSTEMICS FOR CONTROL OF CATTLE GRUBS, *HYPODERMA* SPP.

Systemic	Treatment method	Ref.
Crufomate	i.m., feed	91
	Spray	92, 99
	Feed, salt, spray	94
	Pouron	97
Fenthion	Spray	92
Coumaphos	Spray	92
	Spray, spray-dip, dip	95
	Dip	98
Dowco® 109	s.c., oral, feed, spray	93
	Spray	95
Dowco® 105	s.c., oral	93

1962

Systemic	Treatment method	Ref.
Coumaphos	Spray, pouron, i.m.	100
	Spray, pouron	101
	Pouron	105
	Backrubber	106
Crufomate	Backrubber	106
	Spray, pouron	101, 103, 105
	Dip, pouron	104
Fenthion	Spray, pouron, i.m.	101
	Backrubber	106
	i.m.	102
	Spray, pouron	105
Famphur	Pouron, i.m.	101
	i.m.	102
Ronnel	Oral	103
Trichlorfon	Pouron, spray	105
Menazon	Feed, spray	107

1963

Systemic	Treatment method	Ref.
BAY 9018	Drinking water	108
Ronnel	Feed, mineral	109
Chlorfenvinphos	Spray	110
BAY 37342	Spray, pouron	110
Trichlorfon	Pouron	110
Famphur	i.m.	110
	Oral	111
Fenthion	Pouron	110, 111
Crufomate	Dip	110
	Pouron	111
Coumaphos	Pouron	111

1965

Systemic	Treatment method	Ref.
Coumaphos	Spray, spray-dip	112
	Salt	113
Ronnel	Mineral	114
Crufomate	Pouron, spray	115

Table 1 (continued)
TESTS WITH SYSTEMICS FOR CONTROL OF
CATTLE GRUBS, *HYPODERMA* SPP.

Systemic	Treatment method	Ref.
1966		
BAY 37342	Pouron	116
Coumaphos	Pouron	116
Fenthion	Pouron, spray	116
Phosmet	Spray	116
Dichlofenthion	Pouron	116
Ronnel	Pouron	116
Crufomate	Pouron, spray	116
Chlorfenvinphos	Spray	116
Stauffer® R-2371	Pouron	116
Trichlorfon	Pouron, spray	116
1967		
Coumaphos	Pouron, brushon	117
	Pouron	118
	Feed	122, 123
Trichlorfon	Pouron	118, 120, 123
Fenthion	Feed, water	118
	Pouron, feed	120, 123
	Feed	122
Phosmet	Spray, pouron	119
Crufomate	Pouron, spray	119
Ronnel	Mineral	121
Maretin	Feed	122
1968		
Crufomate	Pouron	124
Fenthion	Dust bag	124
Coumaphos	Dust bag	124
Stirofos	Pouron	125
Shel® SD-8436	Pouron	125
Shell® SD-8448	Pouron	125
1969		
Coumaphos	Spray	126
Crufomate	Pouron	127
1970		
Crufomate	Pouron, spray	128
Phosmet	Spray, pouron	128
Coumaphos	Pouron, spray	128
Fenthion	Pouron	128
Trichlorfon	Pouron	128
1971		
Phosmet	Dust bag	129

Table 1 (continued)
TESTS WITH SYSTEMICS FOR CONTROL OF
CATTLE GRUBS, *HYPODERMA* SPP.

Systemic	Treatment method	Ref.
	1972	
Phosmet	Dust bag	130
Coumaphos	Dust bag	130
Phosmet	Pouron, spray	131
Crufomate	Pouron, spray	131
Fenthion	Pouron	131
Trichlorfon	Pouron	131
Ronnel	Salt	132
	1973	
Fenthion	Feed, pouron, water	133
	Pouron, spoton	134
Coumaphos	Pouron	133
Trichlorfon	Pouron	133
Crufomate	Pouron, spoton	134
Phosmet	Pouron	134

mercially available products while others were not. It is interesting to note that trichlorfon, which was extensively tested and used in Europe, was not evaluated in the U.S. until a number of other systemics had become commonly available.

Of special significance during this period was the introduction by Rogoff and Kohler[82] of the pouron treatment methods in which a small, measured volume of systemic insecticide per unit body weight, usually 15 or 30 cm^3/45 kg, was poured onto the backline of cattle. Such a treatment was as effective as a whole body spray and was less time consuming and easier to apply.

Carbaryl, a carbamate, was not effective systemically when given orally or parenterally to cattle and as a spray failed to control cattle grub larvae in warbles.[135] Back treatments of naled sprays controlled larvae in warbles, but the treatments were not considered to be systemically active.[136]

During this period, a series of papers[137-149] presented data on screening tests in the guinea pig-multiple arthropod test and on preliminary and secondary small-scale tests with 213 systemics against cattle grub larvae in cattle. Since 1976, the results of similar tests with new and commercially available systemics have been reported annually in *Insecticide and Acaricide Tests*.

Another significant advance in the technology of the treatment of cattle with systemics was the development of the spoton treatment technique by Loomis et al.[134] A very small volume of concentrated insecticide is applied to a single spot on the back of an animal at a specific volume to weight relationship, usually 1 to 2 cm^3/45 kg.

A few additional tests with ''standard'' systemics were published after 1973. A pouron of trichlorfon or spray of crufomate afforded excellent control of cattle grub larvae.[150] Famphur was effective when given as a pouron or as an intramuscular injection.[151] A flowable formulation of coumaphos controlled cattle grub larvae when used in a dipping vat, and the formulation had excellent vat management characteristics.[152] Pourons of famphur were only partially effective systemically.[153]

Dilutions of the label-listed dosages of commercially available systemics were applied to several groups of cattle and the data on effectiveness against cattle grub larvae were subjected to probit analysis. Label-listed dosages of coumaphos spray, phosmet spray, or pouron and trichlorfon spray all exceeded the calculated LC_{90}.[154] In further tests with titrated dosages of labeled systemics,[155] label-listed dosages of crufomate pouron, fenthion pouron, trichlorfon pouron, and phosmet spray or pouron and the maximum dosage of fenthion spoton exceeded the calculated LC_{90} dosages. However, the label-listed dosages of coumaphos pouron or famphur pouron did not exceed the calculated LC_{90} dosages.

D. Eradication of Cattle Grubs

The effectiveness of systemics stimulated new thinking on the use of chemicals to eradicate cattle grubs. Graham and Drummond[156] reviewed the past technologies, such as extraction of larvae and rotenone treatment of warbles that were used to eradicate cattle grubs, and speculated that appropriate use of systemics would allow for the eradication of cattle grubs from circumscribed areas. Six annual treatments with systemics lowered the cattle grub larval population in an isolated herd of cattle in Canada from 30.2 to 0.2 larvae per calf, but when the treatments were stopped in the 7th year, numbers of larvae increased by tenfold, indicating the ability of cattle grub populations to increase rapidly.[157] Crufomate pouron was used to treat native cattle and calves imported to Santa Rosa Island, California, and in 4 years the cattle grub larval population had dropped from 22.6 larvae per animal to only 1 larva found in 977 cattle.[158] Three consecutive yearly treatments of cattle in an area of Alberta with coumaphos or crufomate sprays reduced numbers of larvae in cattle in a 12,900-ha central zone to zero, and populations were almost that low in a surrounding 8-km-wide buffer zone.[159]

The use of animal systemic insecticides to eradicate cattle grubs, which has received much more attention in Europe than in North America, was the subject of a symposium in 1975.[160] In Wetaskiwin County, Alberta, Canada,[161] years of treatments lowered cattle grub populations, but eradication was not accomplished. It was generally concluded[162] that eradication was technologically feasible, but in most areas human and organizational problems must be overcome before eradication can be accomplished.

In Chapter 20, we briefly described a large-scale pilot test in which some cattle in the U.S. and Canada are being treated with systemics in order to lower populations of cattle grubs. In addition, sterile heel flies are being released within limited zones of the areas containing treated cattle to determine if the sterile insect technique can be used to further decrease or eradicate cattle grub populations.

E. Other Treatment Technologies

A drinking water treatment of methoprene, an insect growth regulator, did not prevent cattle grub larvae from reaching backs of cattle but did prevent adults from eclosing from pupae collected from treated cattle.[154] Methoprene, given to cattle as a water treatment, a feed treatment, or as a sustained-release bolus when animals had cattle grub larvae in their backs, caused 62 to 100% inhibition of eclosion of adults, but the treatment was less effective when started after cattle grub larvae had begun to leave the backs of the animals.[163]

Dichlorvos-impregnated plastic strips applied to legs of cattle during the heel fly season prevented the appearance of cattle grub larvae in backs of treated cattle.[164] In later tests, the dichlorvos treatments placed on legs after the end of heel fly season still controlled cattle grub larvae, thus demonstrating the systemic activity of dichlorvos.[165]

Of special interest is the effectiveness of subcutaneous injections of ivermectin, a chemically modified form of a fermentation product of *Streptomyces avermitilis,* which was exceptionally active as a systemic insecticide for the control of cattle grub larvae at extremely low dosages. The LD_{90} was calculated to be about 0.1 μg/kg.[155] Ivermectin is systemically active against a variety of arthropod pests of livestock.[166]

IV. OVERVIEW AND CURRENT TECHNOLOGY

In North America, cattle grubs have been recognized as an important pest of cattle since before the turn of the century. The use of rotenone treatments to kill larvae in warbles was a significant advance in the control of *Hypoderma* spp., and rotenone was used for 30 years to control cattle grub larvae.

A turning point in the control of cattle grubs came with the discovery and use of animal systemic insecticides which killed larvae before they could damage hides and cause trim loss of meat at slaughter. Soon a number of treatment methodologies were developed to administer a variety of systemics. A significant trend in treatment methodology was the reduction in the volume of dermal treatment applied to cattle — dip, spray, pouron to spoton. The recent commercial availability of ivermectin which is systemically active as a subcutaneous injection is another significant advance in current technology for the control of cattle grubs.

The integrated sterile male technique pilot test currently underway could provide solutions to obstacles that stand in the way of the creation of grub-free areas. In these areas, cattle would not have to be treated annually as is the situation now. Cattle from such areas should command a premium at sales because of the fact that they would not have to be treated for the control of cattle grubs.

REFERENCES

1. **Osborn, H.,** Insects affecting domestic animals: an account of the species of importance in North America, with mention of related forms occurring on other animals, *U.S. Dep. Agric. Bull.*, 5, 1896.
2. **Riley, C. V.,** The ox bot in the United States, *Insect Life*, 4, 302, 1892.
3. **Marlatt, C. L.,** The ox warble, *U.S. Dep. Agric. Bur. Entomol. Circ.*, 25, 1897.
4. **Imes, M. and Schneider, F. L.,** Experimental treatment of cattle to prevent ox warble infestation, *J. Am. Vet. Med. Assoc.*, 59, 722, 1921.
5. **Imes, M.,** Summary of results of field trials by the U.S. Bureau of Animal Industry on ox-warble control, *J. Parasitol.*, 13, 42, 1926.
6. **Bishopp, F. C., Laake, E. W., Brundrett, H. M., and Wells, R. W.,** The cattle grubs or ox warbles, their biologies and suggestions for control, *U.S. Dep. Agric. Dept. Bull.*, 1369, 1926.
7. **Wells, R. W., Bishopp, F. C., and Laake, E. W.,** Derris as a promising insecticide, *J. Econ. Entomol.*, 15, 90, 1922.
8. **Bishopp, F. C., Laake, E. W., and Wells, R. W.,** Cattle grubs or heel flies with suggestions for their control, *U.S. Dep. Agric. Farmers' Bull.*, 1596, 1929.
9. **Bishopp, F. C., Laake, E. W., Wells, R. W., and Peters, H. S.,** Experiments with insecticides against cattle grubs, *Hypoderma* spp., *J. Econ. Entomol.*, 23, 852, 1930.
10. **Stotchik, J.,** Report on brine treatment of *Hypoderma* larvae in the backs of cattle, *J. Am. Vet. Med. Assoc.*, 86, 488, 1935.
11. **Bishopp, F. C., Laake, E. W., and Wells, R. W.,** Cattle grubs or heel flies with suggestions for their control, *U.S. Dep. Agric. Farmers' Bull.*, 1596, 1936.
12. **Gibson, A. and Twinn, C. R.,** Warble fly control in Canada, *Sci. Agric.*, 17, 179, 1936.
13. **Smith, C. E., Livengood, E., and Roberts, I. H.,** The value and relative effectiveness of preparations of rotenone, derris powder and cube powder as larvicides for cattle grubs, *J. Am. Vet. Med. Assoc.*, 99, 391, 1941.
14. **Wells, R. W.,** The use of power sprayers in the control of cattle grubs, *J. Econ. Entomol.*, 35, 112, 1942.
15. **Laake, E. W.,** Dry application of cube or derris in combination with wettable sulfur for the control of cattle grubs, *J. Econ. Entomol.*, 35, 112, 1942.
16. **Laake, E. W., Bishopp, F. C., and Wells, R. W.,** Cattle grubs, or heel flies, *U.S. Dep. Agric. Yearb. Agric.*, 612, 1942.
17. **Stewart, M. A.,** Rotenone and ox warble control, *J. Econ. Entomol.*, 37, 756, 1944.

18. **Snipes, B. T., Cooper, R. S., and Clark, S. W.,** Comparative effectiveness of variations in spray pressure, rotenone concentration, sulfur content, diluents and application methods in cattle grub control, *J. Econ. Entomol.,* 41, 635, 1948.
19. **Furman, D. P. and Douglas, J. R.,** Comparative evaluations of insecticides for cattle grub control, *J. Econ. Entomol.,* 41, 783, 1948.
20. **Douglas, J. R. and Furman, D. P.,** Comparative evaluation of rotenone formulations for cattle grub control, *J. Econ. Entomol.,* 42, 884, 1949.
21. **Baker, A. W., Kingscote, A. A., and Allan, W. C.,** Warble fly control in Ontario, *Annu. Rep. Entomol. Soc. Ont.,* 81, 76, 1950.
22. **McGregor, W. S., Smith, C. L., and Richards, R.,** Comparison of high and low spray pressures for control of cattle grubs, *J. Econ. Entomol.,* 45, 740, 1952.
23. **Roberts, I. H., Lofgren, J. A., and Berndt, W. L.,** Tests with insecticide formulations for the destruction of cattle grubs, *J. Econ. Entomol.,* 45, 909, 1952.
24. **Bishopp, F. C., Laake, E. W., and Wells, R. W.,** Cattle grubs or heel flies with suggestions for their control, *U.S. Dep. Agric. Farmers' Bull.,* 1596, 1949.
25. **Scharff, D. K.,** Cattle grubs their biologies, their distribution, and experiments in their control, *Mont. State Coll. Agric. Exp. Stn. Bull.,* 471, 1950.
26. **Laake, E. W. and Roberts, I. W.,** Cattle grubs, *U.S. Dep. Agric. Yearb. Agric.,* 672, 1952.
27. **Baker, A. W., Kingscote, A. A., and Allan, W. C.,** Five years progress in the control of warble fly in Ontario 1951—1955, *Annu. Rep. Entomol. Soc. Ont.,* 86, 1955.
28. **Telford, H. S.,** Insecticides for cattle grub control, *J. Econ. Entomol.,* 40, 928, 1947.
29. **Smith, C. L. and Richards, R.,** New insecticides for control of the cattle grub, *J. Econ. Entomol.,* 47, 712, 1954.
30. **Roth, A. R. and Eddy, G. W.,** Tests with some phosphorus compounds against cattle grubs, *J. Econ. Entomol.,* 48, 201, 1955.
31. **Matthysse, J. G.,** Grub control on dairy cattle in the Northeast, *J. Econ. Entomol.,* 38, 442, 1945.
32. **Graham, O. H.,** An attempt to protect cattle from grub infestation by use of insecticides, *J. Econ. Entomol.,* 42, 837, 1949.
33. **Raun, E. S.,** Use of synergized pyrethrins to prevent oviposition by cattle grubs, *J. Econ. Entomol.,* 48, 603, 1955.
34. **Knapp, F. W.,** Prevention of cattle grub infestation in lactating dairy cows by use of daily applications of crotoxyphos, *J. Econ. Entomol.,* 65, 466, 1972.
35. **Roberts, I. H. and Lindquist, A. W.,** Cattle grubs, *U.S. Dep. Agric. Yearb. Agric.,* 300, 1956.
36. **Bushland, R. C., Radeleff, R. D., and Drummond, R. O.,** Development of systemic insecticides for pests of animals in the United States, *Annu. Rev. Entomol.,* 8, 215, 1963.
37. **Worden, A. N.,** The dosing of warble-infested cattle with anthelmintics, *Vet. Rec.,* 65, 586, 1953.
38. **Schwartz, B., Porter, D. A., and Herlich, H.,** Effects of free-choice ingestion of phenothiazine on the incidence of cattle grub, *Hypoderma lineatum, Vet. Med.,* 49, 405, 1954.
39. **Riedel, B. B., Owen, J., Morrow, G. E., and McCrory, H. F.,** Phenothiazine administered daily for the control of cattle grubs, *Hypoderma* spp., *Trans. Am. Microbiol. Soc.,* 74, 358, 1955.
40. **Cobbett, N. G., Peterson, H. O., and Jones, E. M.,** Tests involving the oral administration of phenothiazine, hexachloroethane and di-n-butyltin dilaurate for the control of cattle grubs, *Vet. Med.,* 52, 69, 1957.
41. **Roberts, I. H., Mansfield, M. E., and Cmarik, G. F.,** Ineffectiveness against cattle grubs of phenothiazine and stilbesterol in daily diet of fattening steers, *J. Econ. Entomol.,* 50, 808, 1957.
42. **Kohler, P. H. and Rogoff, W. M.,** Studies with phenothiazine and hypolin for the control of cattle grubs, *J. Econ. Entomol.,* 52, 1223, 1959.
43. **Penny, R. H. C.,** Warble-fly infestation, *Vet. Rec.,* 66, 890, 1954.
44. **Weintraub, J. and Robertson, R. H.,** Failure of lithium antimony thiomalate to control warble grubs [*Hypoderma lineatum* (De Vill.) and *H. bovis* (L.)], *Vet. Rec.,* 74, 257, 1962.
45. **McGregor, W. S., Radeleff, R. D., Claborn, H. V., and Bushland, R. C.,** Dieldrin, aldrin & lindane systemic insecticides against livestock pests, *Agric. Chem.,* 10, 34, 1955.
46. **Roth, A. R. and Johnson, J. B.,** Tests with dieldrin as a systemic against cattle grubs, *J. Econ. Entomol.,* 48, 761, 1955.
47. **McGregor, W. S., Radeleff, R. D., and Bushland, R. C.,** Some phosphorus compounds as systemic insecticides against cattle grubs, *J. Econ. Entomol.,* 47, 465, 1954.
48. **Roth, A. R. and Eddy, G. W.,** Tests with Dow ET-57 against cattle grubs in Oregon, *J. Econ. Entomol.,* 50, 244, 1957.
49. **McGregor, W. S. and Bushland, R. C.,** Tests with Dow ET-57 against two species of cattle grubs, *J. Econ. Entomol.,* 50, 246, 1957.
50. **Marquardt, W. C. and Fritts, D. H.,** Control of cattle grubs by an orally administered organic phosphorous compound, *J. Am. Vet. Med. Assoc.,* 131, 562, 1957.

51. **Raun, E. S. and Herrick, J. B.**, Feedlot tests of the efficacy of Dow ET-57 (Trolene) for control of cattle grubs, *J. Am. Vet. Med. Assoc.*, 131, 421, 1957.

52. **Raun, E. S. and Herrick, J. B.**, Clinical test of the efficacy of Dow ET-57 for grub control in cattle, *J. Econ. Entomol.*, 50, 832, 1957.

53. **Adkins, T. R., Jr.**, Field evaluations of Dow ET-57 as a systemic insecticide for the control of the common cattle grub in Alabama, *J. Econ. Entomol.*, 50, 474, 1957.

54. **Jones, R. H., Brundrett, H. M., and Radeleff, R. D.**, Ranch tests against cattle grubs with the systemic insecticide Dow ET-57, *Agric. Chem.*, 12, 45, 1957.

55. **Brundrett, H. M., McGregor, W. S., and Bushland, R. C.**, Systemic cattle grub control with Bayer 21/199 sprays, *Agric. Chem.*, 12, 36, 1957.

56. **Graham, O. H.**, Tests with Bayer 21/199 for the control of cattle grubs, *J. Econ. Entomol.*, 51, 359, 1958.

57. **Knapp, F. W., Terhaar, C. J., and Roan, C. C.**, Field studies with feed and bolus formulations of Dow ET-57 for control of cattle grubs, *J. Econ. Entomol.*, 51, 119, 1958.

58. **Hewitt, R., Emro, J., Entwistle, J., Pankavich, J., Thorson, R., Wallace, W., and Waletzky, E.**, Carbamoyl alkyl phosphorodithioates as chemotherapeutic agents: effects of dimethoate against grubs in cattle, *J. Econ. Entomol.*, 51, 445, 1958.

59. **Burns, E. C. and Goodwin, E. E.**, Tests with Dow ET-57 and Bayer 21/199 against cattle grubs in Southwest Louisiana, *J. Econ. Entomol.*, 51, 545, 1958.

60. **Turner, E. C., Jr. and Gaines, J. A.**, Systemic insecticides for control of cattle grubs in Virginia, *J. Econ. Entomol.*, 51, 582, 1958.

61. **Neel, W. W.**, Field tests with systemic insecticides for the control of cattle grubs, *J. Econ. Entomol.*, 51, 793, 1958.

62. **Wade, L. L. and Colby, R. W.**, Treatment time with Dow ET-57 for cattle grub control, *J. Econ. Entomol.*, 51, 808, 1958.

63. **DeFoliart, G. R., Glenn, M. W., and Robb, T. R.**, Field studies with systemic insecticides against cattle grubs and lice, *J. Econ. Entomol.*, 51, 876, 1958.

64. **Roth, A. R. and Eddy, G. W.**, Tests with a new organophosphorus compound (Dowco 109) against cattle grubs in Oregon, *J. Econ. Entomol.*, 52, 169, 1959.

65. **Jones, C. M. and Matsushima, J.**, Effects of ronnel on control of cattle grubs and weight gains of beef cattle, *J. Econ. Entomol.*, 52, 488, 1959.

66. **Kohler, P. H., Rogoff, W. M., and Duxbury, R.**, Continuous individual feeding of systemic insecticides for cattle grub control, *J. Econ. Entomol.*, 52, 1222, 1959.

67. **Khan, M. A., Thompson, C. O. M., and Pelham, W. L.**, Co-Ral sprays for systemic control of the cattle grubs *Hypoderma bovis* L. and *H. lineatum* de Vill., *Can. J. Anim. Sci.*, 39, 115, 1959.

68. **Harris, E. D., Jr., Genung, W. G., and Chapman, H. L., Jr.**, Comparison of two systemic insecticides and the dates of application for cattle grub control in the Everglades, *J. Econ. Entomol.*, 52, 425, 1959.

69. **Rogoff, W. M. and Kohler, P. H.**, Free-choice administration of ronnel in a mineral mixture for the control of cattle grubs, *J. Econ. Entomol.*, 52, 958, 1959.

70. **Weintraub, J., Rich, G. B., and Thompson, C. O. M.**, Timing the treatment of cattle with trolene for systemic control of the cattle grubs *Hypoderma lineatum* (De vill.) and *H. bovis* (L.) in Alberta and British Columbia, *Can. J. Anim. Sci.*, 39, 50, 1959.

71. **Weintraub, J., Thompson, C. O. M., and Qually, M. C.**, Low-level feeding of trolene for control of the cattle grubs *Hypoderma lineatum* (De Vill.) and *H. bovis* (L.), *Can. J. Anim. Sci.*, 39, 58, 1959.

72. **Rich, G. B. and Ireland, H. R.**, Studies of bolus and feed formulation of two systemic insecticides for reduction of cattle warble infestations, (Oestridae: Diptera), in British Columbia, 1957—1958, *Can. J. Anim. Sci.*, 39, 170, 1959.

73. **Drummond, R. O.**, Texas field tests for the control of cattle grubs with sprays of Bayer 21/199, *J. Econ. Entomol.*, 52, 512, 1959.

74. **Drummond, R. O. and Graham, O. H.**, Dowco 109 as an animal systemic insecticide, *J. Econ. Entomol.*, 52, 749, 1959.

75. **Drummond, R. O. and Moore, B.**, Ronnel sprays for systemic control of cattle grubs, *J. Econ. Entomol.*, 52, 1028, 1959.

76. **McGregor, W. S., Ludwig, P. D., and Wade, L. L.**, Progress report on Ruelene for cattle grub control, *Down Earth*, 15, 2, 1959.

77. **Norris, M. G. and Howe, R. G.**, Weight gains and cattle grub control in cattle treated with trolene, *Down Earth*, 15, 4, 1959.

78. **Jones, C. M.**, Cattle grub control with ronnel, *J. Econ. Entomol.*, 52, 524, 1959.

79. **Drummond, R. O.**, Tests with dimethoate for systemic control of cattle grubs, *J. Econ. Entomol.*, 52, 1004, 1959.

80. **Khan, M. A., Connell, R., and Q. Darcel, C. le,** Immunization and parenteral chemotherapy for the control of cattle grubs *Hypoderma lineatum* (De Vill.) and *H. bovis* (L.) in cattle, *Can. J. Comp. Med.,* 24, 177, 1960.

81. **Rogoff, W. M., Kohler, P. H., and Duxbury, R. N.,** The *in vivo* activity of several systemic insecticides against cattle grubs in South Dakota, *J. Econ. Entomol.,* 53, 183, 1960.

82. **Rogoff, W. M. and Kohler, P. H.,** Effectiveness of Ruelene applied as localized "pour-on" and as spray for cattle grub control, *J. Econ. Entomol.,* 53, 814, 1960.

83. **Drummond, R. O. and Moore, B.,** Effects of timing and method of application on efficiency of Co-Ral sprays for cattle grub control, *J. Econ. Entomol.,* 53, 729, 1960.

84. **Khan, M. A.,** Application of Co-Ral for systemic control of cattle grubs *Hypoderma lineatum* (De Vill.) and *H. bovis* (L.), *Can. J. Anim. Sci.,* 40, 114, 1960.

85. **Rich, G. B.,** Free-choice feeding of Trolene for reduction of cattle warble infestations (Oestridae: Diptera), *Can. J. Anim. Sci.,* 40, 30, 1960.

86. **Raun, E. S. and Herrick, J. B.,** Organophosphate systemics as sprays and feed additives for cattle grub control, *J. Econ. Entomol.,* 53, 125, 1960.

87. **Thurber, H. E. and Peterson, G. D., Jr.,** Feed lot tests with ronnel for control of cattle grubs, *J. Econ. Entomol.,* 53, 339, 1960.

88. **Knapp, F. W., Terhaar, C. J., and Roan, C. C.,** Systemic insecticides for cattle grub control, *J. Econ. Entomol.,* 53, 541, 1960.

89. **Marquardt, W. C., Lovelace, S. A., and Fritts, D. H.,** Spray treatment of calves with Bayer 21/199 for control of cattle grubs and lice in Montana, *J. Am. Vet. Med. Assoc.,* 137, 589, 1960.

90. **Drummond, R. O.,** Tests with sprays of General Chemical 4072 for systemic control of cattle grubs, *J. Econ. Entomol.,* 54, 1047, 1961.

91. **Rich, G. B. and Ireland, H. R.,** An appraisal of Ruelene and Trolene against cattle grub infestation (Oestridae: Diptera), *Can. J. Anim. Sci.,* 41, 115, 1961.

92. **Roth, A. R. and Eddy, G. W.,** Field tests with new cattle grub systemics, *J. Econ. Entomol.,* 54, 203, 1961.

93. **Weintraub, J. and Thompson, C. O. M.,** Comparison of ronnel, Dowco 109, and Dowco 105 for systemic control of cattle grubs in Alberta, *J. Econ. Entomol.,* 54, 79, 1961.

94. **Kohler, P. H. and Rogoff, W. M.,** Ruelene administered free-choice in a mineral mixture for cattle grub control, *J. Econ. Entomol.,* 54, 278, 1961.

95. **Raun, E. S. and French, F. E.,** Practical application methods for systemic cattle grub control, *J. Econ. Entomol.,* 54, 428, 1961.

96. **Marquardt, W. C. and Lovelace, S. A.,** A comparison of dimethoate administered as an injection and in supplemental feed for control of cattle grubs, *J. Econ. Entomol.,* 54, 252, 1961.

97. **Harvey, T. L. and Brethour, J. R.,** Effectiveness of Ruelene and ronnel for ear tick compared with cattle grub control, *J. Econ. Entomol.,* 54, 814, 1961.

98. **Simco, J. S. and Lancaster, J. L., Jr.,** Control of cattle grubs and horn flies by summer dipping with Co-Ral, *J. Econ. Entomol.,* 54, 208, 1961.

99. **Howe, R. G. and Ludwig, P. D.,** Top line spraying of cattle with Ruelene for control of cattle grubs, *Down Earth,* 17, 19, 1961.

100. **Drummond, R. O. and Graham, O. H.,** Low-volume dermal applications and injections of Co-Ral for systemic control of cattle grubs, *J. Econ. Entomol.,* 55, 255, 1962.

101. **Kohler, P. H. and Rogoff, W. M.,** Control of cattle grubs by pour-on, injection, and spray, *J. Econ. Entomol.,* 55, 539, 1962.

102. **Marquardt, W. C. and Hawkins, W. W., Jr.,** Control of cattle grubs by the intramuscular injection of Bayer 29493 or CL 38023, *Cornell Vet.,* 52, 228, 1962.

103. **Baird, D. M., McCampbell, H. C., Ciordia, H., White, P. E., and Bizzell, W. E.,** Two systemic insecticides for the control of cattle grubs and observations on their effect on internal parasites, *Ga. Vet.,* 14, 9, 1962.

104. **Scharff, D. K. and Ludwig, P. D.,** Cattle grub control with Ruelene as a dip and a pour-on treatment, *J. Econ. Entomol.,* 55, 191, 1962.

105. **Turner, E. C., Jr.,** Spray and pour-on application of systemic insecticides for control of cattle grubs in Virginia, *J. Econ. Entomol.,* 55, 564, 1962.

106. **Brethour, J. R. and Harvey, T. L.,** Effects of certain systemic insecticides in backrubbers for cattle grub control, *J. Econ. Entomol.,* 55, 811, 1962.

107. **Goulding, R. L.,** Menazon as a systemic insecticide in cattle, *J. Econ. Entomol.,* 55, 577, 1962.

108. **Dobson, R. C. and Sanders, D. P.,** Cattle grub control by the addition of a systemic insecticide to drinking water, *J. Econ. Entomol.,* 56, 717, 1963.

109. **Medley, J. G., Drummond, R. O., and Graham, O. H.,** Field tests with low-level feeding of ronnel for control of cattle grubs and horn flies, *J. Econ. Entomol.,* 56, 500, 1963.

110. **Drummond, R. O.,** Small-scale field tests in Texas with six systemic insecticides for the control of cattle grubs, *J. Econ. Entomol.,* 56, 632, 1963.

111. **Neel, W. W., Blount, C. L., and Kilby, W. W.,** Systemic insecticides applied as a topical pour-on and as an oral drench for cattle grub control, *J. Econ. Entomol.,* 56, 101, 1963.

112. **Drummond, R. O., Whetstone, T. M., and Ernst, S. E.,** Control of cattle grubs with coumaphos applied by sprayer and spray-dip machine, *J. Econ. Entomol.,* 58, 1017, 1965.

113. **Knapp, F. W.,** The effect of free-choice coumaphos salt mixtures on cattle and cattle parasites, *J. Econ. Entomol.,* 58, 197, 1965.

114. **Knapp, F. W.,** Free choice feeding of ronnel mineral block and granules for face fly, horn fly, and cattle grub control, *J. Econ. Entomol.,* 58, 836, 1965.

115. **Riehl, L. A., Addis, D. G., Burgess, J. B., and Deal, A. S.,** Trials of Ruelene for cattle grub control in Southern California, *J. Econ. Entomol.,* 58, 361, 1965.

116. **Drummond, R. O. and Graham, O. H.,** Dermal application of ten systemic insecticides to cattle for the control of the common cattle grub, *J. Econ. Entomol.,* 59, 723, 1966.

117. **Roth, A. R. and Rogoff, W. M.,** Comparative efficiency of coumaphos applications on various body areas by brush-on or pour-on for the control of cattle grubs, *J. Econ. Entomol.,* 60, 1754, 1967.

118. **Burgess, T. D., Allan, W. C., and Mozier, J.,** Warble fly larvae control study, *Proc. Entomol. Soc. Ont.,* 97, 117, 1967.

119. **Rogoff, W. M., Brody, G., Roth, A. R., Batchelder, G. H., Meyding, G. D., Bigley, W. S., Gretz, G. H., and Orchard, R.,** Efficacy, cholinesterase inhibition, and residue persistence of Imidan for the control of cattle grubs, *J. Econ. Entomol.,* 60, 640, 1967.

120. **Hagen, A. F.,** Systemic insecticides and late-season application for cattle grub control in western Nebraska, *J. Econ. Entomol.,* 60, 590, 1967.

121. **Knapp, F. W., Bradley, N. W., and Templeton, W. C., Jr.,** Effect of ronnel mineral block (Rid-Ezy®) on control of cattle grubs and weight gain of beef cattle, *J. Econ. Entomol.,* 60, 1455, 1967.

122. **Cox, D. D., Allen, A. D., and Maurer, E. M.,** Control of cattle grubs with organic phosphorus compounds administered in feed, *J. Econ. Entomol.,* 60, 105, 1967.

123. **Cox, D. D., Mullee, M. T., and Allen, A. D.,** Cattle grub control with feed additives (coumaphos and fenthion) and pour-ons (fenthion and trichlorfon), *J. Econ. Entomol.,* 60, 522, 1967.

124. **Matthysse, J. G., Lloyd, J. E., Butler, J. F., and Tillapaugh, K.,** Cattle grub control by dust bag application of coumaphos in summer, *J. Econ. Entomol.,* 61, 311, 1968.

125. **Rogoff, W. M., Roth, A. R., Gretz, G. H., Bigley, W. S., and Orchard, R.,** Evaluation of Shell SD 8447, SD 8448, and SD 8436 as candidate systemic insecticides for control of common and northern cattle grubs, *J. Econ. Entomol.,* 61, 487, 1968.

126. **Collins, R. C., Dewhirst, L. W., and Carruth, L. A.,** The cattle grub problem in Arizona. I. Timing of adult activity of the common cattle grub, *J. Econ. Entomol.,* 62, 652, 1969.

127. **Landram, J. F., Ludwig, P. D., Bucek, O. C., Swart, R. W., and McGregor, W. S.,** The effect on cattle grubs, internal parasites, and weight gains in feedlot cattle treated topically with crufomate, *Pract. Nutr.,* 3, 9, 1969.

128. **Loomis, E. C., Crenshaw, G. L., Bushnell, R. B., and Dunning, L. L.,** Systemic insecticide study on livestock in California, 1965—67. I. Cattle grub control, *J. Econ. Entomol.,* 63, 1237, 1970.

129. **Lloyd, J. E.,** Cattle grub control in Wyoming with a late-summer dust-bag application of prolate, *J. Econ. Entomol.,* 64, 899, 1971.

130. **Hayes, B. W., Janes, M. J., and Beardsley, D. W.,** Dust bag treatments in improved pastures to control horn flies and cattle grubs, *J. Econ. Entomol.,* 65, 1368, 1972.

131. **Loomis, E. C., Crenshaw, G. L., and Dunning, L. L.,** Systemic insecticide study on livestock in California, 1967—68. II. Evaluation of Imidan® for cattle grub control, *J. Econ. Entomol.,* 65, 450, 1972.

132. **Colby, R. W.,** Trolene 18 insecticidal salt premix for lice and grub control, *Pract. Nutr.,* 6, 5, 1972.

133. **Campbell, J. B., Woods, W., Hagen, A. F., and Howe, E. C.,** Cattle grub insecticide efficacy and effects on weight-gain performance on feeder calves in Nebraska, *J. Econ. Entomol.,* 66, 429, 1973.

134. **Loomis, E. C., Dunning, L. L., and Riehl, L. A.,** Control of *Hypoderma lineatum* and *H. bovis* in California, 1970—72, using crufomate, fenthion, and Imidan in new low-volume and usual pour-on formulations, *J. Econ. Entomol.,* 66, 439, 1973.

135. **Khan, M. A., Avery, R. J., and Dueck, H. P.,** Toxicity of sevin (1-naphthyl-*n*-methyl-carbamate) to cattle grubs, lice, and cattle, *Can. J. Comp. Med. Vet. Sci.,* 26, 234, 1962.

136. **Goulding, R. L. and Taylor, N. O.,** Effects of topical applications of dibrom upon cattle lice and cattle grubs, *J. Econ. Entomol.,* 55, 744, 1962.

137. **Drummond, R. O.,** Preliminary evaluation of animal systemic insecticides, *J. Econ. Entomol.,* 53, 1125, 1960.

138. **Drummond, R. O.,** Further evaluation of animal systemic insecticides, 1961, *J. Econ. Entomol.,* 55, 398, 1962.

139. **Drummond, R. O.**, Further evaluation of animal systemic insecticides, 1962, *J. Econ. Entomol.*, 56, 831, 1963.

140. **Drummond, R. O.**, Further evaluation of animal systemic insecticides, 1963, *J. Econ. Entomol.*, 57, 741, 1964.

141. **Drummond, R. O.**, Further evaluation of animal systemic insecticides, 1964, *J. Econ. Entomol.*, 58, 773, 1965.

142. **Drummond, R. O.**, Further evaluation of animal systemic insecticides, 1965, *J. Econ. Entomol.*, 59, 1049, 1966.

143. **Drummond, R. O.**, Further evaluation of animal systemic insecticides, 1966, *J. Econ. Entomol.*, 60, 733, 1967.

144. **Drummond, R. O.**, Further evaluation of animal systemic insecticides, 1967, *J. Econ. Entomol.*, 61, 1261, 1968.

145. **Drummond, R. O. and Gladney, W. J.**, Further evaluation of animal systemic insecticides, 1968, *J. Econ. Entomol.*, 62, 934, 1969.

146. **Drummond, R. O., Darrow, D. I., and Gladney, W. J.**, Further evaluation of animal systemic insecticides, 1969, *J. Econ. Entomol.*, 63, 1103, 1970.

147. **Drummond, R. O., Darrow, D. I., and Gladney, W. J.**, Further evaluation of animal systemic insecticides, 1970, *J. Econ. Entomol.*, 64, 1166, 1971.

148. **Drummond, R. O., Darrow, D. I., and Gladney, W. J.**, Further evaluation of animal systemic insecticides, 1971, *J. Econ. Entomol.*, 65, 745, 1972.

149. **Drummond, R. O. and Whetstone, T. M.**, Cattle grubs: evaluation of new animal systemic insecticides, 1971—72, *J. Econ. Entomol.*, 67, 237, 1974.

150. **Smith, D. L.**, Weight gain in calves in response to control of cattle grubs with insecticides, *Manit. Entomol.*, 10, 5, 1976.

151. **Loomis, E. C. and Schock, R. C.**, Comparison of famphur (Warbex®) pour-on and intramuscular injectable formulations for cattle grub control, California, 1975—1976, *J. Med. Entomol.*, 14, 649, 1978.

152. **Ronald, N. C.**, Evaluation of Bay VB9328 flowable (coumaphos) in a dip vat: efficacy against the common cattle grub, *Hypoderma lineatum*, with observations on mixing and settling characteristics, *Southwest Vet.*, 34, 109, 1981.

153. **Khan, M. A. and Kozub, G. C.**, Systemic control of cattle grubs (*Hypoderma* spp.) in steers treated with Warbex® and weight gains associated with grub control, *Can. J. Comp. Med.*, 45, 15, 1981.

154. **Drummond, R. O., Whetstone, T. M., Shelley, B. K., and Barrett, C. C.**, Common cattle grub: control with animal systemic insecticides, *J. Econ. Entomol.*, 70, 176, 1977.

155. **Drummond, R. O.**, Control of larvae of the common cattle grub (Diptera: Oestridae) with animal systemic insecticides, *J. Econ. Entomol.*, 77, 402, 1984.

156. **Graham, O. H. and Drummond, R. O.**, The potential of animal systemic insecticides for eradicating cattle grubs, *Hypoderma* spp., *J. Econ. Entomol.*, 60, 1050, 1967.

157. **Rich, G. B.**, Systemic treatments for control of cattle grubs *Hypoderma* spp. in an isolated range herd, *Can. J. Anim. Sci.*, 45, 165, 1965.

158. **Riehl, L. A., Lembright, H. W., and Ludwig, P. D.**, Area population control of heel flies by Ruelene pour-on application annually to cattle, *J. Econ. Entomol.*, 58, 1, 1965.

159. **Khan, M. A.**, Extermination of cattle grubs (*Hypoderma* spp.) on a regional basis, *Vet. Rec.*, 83, 97, 1968.

160. **Khan, M. A.**, Eradication of hypodermosis, *Vet. Parasitol.*, 3, 205, 1977.

161. **Khan, M. A.**, The feasibility of exterminating warble flies (*Hypoderma* spp.) on a regional basis, *Vet. Parasitol.*, 3, 217, 1977.

162. **Khan, M. A., Weintraub, J., and Croome, G. C. R.**, Progress in extermination of cattle grubs (*Hypoderma* spp.): summary of the symposium, *Vet. Parasitol.*, 3, 271, 1977.

163. **Barrett, C. C., Miller, J. A., Drummond, R. O., and Pickens, M. O.**, Effect of methoprene on eclosion of the common cattle grub and the northern cattle grub, *Southwest. Entomol.*, 3, 232, 1978.

164. **Hunt, L. M., Beadles, M. L., Shelley, B. K., Gilbert, B. N., and Drummond, R. O.**, Control of cattle grubs with dichlorvos-impregnated strips attached to legs of cattle, *J. Econ. Entomol.*, 73, 32, 1980.

165. **Miller, J. A., Kunz, S. E., and Beadles, M. L.**, Efficacy and mode of action of insecticide-impregnated ear tags and leg bands for control of cattle grubs, *Southwest. Entomol.*, 6, 265, 1981.

166. **Drummond, R. O.**, Effectiveness of Ivermectin for control of arthropod pests of livestock, *Southwest. Entomol.*, Suppl. 7, 34, 1985.

Chapter 9

CONTROL OF LICE ON CATTLE*

I. INTRODUCTION

In the U.S. and Canada, cattle are infested with one species of biting lice, the cattle biting louse◆, *Bovicola bovis* (Linnaeus) (previously known as *Damalinia bovis* or *Trichodectes scalaris*), and four species of sucking lice: the shortnosed cattle louse◆, *Haematopinus eurysternus* (Nitzsch); the longnosed cattle louse◆, *Linognathus vituli* (Linnaeus); the little blue louse, *Solenopotes capillatus* Enderline; and, in limited geographical areas of the southern U.S., the cattle tail louse◆, *Haematopinus quadripertusus* Fahrenholz. Biting lice irritate their hosts, causing them to rub and scratch, which may lead to a general loss of vitality and productivity. Sucking lice are hematophagus and can cause anemia and loss in condition and productivity. Some cattle that are very highly tolerant of large infestations of shortnosed cattle lice are called "carriers" and serve as sources of infestation of other cattle in a herd. The only technology available for the control of lice is the treatment of cattle with insecticides.

II. EARLY TREATMENT TECHNOLOGY

In 1896, Osborn[1] listed the following treatments to control sucking lice on cattle: washes of plant extracts, especially those of *Delphinium* spp., carbolic acid, and tobacco; ointments containing mercury, kerosene, and lard; road dust or ashes; and fumigation with sulfur or tobacco smoke. Treatments for biting lice were washes of kerosene emulsion or a tobacco decoction and fumigation with sulfur.

The first edition of *U.S. Dep. Agric. Farmers' Bulletin* No. 909 in 1918[2] listed three methods used to apply a variety of chemicals to cattle to control lice: (1) hand application of dusts of naphthalene or pyrethrins, of washes of kerosene and cottonseed oil, kerosene and lard, crude petroleum, or any of the chemicals used as dips, (2) spraying of any of the chemicals used as dips, and (3) dipping in arsenic, coal-tar creosote, or nicotine. Biting lice were easily controlled by a number of treatments (even soap and water killed all stages except eggs), and sodium fluoride was effective as a spray or dust.[3] Other effective treatments included rotenone dust,[4] finely powdered inert dusts,[5] and sprays of a white oil emulsion known as Volck.[6,7] The 1940 edition of Bulletin No. 909[8] was the same as the earlier editions but added rotenone dust and spray as effective treatments and eliminated greases from the list of suggested treatments. Matthysse[9] presented an excellent, comprehensive review of information on the older materials applied to cattle, tested a number of chemicals as dusts, and concluded that rotenone dust was the most effective treatment.

III. ORGANOCHLORINE TREATMENTS

Use of sprays, washes, dips, and dusts of chlorinated hydrocarbon insecticides for louse control began at the end of World War II. Early tests with DDT were not very promising.[9] Benzene hexachloride (BHC) and lindane controlled adults, nymphs, and eggs.[10,11] DDT sprays controlled the cattle tail louse, observed in Florida for the first time in 1945.[12] DDT

---

* Common names of insects and acarines, as listed in *Common Names of Insects and Related Organisms* (published by the Entomological Society of America), are marked with a ◆ the first time they are cited preceding the scientific name.

sprays and dips controlled both biting and sucking lice.[13,14] The 1947 edition of Bulletin No. 909[15] listed a number of older materials as well as the use of DDT dusts, washes, sprays, and dips to control lice. Bishopp and Knipling[16] and Knipling[17] reviewed current research on control of arthropod pests of livestock and reported eradication of lice with one thorough spraying or dipping with DDT and excellent control of lice and eggs with BHC with a low gamma isomer concentration; chlordane, toxaphene, methoxychlor, and TDE were as effective as DDT. These reports also raised the issue of the problems of residues of chlorinated hydrocarbon insecticides in tissues and milk of treated animals.

A single spray application of chlordane or two applications of lindane or rotenone gave season-long control of sucking and biting lice.[18] The 1953 edition of Bulletin No. 909[19] recommended dusts, washes, and sprays of DDT, BHC, lindane, chlordane, and toxaphene but limited recommended dips to arsenic, coal-tar creosote, nicotine, rotenone, and DDT, because the other chlorinated hydrocarbon insecticides had not been tested sufficiently in dips. This bulletin first mentions the appearance of *H. quadripertusus* in Puerto Rico, Texas, and Florida and its control with DDT. In general, chlorinated hydrocarbon insecticides were effective, but not all provided complete control with one application. Their use in dairy barns and on dairy cattle was eliminated or severely restricted because of residues in milk. Their use on beef cattle was contingent upon observing long intervals between treatment and slaughter in order for residues in tissues to be depleted below approved levels.

In order to control lice on cattle without gathering animals for treatment, a self-treatment rubbing device was used[20] to apply chlordane in fuel oil to cattle in feedlots or small pastures. DDT, methoxychlor, and toxaphene were also effective when applied by this technique.[21] This backrubber was a slight modification of a cable-type backrubber developed earlier[22] to apply insecticides to cattle to control the horn fly*, *Haematobia irritans* (Linnaeus). Backrubbers provided inexpensive louse control when used free choice by cattle when installed near feed boxes, salt licks, or watering places, or by forced use when devices were hung in places where cattle had to pass under them daily. Chlordane, toxaphene, methoxychlor, lindane, DDT, and malathion were effective in backrubbers.[23,24] The 1956 *Yearbook of Agriculture*[25] reviewed materials and methods used to control lice on beef and dairy cattle.

IV. ORGANOPHOSPHORUS TREATMENTS

The introduction of the organophosphorus insecticides in the late 1950s and early 1960s provided a variety of additional insecticides that controlled lice at low concentrations.[26] Insecticides found effective as body sprays in field tests were malathion,[27,28] coumaphos and Dowco® 109,[29,30] chlorfenvinphos,[31] naled,[32] malathion, ronnel, and coumaphos,[33] crotoxyphos, coumaphos, fenthion, and malathion,[34] and coumaphos and trichlorfon.[35] Carbaryl, a carbamate, as a spray controlled sucking and biting lice.[36] In limited trials, American Cyanamid 12503, General Chemical 3582, famphur, and Bayer 37342 were as effective as methoxychlor (the standard treatment) when sprayed onto the muzzles of cattle for control of the little blue louse.[37] Malathion sprays successfully eradicated biting and sucking lice from a closed herd of cattle.[38]

High-volume sprays of coumaphos, diazinon, crotoxyphos, or carbaryl controlled biting and sucking lice on stanchioned dairy cattle. Low-volume (60 to 240 mℓ per cow) mist applications (the technique of Matthysse and Marshall[39]) of emulsions or oil solutions of several organophosphorus insecticides or rotenone were also effective.[40]

The volume of treatment, but not amount of the active ingredient of insecticide, used to control lice was further reduced when the pouron technique was used[41] to apply ronnel, coumaphos, famphur, or crufomate to cattle to significantly reduce populations of sucking lice. Crufomate and fenthion pourons reduced populations of both sucking and biting lice.[40] Louse control was obtained by use of the spoton technique in which a few cubic centimeters of a highly concentrated insecticide were applied to a single spot on the back. Insecticides effective when applied by the pouron or spoton techniques included fenthion,[42] ronnel,[43] phosmet,[44] chlorpyrifos,[45-47] chlorpyrifos, ronnel, and famphur,[48] and methidathion, fenthion, and famphur.[49] Ronnel pouron or coumaphos dust gave excellent louse control.[50] Issues of *Insecticide and Acaricide Tests* and *Pesticide Research Reports* (Agriculture Canada) during 1977 to 1980 contain a large number of articles on the use of pouron or spoton techniques to apply organophosphorus insecticides to cattle for lice control.

V. OTHER TREATMENT TECHNOLOGIES

A. Dermal Treatments

Sprays of three insect juvenile hormone mimics, RO 06-9550, RO 08-4314, and RO 20-3600, reduced numbers of shortnosed cattle lice but did not eradicate the populations.[51]

Permethrin as a spray or pouron controlled shortnosed cattle lice on heavily infested cows.[52] Permethrin as a dust or spray and cypermethrin as a pouron also controlled cattle biting lice, short- and longnosed cattle lice, but two treatments of permethrin were required for adequate control.[53] Most issues of *Insecticide and Acaricide Tests* since 1981 contain results of tests with the pyrethroids to control lice on cattle.

B. Insecticide-Impregnated Ear Tags

Harvey and Ely[54] confined cattle singly in a shed and exposed them to vapors of dichlorvos from dichlorvos-impregnated resin strips. As little as 3 hr of exposure controlled shortnosed cattle lice on lightly infested animals, but 12 to 24 hr of exposure was necessary to control lice on heavily infested animals. Insecticide-impregnated ear tags containing fenvalerate,[55] developed for the control of ticks and horn flies on cattle, were found to be effective against shortnosed cattle lice. Recent issues of *Insecticide and Acaricide Tests* contain results of tests with ear tags impregnated with chlorpyrifos, stirofos, cypermethrin, flucythrinate, or permethrin for the control of lice. Generally, insecticide-impregnated ear tags gradually reduced but did not completely control populations of sucking and biting lice.

C. Systemic Insecticides

Some control of lice on cattle has been obtained with the oral or percutaneous administration of animal systemic insecticides. Feeding of sulfur to calves did not reduce louse populations.[56] Single oral or multiple daily (short-term) feed treatments with early systemics, ronnel, Dowco®109, and dimethoate, did not control sucking lice.[57] Three oral treatments of high dosages of ronnel were effective, but low-dosage daily feed treatments did not provide complete control of *H. eurysternus*.[58] Little additional research on the use of systemics for louse control was conducted until recently.

A single subcutaneous injection of nifluridide, an experimental benzimidazole systemic, eliminated longnosed cattle lice but not biting lice on cattle.[59] An important advance in the control of lice systemically has been the appearance of ivermectin as an animal systemic insecticide. A single subcutaneous injection of ivermectin is highly effective against sucking lice and also, in some reports, against biting lice (see Drummond[60] for a review of ivermectin in livestock). As reported in *Insecticide and Acaricide Tests* in 1983 to 1984, intramuscular injections of famphur gave short-term control of sucking lice, but an oral paste of famphur appeared to be more effective systemically.

VI. OVERVIEW AND CURRENT TECHNOLOGY

In general, control of lice depends upon the treatment of cattle dermally with an appropriate insecticide to kill all the motile stages and have sufficient residual effectiveness to kill newly emerged nymphs. Two treatments 7 to 10 days apart of a less effective insecticide may be necessary to control lice.

The use of oils, dusts, sprays, and dips of a variety of chemicals provided control of biting and sucking lice on cattle at the turn of the century. Chlorinated hydrocarbon insecticides replaced earlier treatments after World War II. In the 1960s, organophosphorus insecticides replaced many of the organochlorine compounds. In the 1980s, pyrethroid insecticides were also available for the control of lice.

Changes in treatment technology occurred with the use of the self-application backrubber to apply insecticides. The pouron treatment provided louse control and was easy to administer; treatment volume was further reduced with the advent of the spoton treatment. Insecticide-impregnated ear tags afford some control of lice on cattle but results are not consistent.

A recent development in the technology of the control of sucking lice on cattle is the treatment of cattle with subcutaneous injections of a highly active systemic insecticide, ivermectin, which is now commercially available.

REFERENCES

1. **Osborn, H.**, Insects affecting domestic animals: an account of the species of importance in North America with mention of related forms occurring on other animals, *U.S. Dep. Agric. Bull.*, 5, 1896.
2. **Imes, M.**, Cattle lice and how to eradicate them, *U.S. Dep. Agric. Farmers' Bull.*, 909, 1918.
3. **Bishopp, F. C. and Wood, H. P.**, Preliminary experiments with sodium fluoride and other insecticides against biting and sucking lice, *Psyche*, 24, 187, 1917.
4. **Wells, R. W., Bishopp, F. C., and Laake, E. W.**, Derris as a promising insecticide, *J. Econ. Entomol.*, 15, 90, 1922.
5. **Shull, W. E.**, Control of the cattle louse, *Bovicola bovis* Linn. (Mallophaga, Trichodectidae), *J. Econ. Entomol.*, 25, 1208, 1932.
6. **Bruce, W. G.**, The use of Volck against external parasites of domestic animals, *J. Kans. Entomol. Soc.*, 1, 74, 1928.
7. **Caler, H. L.**, Volck special emulsion number 2 as a control for external parasites of animals, *J. Kans. Entomol. Soc.*, 4, 77, 1931.
8. **Imes, M.**, Cattle lice and how to eradicate them, *U.S. Dep. Agric. Farmers' Bull.*, 909, 1940.
9. **Matthysse, J. G.**, Cattle lice their biology and control, *Cornell Univ. Agric. Exp. Stn. Bull.*, 832, 1946.
10. **Wells, R. W. and Barrett, W. L., Jr.**, Benzene hexachloride as an ovicide for the short-nosed ox louse, *J. Econ. Entomol.*, 39, 816, 1946.
11. **Furman, D. P.**, Benzene hexachloride to control cattle lice, *J. Econ. Entomol.*, 40, 672, 1947.
12. **Bruce, W. G.**, The tail louse, a new pest of cattle in Florida, *J. Econ. Entomol.*, 40, 590, 1947.
13. **Kemper, H. E., Cobbett, N. G., Roberts, I. H., and Peterson, H. O.**, DDT emulsions for the destruction of lice on cattle, sheep and goats, *Am. J. Vet. Res.*, 9, 373, 1948.
14. **Snipes, B. T.**, Beef cattle freed of lice in one treatment control, *Agric. Chem.*, 3, 30, 1948.
15. **Imes, M.**, Cattle lice and how to eradicate them, *U.S. Dep. Agric. Farmers' Bull.*, 909, 1947.
16. **Bishopp, F. C. and Knipling, E. F.**, Insecticides applied on livestock, *Ind. Eng. Chem.*, 40, 713, 1948.
17. **Knipling, E. F.**, Livestock insects and their control, with comments on the new insecticides, *Proc. 52 Annu. Meet. U.S. Livestock Sanit. Assoc.*, 94, 1948.
18. **Lancaster, J. L., Jr.**, One application control for cattle lice, *J. Econ. Entomol.*, 44, 718, 1951.
19. **Kemper, H. E. and Peterson, H. O.**, Cattle lice and how to eradicate them, *U.S. Dep. Agric. Farmers' Bull.*, 909, 1953.
20. **Hoffman, R. A.**, Self-treatment rubbing devices for louse control on cattle, *J. Econ. Entomol.*, 47, 701, 1954.
21. **Hoffman, R. A.**, The effectiveness and limitations of homemade self-treatment rubbing devices for louse control on cattle, *J. Econ. Entomol.*, 47, 1152, 1954.
22. **Rogoff, W. M. and Moxon, A. L.**, Cable type back rubbers for horn fly control on cattle, *J. Econ. Entomol.*, 45, 329, 1952.
23. **Neel, W. W.**, Tests with self-treating devices for the control of lice on cattle in Mississippi, *J. Econ. Entomol.*, 49, 138, 1956.

24. **Gressette, F. R., Jr. and Goodwin, W. J.,** Cattle louse control with treated rubbing devices and their distribution in South Carolina, *J. Econ. Entomol.,* 49, 236, 1956.

25. **Smith, C. L. and Roberts, I. H.,** Cattle lice, *U.S. Dep. Agric. Yearb. Agric.,* 307, 1956.

26. **Smith, C. L. and Richards, R.,** Evaluations of some new insecticides against lice on livestock and poultry, *J. Econ. Entomol.,* 48, 566, 1955.

27. **DeFoliart, G. R.,** Lice control on northern range herds with residual sprays, *J. Econ. Entomol.,* 50, 618, 1957.

28. **Anthony, D. W.,** Tests with DDT, lindane and malathion for control of the long-nosed cattle louse *Linognathus vituli* (L.), *J. Econ. Entomol.,* 52, 782, 1959.

29. **DeFoliart, G. R., Glenn, M. W., and Robb, T. R.,** Field studies with systemic insecticides against cattle grubs and lice, *J. Econ. Entomol.,* 51, 876, 1958.

30. **Marquardt, W. C., Lovelace, S. A., and Fritts, D. H.,** Spray treatment of calves with Bayer 21/199 for control of cattle grubs and lice in Montana, *J. Am. Vet. Med. Assoc.,* 137, 589, 1960.

31. **Hoffman, R. A. and Drummond, R. O.,** Control of lice on livestock and parasites on poultry with General Chemical 4072, *J. Econ. Entomol.,* 54, 1052, 1961.

32. **Goulding, R. L. and Taylor, N. O.,** Effects of topical applications of Dibrom upon cattle lice and cattle grubs, *J. Econ. Entomol.,* 55, 744, 1962.

33. **Shemanchuk, J. A., Haufe, W. O., and Thompson, C. O. M.,** Effects of some insecticides on infestations of the short-nosed cattle louse, *Can. J. Anim. Sci.,* 43, 56, 1963.

34. **Roberts, J. E., Baird, D. M., and White, P. E.,** Georgia station trials examine population and control of cattle lice and grubs, *Ga. Agric. Res.,* 5, 6, 1964.

35. **Knapp, F. W.,** Low concentration of coumaphos and trichlorfon spray treatments for control of the cattle lice *Solenopotes capillatus* and *Bovicola bovis, J. Econ. Entomol.,* 58, 585, 1965.

36. **Khan, M. A., Avery, R. J., and Dueck, H. P.,** Toxicity of Sevin (1-naphthyl-*n*-methyl-carbamate) to cattle grubs, lice, and cattle, *Can. J. Comp. Med. Vet. Sci.,* 26, 234, 1962.

37. **Roberts, R. H.,** Preliminary tests with insecticides for the control of the little blue cattle louse, *J. Econ. Entomol.,* 57, 42, 1964.

38. **Anthony, D. W., Mott, L. O., and Mills, G. D.,** Cattle lice eradication studies — a 3-year evaluation, *J. Am. Vet. Med. Assoc.,* 142, 130, 1963.

39. **Matthysse, J. G. and Marshall, J.,** The importance, relation to foot rot, and control of *Chorioptes bovis* on cattle and sheep, in *Advances in Acarology,* Vol. 1, Naegele, J. A., Ed., Cornell University Press, Ithaca, N.Y., 1963, 39.

40. **Matthysse, J. G., Pendleton, R. F., Padula, A., and Nielsen, G. R.,** Controlling lice and chorioptic mange mites on dairy cattle, *J. Econ. Entomol.,* 60, 1615, 1967.

41. **Rich, G. B.,** Pour-on systemic insecticides for the protection of calves from *Linognathus vituli, Can. J. Anim. Sci.,* 46, 125, 1966.

42. **Roberts, J. E., Sr.,** Control of lice on beef cattle with 20% Tiguvon spotton and 3% Tiguvon pouron, *Va. J. Sci.,* 24 (Abstr.), 111, 1973.

43. **McGregor, W. S.,** New developments for controlling cattle lice, *Down Earth,* 28, 11, 1973.

44. **Khan, M. A.,** Effectiveness of phosmet for integrated control of cattle grubs and cattle lice, in Research Highlights — 1979, Croome, G. C. R. and Wilson, D. B., Eds. Agriculture Canada Research Station, Lethbridge, Alberta, 1980, 67.

45. **Knapp, F. W. and Christensen, C.,** Dursban 44 insecticide as a spot treatment for cattle lice, *Down Earth,* 36, 14, 1979.

46. **McMartin, K. D.,** Control of cattle lice with a low volume pour-on formulation of chlorpyrifos, *Down Earth,* 33, 18, 1977.

47. **Khan, M. A.,** Dursban 44 for winter control of lice on range cows, in Research Highlights — 1980, Croome, G. C. R. and Atkinson, T. G., Eds., Agriculture Canada Research Station, Lethbridge, Alberta, 1981, 51.

48. **Loomis, E. C., Webster, A. N., and Lobb, P. G.,** Trials with chlorpyrifos (Dursban) as a systemic insecticide against the cattle louse, *Vet. Rec.,* 98, 168, 1976.

49. **Hart, R. J., Cavey, W. A., Moore, B., and Strong, M. B.,** Efficiency and safety of methidathion applied as a pour-on systemic insecticide for control of cattle lice, *Aust. Vet. J.,* 55, 575, 1979.

50. **Wright, R. E.,** Efficacy of ronnel as a pour-on and coumaphos as a dust for control of cattle lice, *Can. Entomol.,* 108, 83, 1976.

51. **Meleney, W. P. and Roberts, I. H.,** Insect juvenile hormone mimics against the short-nosed cattle louse, *Haematopinus eurysternus* Denny (Anoplura), and their effect on warbles of *Hypoderma* sp. Latr. (Diptera:Oestridae), *J. Parasitol.,* 61, 956, 1975.

52. **Khan, M. A.,** Permethrin for combined control of cattle lice and cattle grubs, in Research Highlights — 1978, Croome, G. C. R. and Holmes, N. D., Eds., Agriculture Canada Research Station, Lethbridge, Alberta, 1979, 65.

53. **Madder, D. J. and Surgeoner, G. A.,** Effect of permethrin, cypermethrin and chlorpyrifos on louse populations of beef cattle, *Proc. Entomol. Soc. Ont.,* 110, 29, 1979.

54. **Harvey, T. L. and Ely, D. G.,** Controlling short-nosed cattle lice with dichlorvos resin strips, *J. Econ. Entomol.,* 61, 1128, 1968.

55. **Khan, M. A.,** Bovaid ear tags for control of cattle lice, in Research Highlights — 1983, Sears, L. J. L. and Wilson, D. B., Eds., Agriculture Canada Research Station, Lethbridge, Alberta, 1984, 44.

56. **Babcock, O. G. and Boughton, I. B.,** Sulfur-feeding tests for the control of ectoparasites of animals, *J. Am. Vet. Med. Assoc.,* 103, 209, 1943.

57. **DeFoliart, G. R., Glenn, M. W., and Robb, T. R.,** Field studies with systemic insecticides against cattle grubs and lice, *J. Econ. Entomol.,* 51, 876, 1958.

58. **Shemanchuk, J. A., Haufe, W. O., and Thompson, C. O. M.,** Effects of some insecticides on infestations of the short-nosed cattle louse, *Can. J. Anim. Sci.,* 43, 56, 1963.

59. **Boisvenue, R. J. and Clymer, B. C.,** Systemic activity of nifluridide against sucking lice and the common scabies mite on cattle, *Vet. Parasitol.,* 11, 253, 1982.

60. **Drummond, R. O.,** Effectiveness of Ivermectin for control of arthropod pests of livestock, *Southwest. Entomol.,* Suppl.7, 34, 1985.

Chapter 10

CONTROL OF MITES ON CATTLE*

I. INTRODUCTION

Cattle are infested with several species of mites which cause a skin disease called mange, scab, scabies, or itch. The most important species are the sheep scab mite♦, *Psoroptes ovis* (Hering), which can cause severe body mange in cattle; the itch mite♦, *Sarcoptes scabiei* (DeGeer), which tunnel into the epidermis of the skin; *Chorioptes bovis* (Hering), which usually feeds on epidermal debris, but which may cause feeding lesions on cattle; and the cattle follicle mite♦, *Demodex bovis* Stiles, found in hair follicles and sebaceous glands in the skin of cattle. Two species of lesser importance are *Psorergates bos* Johnston, found on the skin of cattle, and *Raillietia auris* (Leidy), found in ears of cattle. A recent review by Meleney[1] provides considerable information on the biology and control of these species.

II. CONTROL OF *PSOROPTES OVIS*

A. Early Treatment Technology

In 1896, Osborn[2] presented detailed information on and illustrations of *P. ovis,* then called *P. communis* Furst, the cause of scab in sheep, with varieties found on cattle and horses. He listed thorough dipping in tobacco or lime-sulfur as the best treatment for most mites affecting livestock. The original issue of *U.S. Dep. Agric. Farmers' Bulletin* No. 152 in 1902,[3] a republication of the *U.S. Dep. Agric. Bureau of Animal Industry Bulletin* No. 40 in 1902,[4] gave details of the preparation of heated lime-sulfur dip and of the use and construction of cage vats and swim-through vats for treating cattle. The 1904 revision of Bulletin No. 152[5] included the use of dips of Beaumont crude oil for the control of mange in cattle. The 1915 revision[6] was the 1904 edition reprinted without change.

U.S. Dep. Agric. Farmers' Bulletin No. 1017[7] in 1918 described the symptoms caused by common or psoroptic scab and recommended multiple spraying or dipping in warm lime-sulfur or nicotine to control psoroptic mange. The 1935 edition of Bulletin No. 1017[8] updated information on mite biology but contained no changes in control technology. The 1953 revision[9] reported that the incidence of psoroptic scab of cattle was decreasing as a result of an eradication program. Official treatment consisted of two sprayings at a 10- to 12-day interval with lindane or benzene hexachloride (BHC) or two dippings in heated lime-sulfur, nicotine, lindane, or BHC.

B. The Eradication Program

A review of the Federal-State program to eradicate psoroptic scabies of cattle showed[10] a decrease in the incidence of psoroptic cattle scabies from 1900 to 1950, until, in 1950 to 1952, no cases were reported and the mite was considered virtually eradicated. However, an outbreak in 1954[11] revealed that the mite had not been eradicated. The 1956 *U.S. Dep. Agric. Yearbook of Agriculture*[12] listed BHC and lindane as effective acaricides and noted that toxaphene was as effective as BHC and lindane.

The program to eradicate or control psoroptic scabies of cattle was reviewed by Meleney and Christy,[13] who described the dynamics of the increase in numbers of cases that started in 1972 and listed the following reasons for the increase: the complexity of the cattle-feeding

---

* Common names of insects and acarines, as listed in *Common Names of Insects and Related Organisms* (published by the Entomological Society of America), are marked with ♦ the first time they are cited preceding the scientific name.

industry, appearance of systemic insecticides that were not as effective as toxaphene or lindane against *P. ovis,* and the addition of coumaphos (in 1974) and phosmet (in 1975), which do not always eradicate mites on a single dipping, to the list of U.S. Department of Agriculture (USDA)-permitted dips. They noted that lindane, a most effective acaricide, was lost from the list in 1979. Toxaphene will no longer be available for use on livestock after 1986. Hourrigan[14] indicated an increase in activity in the eradication program was necessary in order to overcome the problems in detection, reporting, and treatment that prevented eradication. Critical analyses of the program to eradicate psoroptic scabies from cattle were presented by Schubert.[15,16]

C. Recent Treatments

Toxaphene eradicated mites when applied once as a spray, spray-dip, or dip treatment; phosmet and cyhexatin eradicated mites after two dippings; coumaphos did not always eradicate mites after two drippings; crufomate, malathion, and Vendex® were ineffective.[17] Two dippings in phosmet eradicated mites.[18] Dioxathion as a dip was ineffective, but two dippings in amitraz or a flowable formulation of coumaphos and a single dipping in toxaphene eradicated mites.[19] Sprays of two experimental alkyl carbamates were as effective as tox-aphene sprays for the control of *P. ovis* on cattle.[20]

D. Systemic Insecticides

A revolution in the control of psoroptic scabies of cattle came with the discovery and introduction of ivermectin as a systemic parasiticide. Previous studies with the organo-phosphorus systemic, famphur,[21] had shown that daily oral treatments failed to control *P. ovis* on cattle or sheep. Ivermectin, a chemically modified form of a macrocyclic lactone produced by a actinomycete, *Streptomyces avermitilis,*[22,23] is highly effective as a systemic insecticide against a variety of arthropod pests of livestock.[24] A single subcutaneous or intramuscular injection or oral treatment of ivermectin eliminated *P. ovis* infestations from cattle.[25-27] However, the ivermectin treatment does not rapidly kill *P. ovis* and although the fecundity of mites is reduced quickly after treatment, live mites are found on treated cattle for up to 2 weeks posttreatment.[28] In order to prevent spread of live mites from treated cattle to untreated cattle, it is necessary to keep treated cattle isolated for 2 weeks from noninfested cattle.[29] Another systemic, nifluridide, eliminated *P. ovis* from cattle with a single subcu-taneous injection.[30]

III. CONTROL OF *SARCOPTES SCABIEI*

Osborn[2] described the itch mite as a single species with a number of varieties found on different hosts and suggested controlling the species with the dips used to control scab mites. *U.S. Dep. Agric. Farmers' Bulletin* No. 152[3] noted that sarcoptic mange was a serious disease in some livestock but "was not common to cattle". *U.S. Dep. Agric. Farmers' Bulletin* No. 1017[7] reported that the incidence of sarcoptic mange, called "barn itch", was increasing in the U.S. and treatment consisted of four dippings in lime-sulfur or nicotine or one dipping in crude petroleum.

Barn itch was found to be widespread in stanchioned dairy herds in New York and could be controlled with sprays of heated lime-sulfur.[31] In the late 1940s the incidence of sarcoptic mange was increasing in the northeastern states, especially in the winter months. Because dipping was impractical, high-pressure sprayings of lime-sulfur, wettable sulfur, and wettable sulfur plus rotenone (for louse control) weekly for 4 weeks or 2 weekly applications of benzene hexachloride (BHC) eradicated mange.[32] Daily spraying of cattle with a water-miscible, colloidal crude coal tar spray for 1 week eliminated barn itch.[33] A large-scale program in dairy cattle in New York demonstrated that treatment in the fall would control, but not eradicate, mange.[34] Two sprayings of lindane at a 10-day interval controlled but did not eradicate sarcoptic scabies.[35]

The 1953 revision of Bulletin No. 1017[9] and the *U.S. Dep. Agric. Yearbook of Agriculture* in 1956[12] reported that the incidence of sarcoptic mange was increasing in the U.S. Recommended treatments were multiple dippings in lime-sulfur, one dipping in crude petroleum, or two sprayings with BHC or lindane.

In 1975, control of *S. scabiei* in lactating dairy cattle could only be accomplished with expensive and cumbersome treatment with heated lime-sulfur in a spray-dip machine.[36]

Ivermectin as a single subcutaneous injection eliminated infestations of *S. scabiei* in some 13,000 beef cattle in Canada.[37]

IV. CONTROL OF *CHORIOPTES BOVIS*

Osborn[2] listed *Chorioptes symbiotes* Verheyer as single species with several varieties from different hosts and noted that standard dipping treatments controlled this pest. *U.S. Dep. Agric. Farmers' Bulletin* No. 152[3] described symbiotic or tail mange caused by *C. bovis*, noted the lack of contagiousness, and reported that lime-sulfur dip readily controlled the pest. *U.S. Dep. Agric. Farmers' Bulletin* No. 1017[7] discussed chorioptic scab in only seven sentences.

The incidence of chorioptic scabies, commonly called leg or foot mange, increased rapidly in the northeastern states in the late 1940s. Because dipping of cattle was impractical, high-pressure spraying of cattle weekly for 4 weeks with lime-sulfur or wettable sulfur or for 2 weeks with BHC eradicated mange.[32] Two thorough spray treatments with lindane controlled, but did not eradicate, chorioptic scabies.[35] A spray of lindane plus wettable sulfur was more effective than either of the individual ingredients.[38] The 1953 revision of Bulletin No. 1017[9] reported a rapid increase in the incidence of chorioptic scab in the U.S. and that the treatments used for psoroptic and sarcoptic scab would eradicate chorioptic scab. *The U.S. Dep. Agric. Yearbook of Agriculture* in 1956[12] noted that BHC and lindane were more effective than older materials. Whole-body sprays of lindane or localized treatment with benzyl benzoate controlled but did not eradicate chorioptic mange.[39]

Control of *C. bovis* was obtained by spraying cattle with crotoxyphos.[40] High-volume sprays of crotoxyphos or low-volume (240 mℓ per cow) mists of a crotoxyphos emulsion or oil solutions of dichlorvos or dichlorvos plus crotoxyphos controlled chorioptic mange.[41,42]

V. CONTROL OF *DEMODEX BOVIS*

U.S. Dep. Agric. Farmers' Bulletin No. 1017 in 1918[7] described the symptoms of demodectic mange in cattle, suggested killing cattle in the advanced stages of the disease, and treating of the rest of the herd with an approved scabicide. The 1935 revision of this bulletin[8] noted increased interest in demodectic mange of cattle as a result of leather damage caused by the pest. Frequent dipping was believed to delay progress of the disease but not to cure it. The 1953 revision of this bulletin[9] was not different from the 1935 edition. BHC in lanolin ointment or in linseed oil placed on lesions provided some control.[43]

In a comprehensive study on bovine demodicosis in Canada, more than 40% of the cattle and 7% of the calves were infested,[44] but there were no clinical symptoms.[45] When found in nodules or small serum-like scabs or crusts, bovine demodicosis is of considerable interest because of the relationship between infestations and leather defects.[46] One or two sprayings of coumaphos did not reduce the number of lesions.[47] Baker and Fisher[48] confirmed that there was a high incidence of inapparent or subclinical infestations of demodicosis in the U.S. Control of demodicosis in cattle, which generally is not accomplished through treatment with conventional insecticides, was obtained in India by three doses at weekly intervals of orally administered formalin, but not intramuscular injections of benzyl benzoate.[49]

VI. CONTROL OF OTHER MITE PESTS OF CATTLE

Psorergates bos, first identified in New Mexico in 1963[50] and subsequently found on several premises,[51] has been controlled with two treatments of lime-sulfur spray or dip separated by 2 weeks.[52] Ivermectin injections eliminated infestations in bulls in South Africa that were not previously controlled by sprays of flumethrin, a pyrethroid.[53]

Infestations of *Raillietia auris,* first identified in the U.S. in 1872, have been found occasionally in cattle.[54-57] Infestations of *R. auris* have been associated with loss of hearing in cattle.[58] No treatments have been listed for control of this species.

VII. OVERVIEW AND CURRENT TECHNOLOGY

The technology used to apply acaricides to cattle for the control of psoroptic, chorioptic, and sarcoptic mange of cattle was available at the turn of the century. Only thorough dipping in acaricides assured complete treatment of cattle. The program to eradicate *P. ovis* from cattle in the U.S. gradually succeeded in decreasing the incidence of psoroptic mange until the 1950s when the arthropod was virtually eradicated. For a variety of reasons, the incidence of *P. ovis* infestation in cattle has increased. At the present time, there is no official program to eradicate *P. ovis* from cattle in the U.S.

The appearance of Ivermectin, which eliminates psoroptic scab with a single subcutaneous treatment, is a significant event. The use of that treatment with adequate quarantine and surveillance, if fully supported by all facets of the cattle industry, could lead to the eradication of psoroptic scabies from the U.S. However, as long as the incidence of psoroptic scabies in cattle remains low and effective treatments are available, it is unlikely that the cattle industry would call for and support an eradication program.

Sarcoptic scab was not always adequately controlled by the standard technology of dipping and spraying with acaricides. The ivermectin treatment not only eliminates the complications associated with spraying or dipping of cattle in colder weather, but also provides an excellent tool for the control of *S. scabiei.* Unfortunately, sarcoptic scab can be a serious problem in lactating dairy cattle, and ivermectin cannot be used on these animals.

The incidence of chorioptic mange keeps increasing in the U.S., but the infestation can be controlled with treatments of crotoxyphos.

Control of demodectic mange remains a problem in those cases where clinical lesions have developed. Most infestations are subclinical but are of significance to the leather industry. Because defects in the hides that are attributed to demodicosis are not identified until processing at the tannery, there is no economic incentive for cattle producers to be concerned with the treatment of demodectic mange.

REFERENCES

1. **Meleney, W. P.,** Mange mites and other parasitic mites, in *Parasites, Pests and Predators,* Gaafar, W. M., Howard, W. E., and Marsh, R. E., Eds., Elsevier, Amsterdam, 1985, 317.
2. **Osborn, H.,** Insects affecting domestic animals: an account of the species of importance in North America, with mention of related forms occurring on other animals, *U.S. Dep. Agric. Bull.,* 5, 1896.
3. **Hickman, R. W.,** Scabies in cattle, *U.S. Dep. Agric. Farmers' Bull.,* 152, 1902.
4. **Hickman, R. W.,** Scabies in cattle, *U.S. Dep. Agric. Bur. Anim. Ind. Bull.,* 40, 1902.
5. **Hickman, R. W.,** Scabies of cattle, *U.S. Dep. Agric. Farmers' Bull.,* 152, 1904.
6. **Hickman, R. W.,** Scabies of cattle, *U.S. Dep. Agric. Farmers' Bull.,* 152, 1915.
7. **Imes, M.,** Cattle scab and methods of control and eradication, *U.S. Dep. Agric. Farmers' Bull.,* 1017, 1918.

8. **Imes, M.,** Cattle scab and methods of control and eradication, *U.S. Dep. Agric. Farmers' Bull.,* 1017, 1935.
9. **Kemper, H. E. and Peterson, H. O.,** Cattle scab and methods of control and eradication, *U.S. Dep. Agric. Farmers' Bull.,* 1017, 1953.
10. **Graham, O. H. and Hourrigan, J. L.,** Eradication programs for the arthropod parasites of livestock, *J. Med. Entomol.,* 13, 629, 1977.
11. **Kemper, H. E.,** Psoroptic cattle scabies outbreak in 1954, *Proc. U.S. Livestock Sanit. Assoc.,* 58, 288, 1954.
12. **Roberts, I. H. and Cobbett, N. G.,** Cattle scabies, *U.S. Dep. Agric. Yearb. Agric.,* 292, 1956.
13. **Meleney, W. P. and Christy, J. E.,** Factors complicating the control of psoroptic scabies of cattle, *J. Am. Vet. Med. Assoc.,* 173, 1473, 1978.
14. **Hourrigan, J. L.,** Spread and detection of psoroptic scabies of cattle in the United States, *J. Am. Vet. Med. Assoc.,* 175, 1278, 1979.
15. **Schubert, G. O.,** Cattle scabies — past, present, *Proc. Annu. Meet. Livestock Cons. Inst.,* 47, 1980.
16. **Schubert, G. O.,** Scabies eradication, *Proc. Annu. Meet. Livestock Cons. Inst.,* 120, 1981.
17. **Meleney, W. P. and Roberts, I. H.,** Tests with seven established and candidate acaricides against the common scab mite of cattle, *Psoroptes ovis* (Acari: Psoroptidae), *J. Med. Entomol.,* 16, 52, 1979.
18. **Roberts, I. H., Wilson, G. I., and Meleney, W. P.,** Evaluation of phosmet for the control of the common scabies mite on cattle, *J. Am. Vet. Med. Assoc.,* 173, 840, 1978.
19. **Guillot, F. S., Wright, F. C., and Meleney, W. P.,** Efficacy of four acaricides applied as dips for control of the sheep scabies mite, *Psoroptes ovis,* on cattle, *Prevent. Vet. Med.,* 1, 179, 1983.
20. **Kochansky, J. P. and Wright, F. C.,** Synthesis and structure-activity studies on aliphatic carbamates and thiocarbamates toxic to scabies mites, *Psoroptes* spp. (Acari: Psoroptidae), *J. Econ. Entomol.,* 78, 599, 1985.
21. **Roberts, I. H., Meleney, W. P., and Apodaca, S. A.,** Oral famphur for treatment of cattle lice, and against scabies mites and ear ticks of cattle and sheep, *J. Am. Vet. Med. Assoc.,* 155, 504, 1969.
22. **Campbell, W. C.,** An introduction to the avermectins, *N.Z. Vet. J.,* 29, 174, 1981.
23. **Campbell, W. C., Fisher, M. H., Stapley, E. O., Albers-Schonberg, G., and Jacob, T. A.,** Ivermectin: a potent new antiparasitic agent, *Science,* 221, 823, 1983.
24. **Drummond, R. O.,** Effectiveness of Ivermectin for control of arthropod pests of livestock, *Southwest. Entomol.,* Suppl. 7, 34, 1985.
25. **Bailey, V. H.,** Scabies research with injectable Ivermectin, *Proc. Annu. Meet. Livestock Cons. Inst.,* 131, 1981.
26. **Pouplard, L. and Detry, M.,** A new systemic antiparasitic agent — Ivermectin, *Ann. Med. Vet.,* 125, 643, 1981.
27. **Meleney, W. P.,** Control of psoroptic scabies on calves with Ivermectin, *Am. J. Vet. Res.,* 43, 329, 1982.
28. **Guillot, F. S. and Wright, F. C.,** Reduced fecundity of *Psoroptes ovis* (Hering) (Acari: Psoroptidae) on calves treated with Ivermectin, *Bull. Entomol. Res.,* 74, 657, 1984.
29. **Guillot, F. S. and Meleney, W. P.,** The infectivity of surviving *Psoroptes ovis* (Hering) on cattle treated with Ivermectin, *Vet. Parasitol.,* 10, 73, 1982.
30. **Boisvenue, R. J. and Clymer, B. C.,** Systemic activity of nifluridide against sucking lice and the common scabies mite on cattle, *Vet. Parasitol.,* 11, 253, 1982.
31. **Baker, D. W.,** Cattle scabies in the Northeastern states, *J. Am. Vet. Med. Assoc.,* 110, 378, 1947.
32. **Schwardt, H. H.,** Diagnosis and control of mange in dairy cattle, *J. Econ. Entomol.,* 42, 444, 1949.
33. **Dunnet, P. L.,** A new therapeutic agent for common dermatoses, *N. Am. Vet.,* 30, 713, 1949.
34. **Baker, D. W. and Howe, I. G.,** Cattle mange in New York State, *J. Am. Vet. Med. Assoc.,* 116, 280, 1950.
35. **Kemper, H. E. and Peterson, H. O.,** Treatment of cattle scabies with lindane, *Vet. Med.,* 47, 453, 1952.
36. **Nusbaum, S. R., Drazek, F. J., Holden, H., Love, T. J., Marvin, J., Rowe, D., and Tyler, L. L.,** *Sarcoptes scabei bovis* — a potential danger, *J. Am. Vet. Med. Assoc.,* 166, 252, 1975.
37. **Lavigne, C. and Smith, H. J.,** Treatment of sarcoptic mange in Canadian cattle with Ivermectin, *Can. Vet. J.,* 24, 389, 1983.
38. **Goodwin, W. J. and Schwardt, H. H.,** Control of the cattle mange mite, *J. Econ. Entomol.,* 45, 122, 1952.
39. **Pullin, J. W.,** Preliminary observations on the incidence, effect and control of chorioptic mange in dairy cattle, *Can. J. Comp. Med. Vet. Sci.,* 20, 107, 1956.
40. **Smith, H. J.,** A preliminary trial on the efficacy of Ciodrin against *Chorioptes bovis* in cattle, *Can. Vet. J.,* 8, 88, 1967.
41. **Matthysse, J. G. and Marshall, J.,** The importance, relation to foot rot, and control of *Chorioptes bovis* on cattle and sheep, in *Advances in Acarology,* Vol. 1, Naegele, J. A., Ed., Cornell University Press, Ithaca, N.Y., 1963, 39.

42. **Matthysse, J. G., Pendleton, R. F., Paula, A., and Nielsen, G. R.,** Controlling lice and chorioptic mange mites on dairy cattle, *J. Econ. Entomol.,* 60, 1615, 1967.
43. **Telford, H. S.,** Benzene hexachloride to control certain insects affecting domestic animals, *J. Econ. Entomol.,* 40, 918, 1947.
44. **Smith, H. J.,** Bovine demodicidosis, I. Incidence in Ontario, *Can. J. Comp. Vet. Med. Sci.,* 25, 165, 1961.
45. **Smith, H. J.,** Bovine demodicidosis. II. Clinical manifestations in Ontario, *Can. J. Comp. Med. Vet. Sci.,* 25, 201, 1961.
46. **Smith, H. J.,** Bovine demodicidosis. III. Its effect on hides and leather, *Can. J. Comp. Med. Vet. Sci.,* 25, 243, 1961.
47. **Smith, H. J.,** Bovine demodicidosis. VI. An attempt at treatment with a systemic organic phosphate insecticide, *Can. J. Comp. Med. Vet. Sci.,* 26, 42, 1962.
48. **Baker, D. W. and Fisher, W. F.,** Demodectic parasites in livestock, *Proc. U.S. Livestock Sanit. Assoc.,* 409, 1966.
49. **Tikaram, S. M., Ruprah, N. S., and Satija, K. C.,** Demodectosis in cattle and its treatment, *Ind. Vet. J.,* 61, 986, 1984.
50. **Johnston, D. E.,** *Psorergates bos,* a new mite parasite of domestic cattle (Acari-Psorergatidae), *Ohio Agric. Exp. Stn. Res. Circ.,* 129, 1964.
51. **Roberts, I. H. and Meleney, W. P.,** Psorergatic acariasis in cattle, *J. Am. Vet. Med. Assoc.,* 146, 17, 1965.
52. **Bergstrom, R. C. and Etherton, S. L.,** Psorergatid mites from cattle in Wyoming, *Vet. Med. Small Anim. Clin.,* 78, 1761, 1983.
53. **Oberem, P. T. and Malan, F. S.,** A new cause of cattle mange in South Africa: *Psorergates bos* Johnston, *J. S. Afr. Vet. Assoc.,* 55, 121, 1984.
54. **Olsen, O. W. and Bracken, F. K.,** Occurrence of the ear mite, *Raillietia auris* (Leidy, 1872), of cattle in Colorado, *Vet. Med.,* 45, 320, 1950.
55. **Menzies, G. C.,** The cattle ear mite, *Raillietia auris* (Leidy, 1872) in Texas, *J. Parasitol.,* 43, 200, 1957.
56. **Schlotthauer, J. C.,** Cattle ear mite *(Raillietia auris)* in Minnesota, *J. Am. Vet. Med. Assoc.,* 157, 1193, 1970.
57. **Heffner, R. S. and Heffner, H. E.,** Occurrence of the cattle ear mite *(Raillietia auris)* in southeastern Kansas, *Cornell Vet.,* 73, 193, 1983.
58. **Heffner, R. S. and Heffner, H. E.,** Effect of cattle ear mite infestation on hearing in a cow, *J. Am. Vet. Med. Assoc.,* 182, 612, 1983.

Chapter 11

CONTROL OF TICKS ON CATTLE*

I. INTRODUCTION

Cattle in the U.S. and Canada are infested with a variety of ticks. Historically, the most important species in the U.S. was the cattle tick*, *Boophilus annulatus* (Say). It and a closely related species, the southern cattle tick*, *B. microplus* (Canestrini), limited in its geographical distribution to south Texas and Florida, were eradicated from the U.S.

Each geographical section of the U.S. has several species of "hard" ticks that are important pests of cattle. In the northwestern U.S. and in Canada, the principal species is the Rocky Mountain wood tick*, *Dermacentor andersoni* Stiles, which is the principal cause of tick paralysis in livestock and humans and a major vector of Rocky Mountain spotted fever. The lone star tick*, *Amlyomma americanum* (Linnaeus), is an important pest of cattle, other livestock, wildlife, and humans in the southeastern third of the U.S. The winter tick*, *D. albipictus* (Packard), a one-host species that is found on cattle, horses, and other large mammals in the fall and winter months, is distributed widely in Canada and the northern tier of states in the U.S. and as far south as Texas. The Gulf Coast tick*, *A. maculatum* Koch, is limited in its distribution to the states along the Gulf Coast but is found as far north as Kansas. It principally attaches to the ears of cattle, and heavy infestations destroy the cartilage of ears causing a condition known as "gotch-ear".

Several other species of ticks found on cattle are of lesser importance. The Pacific Coast tick*, *D. occidentalis* Marx, limited in its distribution to the Pacific Coast, can cause tick paralysis. The American dog tick*, *D. variabilis* (Say), found in the eastern half of the U.S. and Canada, is more a pest of small mammals, dogs, and humans (a vector of Rocky Mountain Spotted Fever) than cattle. The blacklegged tick*, *Ixodes scapularis* (Say), is distributed throughout most of the eastern half of the U.S. and is of limited importance. A closely related species, *I. dammini* Speilman, Clifford, Piesman and Corwin, is found from Massachusetts to Minnesota and is of importance only because it is a vector of Lyme disease and babesiosis of humans.

Two species of "soft" ticks are of importance to livestock. The ear tick*, *Otobius megnini* (Duges), most often called the "spinose" ear tick, infests the ears of cattle and other livestock. Widely distributed throughout the southwestern states, it is also found in other areas of the U.S. and Canada. The pajaroello tick, *Ornithodoros coriaceus* Koch, limited in its geographical distribution to the Pacific Coast of California, is a vector of the agent that causes epizootic bovine abortion. *U.S. Dep. Agric. Agriculture Handbook* No. 485[1] presents a key to the species and a summary of the biology of ticks of veterinary importance.

Generally, ticks on cattle are controlled by the topical application of acaricides directly to the animals by dipping, spraying or other techniques. Tick control has also been obtained experimentally by treating cattle with systemic acaricides. Technologies used for the area control of ticks and chiggers are addressed in Chapter 17. In this chapter, we will review the different technologies used to control several species of ticks on cattle.

---

* Common names of insects and acarines, as listed in *Common Names of Insects and Related Organisms* (published by the Entomological Society of America), are marked with a * the first time they are cited preceding the scientific name.

II. CONTROL OF CATTLE TICKS

A. Early Treatment Technology

Control of the cattle tick has been a subject of importance in the U.S. for nearly 100 years. Even before this species was known to be the vector of the protozoan that causes bovine babesiosis, the cattle tick was the subject of a number of publications around the turn of the century that focused primarily on its control. In 1892, Curtice[2] reported that a kerosene emulsion sprayed onto cattle or oiling cattle with sweet oil or cottonseed oil killed cattle ticks. In 1896, Osborn[3] called the cattle tick the "most important of the American species". He listed tick control measures as sprays of carbolic acid, cottonseed oil, tobacco, sulfur, and their combinations and presented a description of a dipping vat designed by Dr. M. Frances of Texas A & M College. *U.S. Dep Agric. Bureau of Animal Industry Bulletin* No. 78 in 1905[4] reviewed earlier research on *B. annulatus* and its transmission of bovine babesiosis, described a number of other tick species in the U.S., and listed the following tick control measures: picking or brushing ticks off the host (a laborious task to be performed three times per week); smearing or spraying cattle with disinfecting solutions, such as cottonseed oil, fish oil, crude petroleum, kerosene, Beaumont crude oil and coal tar; and dipping cattle in an emulsion of Beaumont crude oil. The initial issue of *U.S. Dep. Agric. Farmers' Bulletin* No. 258 in 1906[5] was a condensed version of Bulletin No. 78.

A classic publication on North American ticks, *U.S. Dep. Agric. Bureau of Entomology Bulletin* No. 72 in 1907,[6] contained an annotated bibliography of the earlier literature on the taxonomy and biology of ticks and presented data on the biology, survival in the field, alternative hosts, and natural parasites and predators of *B. annulatus*.

Early literature in the U.S. emphasized treatment methodology for use in the eradication of *B. annulatus*. In *U.S. Dep. Agric. Farmers' Bulletin* No. 378 in 1909,[7] methods of eradicating the cattle tick included removing cattle from pastures to starve larval ticks and treating cattle by hand spraying or by dipping in crude petroleum emulsions or arsenic. *U.S. Dep. Agric. Bureau of Animal Industry Bulletin* No. 167[8] reported that arsenic dips protected cattle from reinfestation by larvae for 2 to 5 days. During the 1910s and 1920s, there were a number of USDA publications on the use, management, and assay of arsenical dips and vats.[9-11] The original edition of *U.S. Dep. Agric. Farmers' Bulletin* No. 1057 in 1919[12] listed methods of eradication of cattle ticks as freeing pastures of larvae by removing cattle for specific periods of time (pasture spelling) and dipping cattle in a mixture of caustic soda, white arsenic, sal-soda crystals, and pine tar. The 1932[13] and 1940[14] revisions of this bulletin contained no changes in control technology.

B. The Cattle Tick Eradication Program

There are numerous publications on the technology employed by the massive federal-state program to eradicate cattle ticks, *Boophilus* spp., from some 182 million ha of the U.S. The eradication program was reviewed by Graham and Hourrigan.[15] Critical elements of the program were the support of the cattle owners, appropriate laws and regulations and competent local, state, and national professionals who organized and implemented the program. The principal tools of the campaign were dipping of cattle in arsenic, the only official dip material, and vacating pastures to kill larvae.

In most of the U.S. the only species of *Boophilus* was *B. annulatus,* the cattle tick, but the southern cattle tick was found in Florida.[16] In Florida, the continual treatment of cattle and elimination of some deer hosts of this species led to its eradication.

Since 1943, when the tick was declared eradicated from the U.S., a buffer zone and active federal-state quarantine and treatment program has been maintained in Texas from Del Rio to the Gulf Coast in order to prevent the introduction of *B. annulatus* and *B. microplus* from Mexico into the U.S.

C. Organochlorine Treatments

A mixture of DDT and rotenone applied as a spray to cattle was very effective against the southern cattle tick in tropical regions.[17] In tests in Mexico, dips and sprays of DDT, rotenone, and benzene hexachloride (BHC), alone or in combination, were as effective as the standard arsenic dip for control of *B. annulatus,* and both DDT and BHC possessed greater residual effectiveness than rotenone or arsenic against larvae.[18,19] DDT sprays were not as effective as arsenic dips for control of the southern cattle tick, but residues on cattle were toxic to larvae for 1 week, and if used on an appropriate schedule could eradicate the species.[20]

D. Organophosphorus Treatments

In tests with organophosphorus insecticides in Mexico, coumaphos and dioxathion as dips were more effective than arsenic, the standard treatment, or ronnel dips for the control of both *B. microplus* and *B. annulatus.*[21,22] Carbaryl, chlorfenvinphos, toxaphene, and trichlorfon were effective as sprays. Chlorfenvinphos[23] and chlorpyrifos[24] as dips controlled *Boophilus* spp.

In continuing studies in Mexico, criteria and formulae were established in order to evaluate a number of treatments applied to cattle for the control of the cattle tick and the southern cattle tick. In these tests, cattle were artificially infested, treated with sprays or dips and held in stalls so that female ticks could be collected after treatment to determine the effectiveness of the treatments. Effective spray treatments were crotoxyphos, dioxathion, chlorpyrifos, phosmet, stirofos, fenthion, trichlorfon, and a number of experimental compounds; effective dip treatments were chlorpyrifos, dioxathion, chlorfenvinphos, and phosmet.[25-28] Pouron treatments of phosmet and chlorpyrifos gave >90% control of southern cattle ticks, but pouron treatments were not as effective as spray treatments.[29]

Cattle ticks and southern cattle ticks were controlled with dips of a flowable formulation of coumaphos.[30] This formulation had excellent sedimentation and stripping characteristics[31] as well as residual effectiveness against larval ticks.[32] Sprays of crotoxyphos controlled southern cattle ticks.[33]

E. Other Treatment Technologies

Ear tags impregnated with fenvalerate, stirofos, and decamethrin controlled *B. microplus* larvae placed on cattle for as long as 76 days after tags were placed on the cattle.[34] Sprays of amitraz controlled cattle ticks and southern cattle ticks.[35,36] Sprays of permethrin and fenvalerate also controlled the southern cattle tick and the cattle tick.[37,38]

III. CONTROL OF OTHER TICKS OF CATTLE

Although much of the early literature on ticks focused on the cattle tick, control of other tick species was also beginning to be investigated. In their monumental work, Hooker et al.[39] reviewed the literature and presented new data on the life history and bionomics of most of the economically important U.S. ticks. The appropriate technology used to control ticks on cattle was based upon the areas of the animals' bodies that the ticks infested. Ticks in ears could be controlled with oils, such as sweet oil, train oil or fish oil, poured into ears. Ticks on the body were controlled by hand-picking, hand application of coal-tar products, and dipping in standard tick dips.

A. Ear Tick

U.S. Dep. Agric. Farmers' Bulletin No. 980 in 1918[40] specifically addressed the control of the ear tick, *O. megnini,* which was accomplished by placing a mixture of pine tar and cottonseed oil into each ear with a large syringe.

DDT incorporated into a nondrying adhesive applied to the ears of cattle killed many ear ticks and afforded some protection from reinfestation.[41] The ear tick was readily controlled with a mixture of BHC, xylol, and pine oil injected into ears.[42] The 1947 revision of Bulletin No. 980[43] listed ear treatments of BHC-xylene-pine oil, a pyridine-adhesive mixture, and pine tar-cottonseed oil as effective against the ear tick.

The 1952 *Yearbook of Agriculture*[44] suggested controlling the ear tick with ear treatments of BHC-xylene-pine oil. Sprays of toxaphene or a DDT-lindane mixture controlled ear ticks but had to be applied with care. The 1953 revision of Bulletin No. 980[45] listed ear treatments of lindane-pine oil, chlordane-pine oil, pyridine-adhesive, and pine tar-cottonseed oil. Ear ticks were not controlled systemically by ronnel in feed for 4 days or by crufomate as a pour-on, but were controlled by crufomate placed directly into the ears of cattle.[46] Dust of a silica aerogel impregnated with naled applied into the ears of cattle controlled ear ticks.[47] In extensive field tests, the most effective treatments were coumaphos dust or pouron, a coumaphos plus trichlorfon aerosol, and a chlorpyrifos ear wash.[48]

B. Gulf Coast Tick

The Gulf Coast tick is of economic importance because it causes "gotch ear", a name given to the misshapen ears of cattle. Ticks attached to ears were a primary predisposing cause for infestations of the screwworm♦, *Cochliomyia hominivorax* (Coquerel). The tick was not readily controlled by dipping cattle, but hand dressing of ears with pine-tar oil plus benzol or pine-tar oil plus cottonseed oil controlled the Gulf Coast tick.[49,50] DDT in an adhesive formulation applied to ears of cattle controlled Gulf Coast ticks for 3 to 6 weeks[41] and decreased cases of screwworms.[51,52] Full coverage body sprays of DDT were as effective as smear treatments of ears for the control of the Gulf Coast tick.[53] The 1952 *Yearbook of Agriculture*[44] suggested spraying toxaphene or a mixture of lindane and DDT to the ears, necks, and heads of cattle to control Gulf Coast ticks.

The Gulf Coast tick, still a problem in certain areas of Texas and Oklahoma, was controlled by attaching insecticide-impregnated ear tags to ears. These tags released sufficient insecticide to kill attached ticks and prevent reinfestation of ticks and subsequent screwworm infestations. Although several sprays gave good initial control of ticks, residual effectiveness was short, and smears and dusts provided longer residual control. The most effective treatments were ear tags impregnated with dichlorvos, stirofos, fenvalerate, and chlorpyrifos.[54-57] These tags are also labeled for control of ear ticks.

C. Rocky Mountain Wood Tick

The Rocky Mountain wood tick in the Bitter Root Valley of Montana was controlled by dipping all livestock in vats charged with arsenical dip.[58] Mail[59] reviewed the problem of paralysis in humans and animals caused by *D. andersoni* and reported that arsenic dips controlled ticks on cattle but sulfur in the diet of cattle did not control ticks. BHC was effective as a spray for control of *D. andersoni*.[60] *D. andersoni* was controlled by spraying cattle with lindane and chlordane; aldrin and ovex were less effective and dieldrin and Neotran® were ineffective.[61]

Several acaricides were applied as body sprays or as concentrated treatments to the necks and briskets of cattle. Sprays of chlorfenvinphos and crotoxyphos were more effective, and sprays of dioxathion and coumaphos were less effective than the standard toxaphene spray. Concentrated treatments of toxaphene applied to tick-infested areas were more effective than whole body sprays.[62]

In trials presented in Agriculture Canada Pesticide Research Reports from 1977 to 1984, adult Rocky Mountain wood ticks on cattle were controlled with lindane sprays (the standard treatment), permethrin pouron or spray, fenvalerate pouron, phosmet pouron or spray, decamethrin pouron, and chlorpyrifos pouron. Two ear tags of fenvalerate reduced populations by about 50%.

D. Lone Star Tick

BHC applied as a dip or spray killed all stages of the lone star tick on cattle and provided some residual protection against reinfestation.[63] The 1952 *U.S. Dep. Agric. Yearbook of Agriculture*[44] listed sprays of toxaphene and a mixture of lindane and DDT as effective treatments for the lone star tick. Chlordane, strobane and toxaphene sprays controlled adult lone star ticks, but none prevented reinfestation for as long as 1 week posttreatment.[64]

Sprays of coumaphos, malathion, ronnel, dioxathion, carbaryl, and Bayer 22408 were as effective as a spray of toxaphene, the standard treatment, in controlling lone star ticks and preventing reinfestation.[65] Chlorfenvinphos spray was more effective than the toxaphene standard treatment.[66] Crotoxyphos, crufomate, diazinon, fenthion, Methyl Trithion®, and trichlorfon were as effective as the toxaphene standard treatment at 1 week posttreatment.[67] Toxaphene was equally effective when applied as a spray or by a spray-dip machine.[68] Sprays of carbaryl, chlorfenvinphos, chlorpyrifos, coumaphos, phosmet, stirofos, and trichlorfon were as effective as the toxaphene standard treatment; a trichlorfon pouron was only partially effective but "none were so superior as to deserve special note".[69] Lone star ticks on cattle were controlled with sprays of chlordimeform, chlorfenvinphos, coumaphos, iodofenphos, Mobam®, permethrin, and stirofos. Pourons of fenthion and phosmet were also effective, but ear bands, ear tags, or leg bands impregnated with chlorpyrifos, stirofos, or dichlorvos failed to control ticks.[70] Sprays of coumaphos, dioxathion, lindane, malathion, ronnel, stirofos, toxaphene, and toxaphene plus lindane gave significant control of lone star ticks at 1 day but not 1 week posttreatment.[71]

The strategic treatment of cattle with acaricides at 10-day intervals from March to July for the control of lone star ticks reduced numbers of ticks on cattle and in pastures for the following 2 years.[72]

E. Winter Tick

Because the winter tick is found on cattle only in the fall and winter months, usually a single treatment in the fall will control ticks for the remainder of the tick season. The 1952 *Yearbook of Agriculture*[44] suggested sprays of toxaphene or a mixture of DDT and lindane to control this species.

Sprays that were as effective as a toxaphene standard treatment were dioxathion, ronnel, coumaphos, and Bayer 22408, while carbaryl and malathion were less effective.[73] Sprays of chlorfenvinphos were also as effective as sprays of toxaphene.[66] Sprays of fenthion, Methyl Trithion®, crufomate, crotoxyphos, trichlorfon, diazinon, carbophenothion, and dichlofenthion were as effective as the toxaphene standard treatment.[67] Toxaphene was equally effective when applied as a spray or by a spray-dip machine.[68]

IV. SYSTEMIC ACARICIDES

Lindane and dieldrin in peanut oil applied dermally to cattle as unctions or injected subcutaneously controlled southern cattle ticks, but left high residues in tissues.[74] Sulfur in the diet of cattle failed to control *B. microplus*.[75,76] Of several animal systemic acaricides fed to cattle for the control of ticks, the most effective systemic, famphur, controlled the tropical horse tick♦, *Anocentor nitens* (Neumann), *Amblyomma americanum, A. maculatum*, and the American dog tick.[77,78] Famphur given intraruminally to sheep controlled *A. maculatum*.[79] A sustained-release bolus of famphur controlled *A. americanum, A. maculatum*,[80] *B. annulatus*, and *B. microplus*.[81] Injections of Eli Lilly L-27 controlled all stages of the southern cattle tick feeding on cattle at treatment time and provided limited residual activity.[82]

A significant advance, especially in terms of practical, low-dosage administration of systemics for tick control, was evident in the results obtained with ivermectin, which was effective systemically against several species of ticks when given daily subcutaneously or orally to cattle.[83-85] Sustained-release implants of ivermectin[86] provided 40 to 80 days of control of lone star ticks, depending upon the formulation and initial dosage administered to cattle. Drummond[87] reviewed information on the systemic activity of ivermectin for control of a variety of arthropod pests of livestock.

A systemic, closantel, controlled adult lone star ticks when given to cattle orally or subcutaneously.[88] A single subcutaneous injection of nitroxynil, a fasciolicide, affected the engorging and reproduction of *B. microplus* and *Rhipicephalus appendiculatus* Neumann.[89]

V. EXPERIMENTAL CONTROL TECHNOLOGIES

A sex pheromone extracted with hexane from male Gulf Coast ticks was mixed with the acaricide, isobenzan, and placed on a spot on a bovine host. Female ticks, attracted by the pheromone migrated to the spot, were killed by the acaricide.[90] A combination of pheromone with toxaphene was used by Rechav and Whitehead[91] in South Africa to successfully attract and kill nymphs and adults of *A. hebraeum* Koch. In contrast,[92] there was no reduction in mating of American dog ticks after placing pheromone-impregnated collars around necks of dogs. The treatment of dogs, infested with American dog ticks, with an encapsulated or dust formulation of 2,6-dichlorophenol, the tick sex pheromone, caused a significant decrease in mating of ticks attached to the hosts.[93] The combination of 2,6-dichlorophenol with propoxur increased the kill of ticks, especially male ticks, over that of the acaricide alone.[94]

The treatment of American dog ticks topically with precocene-2, an antiallatotropin that disrupts development and reproduction of arthropods, did not induce precocious development, but rather acted as a toxicant to immature stages and impaired feeding and oviposition of adults.[95]

VI. OVERVIEW AND CURRENT TECHNOLOGY

The technology used to control ticks available at the turn of the century, dipping, spraying, and hand application, is still available today for tick control. The dipping of cattle in arsenic plus the removing of cattle from pastures eradicated *Boophilus annulatus* (and *B. microplus*) from the U.S. Identical eradication strategies are employed today except that organophosphorus acaricides replaced arsenic. Amitraz and pyrethroid acaricides are possible future substitutes for the organophosphorus acaricides. The presence of *Boophilus* ticks in Mexico mandates that a continuing program be maintained in Texas to prevent the introduction of ticks into the U.S. and to eradicate introduced ticks.

The ear tick and the Gulf Coast tick can be controlled with a variety of ear treatments as well as insecticide-impregnated ear tags.

Rocky Mountain wood ticks, lone star ticks, and winter ticks have been and can be controlled by spraying cattle with a number of acaricides. Pouron, spoton, and ear tag treatments are not as effective as complete-coverage treatments.

Although systemic acaricides given orally to cattle have controlled a variety of ticks experimentally, none of the treatments has been developed into a practical technology for tick control. The presence of ivermectin, which is effective at an extremely low dosage, allows for further research on low level, sustained-release treatment of cattle for tick control.

Tick attractants and pheromones have been used experimentally, but have not shown great promise as adjuvants for tick control.

REFERENCES

1. **Stickland, R. K., Gerrish, R. R., Hourrigan, J. L., and Schubert, G. O.,** Ticks of veterinary importance, *Agric. Handb.* 485, 1976.
2. **Curtice, C.,** About cattle ticks, *J. Comp. Med. Vet. Arch.,* 13, 9, 1892.
3. **Osborn, H.,** Insects affecting domestic animals: an account of the species of importance in North America, with mention of related forms occurring on other animals, *U.S. Dep. Agric. Bull.,* 5, 1896.
4. **Mohler, J. R.,** Texas fever with mention for its prevention, *U.S. Dep. Agric. Bur. Anim. Ind. Bull.,* 78, 1905.
5. **Mohler, J. R.,** Texas or tick fever and its prevention, *U.S. Dep. Agric. Farmers' Bull.,* 258, 1906.
6. **Hunter, W. D. and Hooker, W. A.,** Information concerning the North American fever tick with notes on other species, *U.S. Dep. Agric. Bur. Entomol. Bull.,* 72, 1907.
7. **Graybill, H. W.,** Methods of exterminating the Texas-fever tick *U.S. Dep. Agric. Farmers' Bull.,* 378, 1909.
8. **Graybill, H. W.,** The action of arsenical dips in protecting cattle from infestation with ticks, *U.S. Dep. Agric. Bur. Anim. Ind. Bull.,* 167, 1913.
9. **Chapin, R. M.,** Laboratory and field assay of arsenical dipping fluids, *U.S. Dep. Agric. Bull.,* 76, 1914.
10. **Chapin, R. M.,** Arsenical cattle dips: methods of preparation and directions for use, *U.S. Dep. Agric. Farmers' Bull.,* 603, 1914.
11. **Graybill, H. W. and Ellenberger, W. P.,** Directions for constructing vats and dipping cattle to destroy ticks, *U.S. Dep. Agric. Bur. Anim. Ind. Circ.,* 207, 1915.
12. **Ellenberger, W. P. and Chapin, R. M.,** Cattle-fever ticks and methods of eradication, *U.S. Dep. Agric. Farmers' Bull.,* 1057, 1919.
13. **Ellenberger, W. P. and Chapin, R. M.,** Cattle-fever ticks and methods of eradication, *U.S. Dep. Agric. Farmers' Bull.,* 1057, 1932.
14. **Ellenberger, W. P. and Chapin, R. M.,** Cattle-fever ticks and methods of eradication, *U.S. Dep. Agric. Farmers' Bull.,* 1057, 1940.
15. **Graham, O. H. and Hourrigan, J. L.,** Eradication programs for the arthropod parasites of livestock, *J. Med. Entomol.,* 13, 629, 1977.
16. **Knapp, J. V.,** Existence of tropical variety of cattle-fever tick (= *Boophilus annulatus,* var. *australis*) complicates tick eradication in Florida, *J. Am. Vet. Med. Assoc.,* 96, 607, 1940.
17. **Squibb, R. L.,** A new method for the control of cattle ticks in tropical regions, *J. Anim. Sci.,* 5, 71, 1946.
18. **Cobbett, N. G.,** Preliminary tests in Mexico with DDT, cube, hexachlorocyclohexane (benzene hexachloride), and combinations thereof, for the control of the cattle fever tick, *Boophilus annulatus, Am. J. Vet. Res.,* 8, 280, 1947.
19. **Cobbett, N. G.,** DDT and DDT combined with benzene hexachloride for the control and eradication of *Boophilus annulatus, Am. J. Vet. Res.,* 9, 270, 1948.
20. **Blakeslee, E. G. and Bruce, W. G.,** DDT to control the cattle tick — preliminary tests, *J. Econ. Entomol.,* 41, 104, 1948.
21. **Drummond, R. O., Graham, O. H., Meleney, W. P., and Diamant, G.,** Field tests in Mexico with new insecticides and arsenic for the control of *Boophilus* ticks on cattle, *J. Econ. Entomol.,* 57, 340, 1964.
22. **Graham, O. H., Drummond, R. O., and Diamant, G.,** The reproductive capacity of female *Boophilus annulatus* collected from cattle dipped in arsenic or coumaphos, *J. Econ. Entomol.,* 57, 409, 1964.
23. **Drummond, R. O., Ernst, S. E., Barrett, C. C., and Graham, O. H.,** Sprays and dips of Shell compound 4072 to control *Boophilus* ticks and larvae of the screw-worm on cattle, *J. Econ. Entomol.,* 59, 395, 1966.
24. **Wade, L. L.,** The efficacy and stability of Dursban® insecticide in dipping vat for control of the southern cattle tick, *J. Econ. Entomol.,* 61, 908, 1968.
25. **Drummond, R. O., Ernst, S. E., Trevino, J. L., and Graham, O. H.,** Insecticides for control of the cattle tick and the southern cattle tick on cattle, *J. Econ. Entomol.,* 61, 467, 1968.
26. **Drummond, R. O., Graham, O. H., Ernst, S. E., and Trevino, J. L.,** Evaluation of insecticides for the control of *Boophilus annulatus* (Say) and *B. microplus* (Canestrini) [Acarina: Ixodidae] on cattle, in *Proc. 2nd Int. Congr. Acarol.,* 493, 1959.
27. **Drummond, R. O., Ernst, S. E., Trevino, J. L., Gladney, W. J., and Graham, O. H.,** *Boophilus annulatus* and *B. microplus* sprays and dips of insecticides for control on cattle, *J. Econ. Entomol.,* 65, 1354, 1972.
28. **Drummond, R. O., Ernst, S. E., Trevino, J. L., Gladney, W. J., and Graham, O. H.,** Tests of acaricides for control of *Boophilus annulatus* and *B. microplus, J. Econ. Entomol.,* 69, 37, 1976.
29. **Loomis, E. C., Noorderhaven, A., and Roulston, W. J.,** Control of the southern cattle tick by pour-on animal systemic insecticides, *J. Econ. Entomol.,,* 65, 1638, 1972.
30. **Davey, R. B. and Ahrens, E. H.,** Control of *Boophilus* ticks on cattle with a flowable formulation of coumaphos, *J. Econ. Entomol.,* 75, 228, 1982.

31. **Ahrens, E. H., Davey, R. B., George, J. E., and Pemberton, J. R.,** Comparison of sedimentation and stripping characteristics of two formulations of coumaphos in cattle dipping vats, *J. Econ. Entomol.,* 75, 665, 1982.

32. **Davey, R. B., Ahrens, E. H., and Pemberton, J. R.,** Residual effectiveness of flowable coumaphos on cattle against *Boophilus annulatus* larvae, *Southwest. Entomol.,* 8, 168, 1983.

33. **Garris, G. I. and George J. E.,** Efficacy of crotoxyphos sprays for the control of the southern cattle tick in Puerto Rico, *J. Agric. Univ. Puerto Rico,* 67, 256, 1983.

34. **Davey, R. B., Ahrens, E. H., and Garza, J., Jr.,** Control of the southern cattle tick with insecticide-impregnated ear tags, *J. Econ. Entomol.,* 73, 651, 1980.

35. **Davey, R. B., Ahrens, E. H., and George, J. E.,** Efficacy of sprays of amitraz against *Boophilus* ticks on cattle, *Prev. Vet. Med.,* 2, 691, 1984.

36. **Garris, G. I. and George, J. E.,** Field evaluation of amitraz applied to cattle as sprays for control of *Boophilus microplus* (Acari: Ixodidae) in the eradication program in Puerto Rico, *Prev. Vet. Med.,* 3, 363, 1985.

37. **Davey, R. B. and Ahrens, E. H.,** Control of *Boophilus* ticks on heifers with two pyrethroids applied as sprays, *Am. J. Vet. Res.,* 45, 1008, 1984.

38. **Garris, G. I. and Zimmerman, R. H.,** Field efficacy of permethrin and fenvalerate applied as sprays to cattle for control of *Boophilus microplus* (Canestrini) (Acari: Ixodidae) in the eradication program in Puerto Rico, *Trop. Pest Manage.,* 31, 120, 1985.

39. **Hooker, W. A., Bishopp, F. C., and Wood, H. P.,** The life history and bionomics of some North American ticks, *U.S. Dep. Agric. Bur. Entomol. Bull.,* 106, 1912.

40. **Imes, M.,** The spinose ear tick and methods of treating infested animals, *U.S. Dep. Agric. Farmers' Bull.,* 980, 1918.

41. **Rude, C. S. and Smith, C. L.,** DDT for control of Gulf Coast and spinose ear ticks, *J. Econ. Entomol.,* 37, 132, 1944.

42. **Kemper, H. E., Roberts, I. H., and Peterson, H. O.,** Hexachlorocyclohexane as an acaricide for the control of the spinose ear tick on cattle, *N. Am. Vet.,* 28, 665, 1947.

43. **Kemper, H. E.,** The spinose ear tick and methods of treating infested animals, *U.S. Dep. Agric. Farmers' Bull.,* 980, 1947.

44. **Knipling, E. F.,** Ticks, lice, sheep keds, mites, *U.S. Dep. Agric. Yearb. Agric.,* 662, 1952.

45. **Kemper, H. E. and Peterson, H. O.,** The spinose ear tick and methods of treating infested animals, *U.S. Dep. Agric. Farmers' Bull.,* 980, 1953.

46. **Harvey, T. L. and Brethour, J. R.,** Effectiveness of Ruelene and ronnel for ear tick compared with cattle grub control, *J. Econ. Entomol.,* 54, 814, 1961.

47. **Tarshis, I. B. and Ommert, W. D.,** Control of the spinose ear tick, *Otobius megnini* (Duges), with an organic phosphate insecticide combined with a silica aerogel, *J. Am. Vet. Med. Assoc.,* 138, 665, 1961.

48. **Drummond, R. O., Whetstone, T. M., and Ernst, S. E.,** Insecticidal control of the ear tick in the ears of cattle, *J. Econ. Entomol.,* 60, 1021, 1967.

49. **Bishopp, F. C. and Hixson, H.,** Biology and economic importance of the Gulf Coast tick, *J. Econ. Entomol.,* 29, 1068, 1936.

50. **Spicer, W. J. and Dove, W. E.,** The screwworm and the Gulf Coast tick in southern Texas, *J. Econ. Entomol.,* 31, 642, 1938.

51. **Matthysse, J. G.,** DDT to control hornflies and Gulf Coast ticks on range cattle in Florida, *J. Econ. Entomol.,* 39, 62, 1946.

52. **Rude, C. S.,** DDT to control the Gulf Coast tick, *J. Econ. Entomol.,* 40, 301, 1947.

53. **Blakeslee, E. B., Tissot, A. N., Bruce, W. G., and Sanders, D. A.,** DDT to control the Gulf Coast tick, *J. Econ. Entomol.,* 40, 664, 1947.

54. **Gladney, W. J.,** Field trials of insecticides in controlled-release devices for control of the Gulf Coast tick and prevention of screwworm in cattle, *J. Econ. Entomol.,* 69, 757, 1976.

55. **Gladney, W. J., Price, M. A., and Graham, O. H.,** Field tests of insecticides for control of the Gulf Coast tick on cattle, *J. Med. Entomol.,* 13, 579, 1977.

56. **Ahrens, E. H., Gladney, W. J., McWhorter, G. M., and Deer, J. A.,** Prevention of screwworm infestation in cattle by controlling Gulf Coast ticks with slow release insecticide devices, *J. Econ. Entomol.,* 70, 581, 1977.

57. **Ahrens, E. H. and Cocke, J.,** Comparative test with insecticide-impregnated ear tags against the Gulf Coast tick, *J. Econ. Entomol.,* 71, 764, 1978.

58. **Hunter, W. D. and Bishopp, F. C.,** The Rocky Mountain spotted fever tick with special reference to the problem of its control in the Bitterroot Valley in Montana, *U.S. Dep. Agric. Bur. Entomol. Bull.,* 105, 1911.

59. **Mail, G. A.,** Tick control with special reference to *Dermacentor andersoni* Stiles, *Sci. Agric.,* 23, 59, 1942.

60. **Gregson, J. D.,** Benzene hexachloride ("666") as an acaricide, *Can. Entomol.,* 201, 1946.
61. **Weintraub, J.,** A preliminary report on acaricides tested for protection against the tick *Dermacentor andersoni* Stiles on cattle, *Proc. Entomol. Soc. B.C.,* 48, 51, 1952.
62. **Roth, A. R. and Eddy, G. W.,** Insecticide control of the Rocky Mountain wood tick on cattle in Wyoming, *J. Med. Entomol.,* 3, 342, 1966.
63. **Portman, R. W.,** Dipping in benzene hexachloride to control *Amblyomma americanum, J. Econ. Entomol.,* 40, 134, 1947.
64. **Brundrett, H. M., Richards, R., and Smith, C. L.,** Tests of toxaphene, chlordane, and strobane against the lone star tick on cattle, *J. Econ. Entomol.,* 48, 223, 1955.
65. **Drummond, R. O., Moore, B., and Wrich, M. J.,** Field tests with insecticides for control of lone star ticks on cattle, *J. Econ. Entomol.,* 53, 953, 1960.
66. **Drummond, R. O.,** Tests with General Chemical 3582 and 4072 for the control of ticks affecting livestock, *J. Econ. Entomol.,* 54, 1050, 1961.
67. **Drummond, R. O. and Medley, J. G.,** Field tests with insecticides for the control of ticks on livestock, *J. Econ. Entomol.,* 58, 1131, 1965.
68. **Drummond, R. O., Whetstone, T. M., and Ernst, S. E.,** Control of ticks on cattle with toxaphene applied by power sprayer and spray race, *J. Econ. Entomol.,* 59, 471, 1966.
69. **Drummond, R. O., Whetsone, T. M., and Ernst, S. E.,** Control of the lone star tick on cattle, *J. Econ. Entomol.,* 60, 1735, 1967.
70. **Drummond, R. O. and Gladney, W. J.,** Acaricides applied to cattle for control of the lone star tick *Southwest. Entomol.,* 3, 96, 1978.
71. **Barnard, D. R. and Jones, B. G.,** Field efficacy of acaricides for control of the lone star tick on cattle in southeastern Oklahoma, *J. Econ. Entomol.,* 74, 558, 1981.
72. **Barnard, D. R., Rogers, G. D., and Jones, B. G.,** Strategic treatment of pastured beef cattle with acaricides: effect on populations of the lone star tick (Acari: Ixodidae), *J. Econ. Entomol.,* 76, 99, 1983.
73. **Drummond, R. O., Moore, B., and Warren, J.,** Tests with insecticides for control of the winter tick, *J. Econ. Entomol.,* 52, 1220, 1959.
74. **Roulston, W. J.,** The effects of some chlorinated hydrocarbons as systemic acaricides against the cattle tick, *Boophilus microplus* (Canestrini), *Aust. J. Agric. Res.,* 7, 608, 1956.
75. **Wilkinson, P. R.,** Factors affecting the distribution and abundance of the cattle tick in Australia: observations and hypotheses, *Acarologia,* 12, 492, 1970.
76. **Utech, K. B. W. and Wharton, R. H.,** Sulphur and the cattle tick *Boophilus microplus, Aust. Vet. J.,* 48, 73, 1972.
77. **Drummond, R. O., Whetstone, T. M., Ernst, S. E., and Gladney, W. J.,** Control of three-host ticks: laboratory tests of systemic insecticides in feed of cattle, *J. Econ. Entomol.,* 65, 1641, 1972.
78. **Gladney, W. J., Ernst, S. E., Dawkins, C. C., Drummond, R. O., and Graham, O. H.,** Feeding systemic insecticides to cattle for control of the tropical horse tick, *J. Med. Entomol.,* 9, 439, 1972.
79. **Teel, P. D., Hair, J. A., and Randolph, T. C., Jr.,** Continuous administration of famphur for control of ticks and bed bugs feeding on ruminants, *J. Econ. Entomol.,* 70, 664, 1977.
80. **Teel, P. D., Hair, J. A., and Stratton, L. G.,** Laboratory evaluation of a sustained-release famphur bolus against Gulf Coast and lone star ticks feeding on Hereford heifers, *J. Econ. Entomol.,* 72, 230, 1979.
81. **Hair, J. A., Gladney, W. J., Davey, R. B., Drummond, R. O., and Teel, P. D.,** Sustained-release famphur bolus for control of *Boophilus* ticks, *J. Econ. Entomol.,* 72, 135, 1979.
82. **Davey, R. B., Garza, J., Jr., and Thompson, G. D.,** Control of *Boophilus microplus* on cattle with injections of Eli Lilly L-27, *Southwest. Entomol.,* 4, 311, 1979.
83. **Drummond, R. O., Whetstone, T. M., and Miller, J. A.,** Control of ticks systemically with Merck MK-933, an avermectin, *J. Econ. Entomol.,* 74, 432, 1981.
84. **Lancaster, J. L., Jr., Kilgore, R. L., and Simco, J. S.,** Efficacy of low level daily doses of Ivermectin in calves against three species of ticks, *Southwest Entomol.,* 7, 116, 1982.
85. **Lancaster, J. L., Jr., Simco, J. S., and Kilgore, R. L.,** Systemic efficacy of Ivermectin MK-933 against the lone star tick *J. Econ. Entomol.,* 75, 242, 1982.
86. **Drummond, R. O. and Miller, J. A.,** Control of ticks systemically with sustained-release implants of Ivermectin, in *Acarology VI,* Vol. 2, Griffiths, D. A. and Bowman, C. E., Eds., Ellis Horwood, Chichester, England, 1984, 1274.
87. **Drummond, R. O.,** Effectiveness of Ivermectin for control of arthropod pests of livestock, *Southwest. Entomol.,* Suppl. 7, 34, 1985.
88. **Drummond, R. O. and Miller, J. A.,** Systemic activity of Closantel for control of lone star ticks, *Amblyomma americanum* (L.), on cattle, *Exp. Appl. Acrol.,* 1, 193, 1985.
89. **Ray, R. J.,** Effects of the anthelmintic nitroxynil upon cattle ticks, in *Acarology VI,* Vol. 2, Griffiths, D. A. and Bowman, C. E., Eds., Ellis Horwood, Chichester, England, 1984, 1269.
90. **Gladney, W. J., Grabbe, R. R., Ernst, S. E., and Oehler, D. D.,** The Gulf Coast tick: evidence of a pheromone produced by males, *J. Med. Entomol.,* 11, 303, 1974.

91. **Rechav, Y. and Whitehead, G. B.,** Field trials with pheromone-acaricide mixtures for control of *Amblyomma hebraeum, J. Econ. Entomol.,* 71, 149, 1978.

92. **Sonenshine, D. E., Silverstein, R. M., and Homsher, P. J.,** Female produced pheromones of Ixodidae, in *Recent Advances in Acarology,* Vol. 2, Rodriquez, J. G., Ed., Academic Press, New York, 1979, 281.

93. **Ziv, M., Sonenshine, D. E., Silverstein, R. M., West, J. R., and Gingher, K. H.,** Use of sex pheromone, 2,6-dichlorophenol, to disrupt mating by American dog tick *Dermacentor variabilis* (Say), *J. Chem. Ecol.,* 7, 829, 1981.

94. **Sonenshine, D. E., Taylor, D., and Corrigan, G.,** Studies to evaluate the effectiveness of sex pheromone-impregnated formulations for control of populations of the American dog tick, *Dermacentor variabilis* (Say) (Acari: Ixodidae), *Exp. Appl. Acarol.,* 1, 23, 1985.

95. **Dees, W. H., Sonenshine, D. E., Breidling, E., Buford, N. P., and Khalil, G. M.,** Toxicity of precocene-2 for the American dog tick, *Dermacentor variabilis* (Acari: Ixodidae), *J. Med. Entomol.,* 19, 734, 1982.

Chapter 12

CONTROL OF ARTHROPOD PESTS OF HORSES*

I. INTRODUCTION

Horses are infested with a variety of lice, ticks, and mites that spend considerable time, if not their entire life cycle, on horses. Lice include the horse sucking louse*, *Haematopinus asini* (Linnaeus), the horse biting louse*, *Bovicola equi* (Denny), and another biting louse, *Trichodetes pilosis* DeGeer. The same species of ticks that attack cattle (see Chapter 11) also infest horses, but two species are of special interest. The winter tick*, *Dermacentor albipictus* (Packard), a one-host species, is found on horses in the U.S. and Canada in the fall and winter. Heavy infestations on horses can cause loss of hair, anemia, and edematous condition called "water belly". The tropical horse tick*, *Anocentor nitens* (Neumann), another one-host species, is found in the ears, nasal diverticulae, and manes of horses in south Texas and Florida and adjacent southeastern states. This tick transmits equine piroplasmosis. The itch mite*, *Sarcoptes scabiei* (DeGeer); the scab mite*, *Psoroptes equi* (Raspail); *Chorioptes bovis* (Hering); and the horse follicle mite*, *Demodex equi* Railliet, live on or in the skin of horses. Chiggers, larvae of trombiculid mites, attach to horses and can cause a transient dermatitis.

Horses are also parasitized by a number of blood-sucking flies (called "biting flies"), especially the stable fly*, *Stomoxys calcitrans* (Linnaeus), the horn fly*, *Haematobia irritans* (Linnaeus), a large variety of horse flies, deer flies, and a number of "small" biting or nuisance flies, such as mosquitoes, biting midges, eye gnats, and black flies. A nonbiting fly, the face fly*, *Musca autumnalis* DeGeer, can cause considerable irritation because of their habit of feeding on or around the eyes and other face areas. Face flies also transmit *Moraxella bovis* (Hauduroy), the etiological agent of "pinkeye" and eyeworms, *Thelazia* spp. The house fly*, *M. domestica* Linnaeus, also feeds on secretions on the face of horses. Occasionally, horses are infested with larvae of the northern cattle grub*, *Hypoderma bovis* (Linnaeus), or the common cattle grub*, *H. lineatum* (Villers). Larvae may form warbles in necks and backs of horses that cause considerable irritation, especially if the warble is located in the skin of the back under the saddle.

Almost all horses in the U.S. are infested with larvae of one or more species of horse bot flies. The horse bot fly*, *Gasterophilus intestinalis* (De Geer), and the throat bot fly*, *G. nasalis* (Linnaeus), are found throughout the U.S., while the nose bot fly*, *G. haemorrhoidalis* (Linnaeus), is limited in its distribution in north-central and northwestern states.

Accumulations of manure, soiled bedding, spoiled feed, and other wastes in the horse environment, such as stalls, stables, and barns, can be the source of large numbers of house flies, stable flies, and other filth-breeding flies which can be a nuisance to horses, their owners, and nearby neighbors. The control of filth-breeding flies in the environment of livestock, including horses, is based on a program of sanitation. That subject is addressed in Chapter 18.

Because the technologies used to control external pests and horse bots differ so greatly, this chapter will be divided into two major sections: (1) control of external arthropod pests of horses, and (2) control of *Gasterophilus* spp. General information on the biology and control of the arthropod pests of horses was recently presented in a chapter in *Livestock Entomology.*[1]

---

* Common names of insects and acarines, as listed in *Common Names of Insects and Related Organisms* (published by the Entomological Society of America), are marked with a * the first time they are cited preceding the scientific name.

II. CONTROL OF EXTERNAL ARTHROPOD PESTS

A review of the literature on the technologies used to control arthropod pests of horses reveals relatively few citations in contrast to the many found for these same pests on cattle. Many of the insecticides and acaricides that control these arthropods on cattle (see Chapters 2 to 11) will also control them on horses. However, the sensitive nature of the skin of horses limits the number of insecticides, solvents, emulsifiers, and oils that can be applied to horses.

A. Flies

For the control of flies, gnats, and mosquitoes, in 1896, Osborn[2] suggested smearing the hair of domestic animals (horses included but not specified) with fish oil, tar, train oil, or axle grease. He listed other insecticidal substances applied to animals as arsenic, carbolic acid, cottonseed oil, kerosene emulsion, pyrethrins powder, sulfur, and tobacco. The 1912 *U.S. Dep. Agri. Yearbook of Agriculture*[3] listed use of smudges and hand applications of oils and greases to protect horses from buffalo gnats. Horse flies and stable flies could be repelled by fish oil, train oil, or tar, and horse nets or burlap wraps placed on the heads and bodies of horses could be used to protect horses from flies. In the 1942 *Yearbook of Agriculture,* a chapter on insect pests of horses and mules[4] listed the elimination or the treatment of breeding and resting grounds to control mosquitos, sand flies, and house flies; gnats were repelled for short periods of time with mixtures of pine tar oil or fish oil soap applied to horses, but no remedies were effective against horse flies.

Following World War II, organochlorine insecticides were found to be effective against external pests of horses. Spraying horses twice daily with DDT gave complete knock-down and kill of stable flies.[5] Sprays of butoxy polypropylene glycol repelled both stable flies and *Tabanus* spp. for 24 hr.[6] Aerosol treatments of deet repelled horse flies from horses for only 1 hr or so, but the heavy applications needed to repel flies caused severe skin reactions and other adverse responses in the horses.[7] The use of repellents on cattle is reviewed and discussed in Chapter 3.

Face flies were controlled on horses fitted with halters constructed of dichlorvos-impregnated plastic strands, but smears of insecticides in mineral oil or corn syrup applied to the face were impractical and ineffective.[8]

Body sprays of carbaryl, coumaphos, crotoxyphos, and malathion controlled horn flies for 1 to 3 weeks, but stable flies were killed at most for 3 days. A spray of pyrethrins plus piperonyl butoxide controlled horn flies for 10 days and stable flies for 7 days.[9]

A variety of body sprays applied to horses in the laboratory were evaluated as toxicants against horse flies by confining field-caught *Tabanus subsimilis* Bellardi and *T. sulcifrons* Macquart in cages on treated horses.[10] Toxaphene, stirofos, chlorpyrifos, chlorfenvinphos, and propoxur were ineffective at 1 day, but the pyrethroids, fenvalerate and permethrin, killed flies for 1 week and ca. 2 weeks, respectively. In similar tests,[11] permethrin caused >90% mortality of the same species of *Tabanus* plus *T. proximus* Walker for 18 days as a spray and for 12 days as a dust.

Stirofos, malathion, crotoxyphos, and methoxychlor in petroleum jelly applied to the ears of horses did not enhance the residual activity of petroleum jelly, which alone gave 3 days protection against the feeding of black flies, predominantly *Simulium vittatum* Zetterstedt.[12]

Low-volume sprays (60 mℓ per animal) of ronnel and wipe-on treatments of ronnel and chlorpyrifos applied at 1- and 2-day intervals provided >90% mortality of stable flies, and the ronnel treatments also repelled stable flies.[13] Spray or rub-on treatments of permethrin controlled stable flies for 7 to 10 days and *Tabanus megalops* Walker for 3 to 6 days. Permethrin-impregnated net blankets were effective for >7 weeks, but were difficult to maintain and keep on horses.[14]

Most issues of *Insecticide and Acaricide Tests* since 1977 have contained one or more reports on the effectiveness of insecticides applied to horses for the control of flies. Mist sprays of a combination of crotoxyphos/pyrethrins/butoxy polypropylene glycol controlled house flies and stable flies. Fenvalerate and stirofos mist sprays, fenvalerate pouron, and permethrin wipe-on controlled stable flies and face flies. Cypermethrin-impregnated plastic strips or permethrin tapes placed on halters controlled flies only on the faces of horses. Flucythrinate- or fenvalerate-impregnated ear tags attached to halters controlled face flies.

The presence and control of cattle grub larvae in the backs of horses was reviewed by Scharff,[15] who prevented the development of cattle grub larvae in horses with a pouron of crufomate.

B. Lice

The 1912 *U.S. Dep. Agric. Yearbook of Agriculture*[3] noted that lice on horses were controlled with commonly used insecticidal dips. Hall[16] reviewed the early literature on lice on horses and listed effective treatments as dusts of sodium fluoride (which did not control sucking lice), oxytoluol, cresol, napththalin, pyrethrins, and sulfur; mercury ointment; and washes of tobacco, fish oil, petroleum, and creolin. Dipping horses in coal-tar dips was commonly used and clipping hair and brushing and currying removed lice and their eggs. The original issue of *U.S. Dep. Agric. Farmers' Bulletin* No. 1493 in 1926[17] described the lice that parasitized horses and presented control measures of hand application of sodium fluoride, oils and greases, fumigation, spraying, and, most effective of all, dipping of horses in arsenic, lime-sulfur, nicotine, and coal-tar creosote. *U.S. Dep. Agric. Circular* No. 148,[18] which superseded Bulletin No. 1493 in 1930, listed the following treatments to control lice: two dippings in arsenic, coal-tar creosote, or nicotine; hand application of sodium fluoride as a dust or wash; and fumigation by burning sulfur. A spray of an emulsion of a white oil, called Volck, killed motile forms of biting and sucking lice, but not eggs.[19] DDT and chlordane sprays controlled biting lice.[20] The 1952 *U.S. Dep. Agric. Yearbook of Agriculture*[21] reported that sprays or dips of DDT eliminated lice from horses.

C. Ticks

U.S. Dep. Agric. Farmers' Bulletin No. 1493 in 1926[17] described the tick pests of horses and reported that the most effective treatments for ticks were dipping horses in arsenic, lime-sulfur, nicotine, or coal-tar creosote. In 1930, *U.S. Dep. Agric. Circular* No. 148[18] superseded Bulletin No. 1493 and reported that the control of ticks was accomplished by treating infested body areas with crude petroleum, kerosene, or other petroleum products. The cattle tick♦, *Boophilus annulatus* (Say), was controlled by dipping horses in the arsenical dips used in the eradication program, and pine tar plus cottonseed oil applied into the ears controlled the ear tick♦, *Otobius megnini* (Duges). The dipping of horses in arsenic controlled tropical horse ticks that were wetted with the dip, but the treatment was not effective against ticks in the false nostrils, ears, and other body areas that were not contacted by the dip.[22] The 1942 *U.S. Dep. Agric. Yearbook of Agriculture,*[4] recommended dipping horses in arsenic or washing with rotenone to control ticks on the bodies of horses. It recommended treating ears with a mixture of pine tar and cottonseed oil to control the ear tick and the Gulf Coast tick♦, *Amblyomma maculatum* Koch, the cause of "gotch-ear".

A DDT wash applied with a sponge controlled winter ticks.[23] DDT paste applied to the ears controlled Gulf Coast ticks, but the treatment caused some skin injury.[24] Chlordane dusts were even more effective than DDT dusts for the control of winter ticks.[25] The 1952 *Yearbook of Agriculture*[21] listed toxaphene, lindane, TDE, and DDT for tick control. The 1956 *U.S. Dep. Agric. Yearbook of Agriculture*[26] stated that toxaphene, lindane, and DDT had largely supplanted rotenone, nicotine, arsenic, and other materials for tick control.

Sprays of carbophenothion, Dilan, chlorfenvinphos, diazinon, crotoxyphos, and toxaphene controlled the winter tick and the blacklegged tick♦, *Ixodes scapularis* Say.[27]

In tests in Mexico and Florida,[28,29] all stages of the tropical horse tick were controlled by insecticides applied in water, mineral oil, or as smears and dusts into horses' ears and false nostrils and applied as aqueous sprays onto the horses' bodies. Of particular interest is the fact that trichlorfon, given in feed for 10 days, afforded complete control of all stages of the tick; oral treatments of fenthion and famphur were less effective. The spraying of horses' bodies with toxaphene and treating of the ears and false nostrils with lindane in vegetable oil controlled tropical horse ticks in Florida and thus controlled the spread of equine piroplasmosis.[30]

D. Mites

In 1904, *U.S. Dep. Agric. Farmers' Bulletin* No. 102[31] noted that psoroptic or sarcoptic scabies on horses could be controlled by the treatments that controlled scabies on cattle, but the skin of horses was sensitive to treatment with Beaumont crude oil. *U.S. Dep. Agric. Farmers' Bulletin* No. 1493 in 1926[17] described psoroptic, chorioptic, and sarcoptic mite pests of horses and listed that two to four dippings in lime-sulfur or nicotine would eradicate mange or scab. In 1930, *U.S. Dep. Agric. Circular* No. 148[18] superseded Bulletin No. 1493 and continued to recommend dipping horses in lime-sulfur or nicotine. Hand treatment with crude petroleum or fumigation with sulfur were also listed, but were less effective than dipping. The 1942 *U.S. Dep. Agric. Yearbook of Agriculture*[32] noted that several dippings (or sprayings which were much less satisfactory) in lime-sulfur or nicotine were necessary in order to eradicate mange.

Chiggers, *Euschoengastia* spp., that formed feeding lesions on horses, were controlled with a methoxychlor wash applied with a large sponge.[33,34] *Psoroptes cuniculi* (Delafond) in the ears of a horse were controlled by three treatments with benzyl benzoate.[35] A review of causes of inflammation of hair follicles of horses[36] stated that no therapeutic agent has been shown to control equine demodicosis. Some cures followed treatment with lime-sulfur, rotenone, lindane, and organophosphorus insecticides.

III. CONTROL OF *GASTEROPHILUS* SPP.

A. Early Treatment Technology

In 1896, Osborn[2] described the stages of the life cycle of horse bots and the injury they cause. He suggested the following control measures: clipping hair to remove eggs, washing egg-infested areas with carbolic acid solution or kerosene, and applying oil or tar to lip hairs to repel ovipositing female *G. haemorrhoidalis*. He stated that control of larvae in the horse's stomach was the work of veterinarians. Carbon disulfide given orally to horses[37] removed bot larvae, but chloroform and oil of chenopodium were ineffective. *U.S. Dep. Agric. Bulletin* No. 597 in 1918[38] presented information on the biology and life history of horse bots and reviewed the early methods used to control horse bot eggs or larvae or to prevent oviposition by flies. It listed the following control measures: oral treatment with carbon disulfide to kill larvae in the gastrointestinal tract, topical application of nicotine sulfate to kill larvae of *G. haemorrhoidalis* attached at the edge of the anus, and washing the horse's body with kerosene or carbolic acid to destroy attached eggs. Repellents of pine tar and other ingredients and mechanical protective devices of leather, burlap, cotton, etc. attached to halters were measures listed to protect horses from ovipositing flies. The original issue of *U.S. Dep. Agric. Farmers' Bulletin* No. 1503[39] in 1926 listed the same control measures and emphasized the benefits of treating horses in the late fall so that horses would be free of bot larvae throughout the winter when flies were not active. *U.S. Dep. Agric. Circular* No. 148[18] in 1930 listed most of the above treatments plus oral treatments of carbon tetrachloride and tetrachlorethylene to control larvae and dermal application of coal-tar creosote to kill eggs.

The application of an undiluted white oil emulsion, called Volck, prevented horse bot eggs from hatching.[19] Warm (>40°C) water applied with a sponge to egg-infested areas of the horse's skin caused >94% of the larvae of *G. intestinalis* to hatch.[40] The 1935 revision of Bulletin No. 1503[41] added the sponging of the body with warm water to hatch eggs and washing the body with kerosene was no longer recommended. The 1941 revision[42] no longer recommended washing the body with coal-tar creosote to destroy eggs.

Toluene was partially effective against horse bot larvae in horses' stomachs when administered orally.[43-45] Lindane, aldrin, dieldrin, chlordane, heptachlor, lead arsenate, and pine oil were ineffective as larvicides when given orally, but toluene and carbon disulfide expelled horse bot larvae.[46]

B. Systemic Insecticides

The advent of practical animal systemic insecticides that controlled *Hypoderma* larvae in cattle stimulated research on the use of systemics to control other parasites of livestock. In the U.S., Drummond et al.[47] found that a single treatment with trichlorfon or dichlorvos by stomach tube or in feed removed horse bot larvae from horses; an intramuscular injection of trichlorfon was only partially effective. Dimethoate was effective orally, via stomach tube or in feed, against *G. nasalis* but less so against *G. intestinalis*.[48] Thiabendazole was ineffective.[49] Butonate, Bayer 37341, and dichlorvos were effective by stomach tube or in feed, and trichlorfon was partially effective as an intramuscular injection or pouron treatment.[50]

Oral treatments of a paste or gel of dichlorvos controlled first instar horse bot larvae in the gingival tissues and tongues of horses.[51-53] Butonate, given orally by stomach tube, was an effective boticide.[54,55] Dichlorvos was highly effective as a resin pellet for feed treatment or as an oral gel.[56,57] Oral treatments of dichlorvos, trichlorfon, and butonate controlled larvae in the mouths and gastrointestinal tracts of horses, but carbon disulfide was active only against larvae in the gastrointestinal tracts.[58]

Further studies on the efficacy and safety of trichlorfon, dichlorvos, and related compounds alone or in combination with a variety of anthelmintics for control of horse bot larvae and helminths in the gastrointestinal tract of horses showed that the anthelmintics alone did not control horse bot larvae, but were effective when combined with the boticides.[59-71]

Warm water scrubs applied weekly throughout the year to stimulate the hatching of bot fly eggs did not affect the numbers of horse bot larvae in the mouths or stomachs of treated ponies, whereas oral treatments of trichlorfon removed all larvae.[72]

Stirofos, fed daily to horses throughout the summer in order to control fly larvae in manure, also caused a >98% reduction of horse bot larvae.[73] Drudge et al.[74] reviewed the efficacy of drugs used for the control of internal parasites in horses and listed only carbon disulfide, trichlorfon, and dichlorvos as approved boticides in current use.

Ivermectin, a chemical derivation of a fermentation product of the fungus, *Streptomyces avermitilis,* controlled horse bot larvae (and a variety of nematode parasites) when given to horses orally by stomach tube,[75] as an intramuscular injection,[76-80] as a subcutaneous injection,[81] or as an oral paste.[82,83] Ivermectin is commercially available as an oral paste treatment for control of horse bot larvae. Recently, oral treatments of a salicylanilide anthelmintic, Closantel,[84,85] controlled horse bot larvae. Multiple treatments during bot fly season prevented infestations of larvae, and a single treatment prevented reinfestation for 2 months after treatment.

IV. OVERVIEW AND CURRENT TECHNOLOGY

Technology used to control external parasites of horses has evolved through the years. Because of the present status of horses as pleasure animals rather than work animals, they have a different relationship to their owners than in the past. Seldom now are horses dipped to control arthropod pests. Insecticides are usually applied as low-volume wipe-ons, washes, and other less violent treatments. Insecticide-impregnated plastic strips are available for attachment to halters and tails of horses to control flies. Pyrethroid insecticides have been shown to be highly effective against biting flies, even horse and deer flies.

However, the technology to provide long-term control of horse flies or deer flies with a single application of insecticide is not available. Such long-term control may not be important with pleasure horses that are handled daily. Horses on the range could benefit from long-term fly control, especially where equine infectious anemia is a problem.

The problem with horse flies, deer flies, stable flies, and most small biting flies is that they are intermittent feeders and visit horses for only short periods of time to feed. Thus, they are exposed to toxicants for a limited time and may not receive a toxic dose. Also, even if all the flies that feed on horses are killed, they are such a small portion of the entire population that there is little reduction of the number of pests that attack horses. Much more needs to be known about the biology, ecology, and behavior of these pests before appropriate control technology can be developed.

Several orally administered boticides are commercially available for the control of horse bot larvae. Some horses may be still treated with boticides in feed or with carbon disulfide administered by a stomach tube for the control of *Gasterophilus* larvae. The most popular technology for control of horse bot larvae is the administration of an effective boticide as an oral paste.

REFERENCES

1. **Knapp, F. W.**, Arthropod pests of horses, in *Livestock Entomology*, Williams, R. E., Hall, R. D., Broce, A. G., and Scholl, P. J., Eds., John Wiley & Sons, New York, 1985, 297.
2. **Osborn, H.**, Insects affecting domestic animals: an account of the species of importance in North America, with mention of related forms occurring on other animals, *U.S. Dep. Agric. Div. Entomol. Bull.*, 5, 1896.
3. **Bishopp, F. C.**, Some important insect enemies of livestock in the United States, *U.S. Dep. Agric. Yearb. Agric.*, 383, 1912.
4. **Bishopp, F. C.**, Some insect pests of horses and mules, *U.S. Dep. Agric. Yearb. Agric.*, 492, 1942.
5. **Blakeslee, E. B.**, DDT as a barn spray in stablefly control, *J. Econ. Entomol.*, 37, 134, 1944.
6. **Granett, P., Haynes, H. L., Connola, D. P., Bowery, T. G., and Barber, G. W.**, Two butoxypoly-propylene glycol compounds as fly repellents for livestock, *J. Econ. Entomol.*, 42, 281, 1949.
7. **Blume, R. R., Roberts, R. H., Eschle, J. L., and Matter, J. J.**, Tests of aerosols of deet for protection of livestock from biting flies, *J. Econ. Entomol.*, 64, 1193, 1971.
8. **Dorsey, C. K.**, Face fly control experiments on quarter horses — 1962—64, *J. Econ. Entomol.*, 59, 86, 1966.
9. **Blume, R. R., Matter, J. J., and Eschle, J. L.**, Biting flies (Diptera: Muscidae) on horses: laboratory evaluation of five insecticides for control, *J. Med. Entomol.*, 10, 596, 1973.
10. **Harris, R. L. and Oehler, D. D.**, Control of tabanids on horses, *Southwest. Entomol.*, 1, 194, 1976.
11. **Bay, D. E., Ronald, N. C., and Harris, R. L.**, Evaluation of a synthetic pyrethroid for tabanid control on horses and cattle, *Southwest. Entomol.*, 1, 198, 1976.
12. **Townsend, L. H., Jr. and Turner, E. C. Jr.**, Field evaluation of several chemicals against ear-feeding black fly pests of horses in Virginia, *Mosq. News*, 36, 182, 1976.
13. **Schmidt, C. D., Matter, J. J., and Meurer, J. H.**, Efficacy of ronnel and chlorpyrifos in controlling biting flies on horses, *Southwest. Entomol.*, 2, 144, 1977.
14. **Lang, J. T., Schreck, C. E., and Pamintuan, H.**, Permethrin for biting-fly (Diptera: Muscidae; Tabanidae) control on horses in central Luzon, Philippines, *J. Med. Entomol.*, 18, 522, 1981.
15. **Scharff, D. K.**, Control of cattle grubs in horses, *Vet. Med./Small Anim. Clin.*, 68, 791, 1973.
16. **Hall, M. C.**, Notes in regard to horse lice, *Trichodectes* and *Haematopinus*, *J. Am. Vet. Med. Assoc.*, 51, 494, 1917.
17. **Imes, M.**, Lice, mange, and ticks of horses, and methods of control and eradication, *U.S. Dep. Agric. Farmers' Bull.*, 1493, 1926.
18. **Schwartz, B., Imes, M., and Wright, W. H.**, Parasites and parasitic diseases of horses, *U.S. Dep. Agric. Circ.*, 148, 1930.

19. **Caler, H. L.,** Volck special emulsion number 2 as a control for external parasites of animals, *J. Kans. Entomol. Soc., 4,* 77, 1931.
20. **Batte, E. G. and Gaines, J. C.,** Comparison of DDT and chlordan for the control of the horse louse, *J. Econ. Entomol., 41,* 830, 1948.
21. **Knipling, E. F.,** Ticks, lice, sheep keds, mites, *U.S. Dep. Agric. Yearb. Agric., 662,* 1952.
22. **Tate, H. D.,** The biology of the tropical cattle tick and other species of tick in Puerto Rico, with notes on the effects on ticks of arsenical dips, *J. Agric. Univ. Puerto Rico, 25,* 1, 1941.
23. **Parish, H. E. and Rude, C. S.,** DDT to control the winter horse tick, *J. Econ. Entomol., 39,* 92, 1946.
24. **Rude, C. S.,** DDT to control the Gulf Coast tick, *J. Econ. Entomol., 40,* 301, 1947.
25. **Knipling, E. F.,** Newer synthetic insecticides, *Soap Sanit. Chem., 23,* 127, 1947.
26. **McIntosh, A. and McDuffie, W. C.,** Ticks that affect domestic animals and poultry, *U.S. Dep. Agric. Yearb. Agric., 157,* 1956.
27. **Drummond, R. O. and Medley, J. G.,** Field tests with insecticides for the control of ticks on livestock, *J. Econ. Entomol., 58,* 1131, 1965.
28. **Drummond, R. O. and Graham, O. H.,** Insecticide tests against the tropical horse tick, *Dermacentor nitens,* on horses, *J. Econ. Entomol., 57,* 549, 1964.
29. **Drummond, R. O. and Ossorio, J. M.,** Additional tests with insecticides for the control of the tropical horse tick on horses in Florida, *J. Econ. Entomol., 59,* 107, 1966.
30. **Taylor, W. M., Bryant, J. E., Anderson, J. B., and Willers, K. H.,** Equine piroplasmosis in the United States — a review, *J. Am. Vet. Med. Assoc., 155,* 915, 1969.
31. **Hickman, R. W.,** Scabies of cattle, *U.S. Dep. Agric. Farmers' Bull., 152,* 1904.
32. **Imes, M.,** Mange in equines, *U.S. Dep. Agric. Yearb. Agric., 476,* 1942.
33. **Annereaux, R. F., Emminger, A. C., and Bills, C. B.,** Infestation of horse with chigger mites, *Bull. Dep. Agric. Calif., 52,* 163, 1963.
34. **Easton, E. R. and Krantz, G. W.,** A *Euschoengastia* species (Acari: Trombiculidae) of possible medical and veterinary importance in Oregon, *J. Med. Entomol., 10,* 225, 1973.
35. **Montali, R. J.,** Ear mites in a horse, *J. Am. Vet. Med. Assoc., 169,* 630, 1976.
36. **Scott, D. W.,** Folliculitis and furunculosis, in *Current Therapy in Equine Medicine,* Robinson, N. E., Ed., W. B. Saunders, Philadelphia, Pa., 1983, 542.
37. **Hall, M. C.,** Notes in regard to bots, *Gasterophilus* spp., *J. Am. Vet. Med. Assoc., 52,* 177, 1917.
38. **Dove, W. E.,** Some biological and control studies of *Gastrophilus haemorrhoidalis* and other bots of horses, *U.S. Dep. Agri. Bull., 597,* 1918.
39. **Bishopp, F. C. and Dove, W. E.,** The horse bots and their control, *U.S. Dep. Agric. Farmers' Bull., 1503,* 1926.
40. **Knipling, E. F. and Wells, R. W.,** Factors stimulating hatching of eggs of *Gasterophilus intestinalis* De Geer and the application of warm water as a practical method of destroying these eggs on the host, *J. Econ. Entomol., 28,* 1065, 1935.
41. **Bishopp, F. C. and Dove, W. E.,** The horse bots and their control, *U.S. Dep. Agric. Farmers' Bull., 1503,* 1935.
42. **Bishopp, F. C. and Dove, W. E.,** The horse bots and their control, *U.S. Dep. Agric. Farmers' Bull., 1503,* 1941.
43. **Todd, A. C., Hansen, M. F., Smith, M. F., and Brown, R. G.,** Action of methyl benzene (toluene) against horse bots, *J. Am. Vet. Med. Assoc., 116,* 369, 1950.
44. **Todd, A. C. and Brown, R. G., Jr.,** Critical tests with toluene for ascarids and bots in horses, *Am. J. Vet. Res., 13,* 198, 1952.
45. **Sinclair, L. R. and Enzie, F. D.,** Toluene against ascarids and bots in horses, *Am. J. Vet. Res., 14,* 49, 1953.
46. **Graham, O. H. and Alford, H. I., Jr.,** The occurrence of *Gasterophilus* spp. in Texas and some tests with insecticides for their control, *J. Econ. Entomol., 44,* 577, 1951.
47. **Drummond, R. O., Jackson, J. B., Gless, E. E., and Moore, B.,** Systemic insecticides for the control of *Gasterophilus* bots in horses, *Agric. Chem., 14,* 41, 1959.
48. **Drudge, J. H., Leland, S. E., Jr., Wyant, Z. N., Elam, G. W., and Lyons, E. T.,** Critical tests with the organic phosphate insecticide, dimethoate, against *Gastrophilus* spp. in the horse, with observations on its anthelmintic action, *Am. J.. Vet. Res., 22,* 1106, 1961.
49. **Drudge, J. H., Szanto, J., Wyant, Z. N., and Elam, G.,** Critical tests of thiabendazole as an anthelmintic in the horse, *Am. J. Vet. Res., 24,* 1217, 1963.
50. **Drummond, R. O.,** Tests with systemic insecticides for the control of *Gasterophilus* larvae in horses, *J. Econ. Entomol., 56,* 50, 1963.
51. **Drudge, J. H. and Lyons, E. T.,** Activity of dichlorvos against horse bots, *Mod. Vet. Pract., 51,* 45, 1970.
52. **Bello, T. R. and Seger, C. L.,** Antiparasitic efficacy of dichlorvos paste formulation against first-instar *Gasterophilus intestinalis* in the tongues of Shetland pony foals, *Am. J. Vet. Res., 33,* 39, 1972.

53. **Drudge, J. H., Lyons, E. T., and Swerczek, T. W.,** Activity of gel and paste formulations of dichlorvos against first instars of *Gasterophilus* spp., *Am. J. Vet. Res., 33,* 2191, 1972.

54. **Smith, J. P. and Bell, R. R.,** Butonate, an organic phorphorous compound as a *Gasterophilus* larvacide in horses, *Southwest. Vet., 21,* 293, 1968.

55. **Voss, J. L. and Hibler, C. P.,** Critical tests of butonate as an ascaricide and boticide in horses, *Am. J. Vet. Res., 32,* 2085, 1971.

56. **Drudge, J. H. and Lyons, E. T.,** Critical tests of a resin-pellet formulation of dichlorvos against internal parasites of the horse, *Am. J. Vet. Res., 33,* 1365, 1972.

57. **Hass, D. K., Albert, J. R., Pillow, B. G., and Brown, L. J.,** Dichlorvos gel formulation as an equine anthelmintic, *Am. J. Vet. Res., 34,* 41, 1973.

58. **Drudge, J. H., Lyons, E. T., and Tolliver, S. C.,** Activity of organophosphorus compounds against oral stages of *Gasterophilus intestinalis* and *Gasterophilus nasalis, Am. J. Vet. Res., 36,* 251, 1975.

59. **Andersen, F. L., Wright, P. D., and Walters, G. T.,** Palatability and efficacy of a powder formulation of thiabendazole and trichlorfon for horses, *J. Am. Vet. Med. Assoc., 162,* 206, 1973.

60. **Rand, H.,** Evaluation of ComBot® (trichlorfon) when combined with phenothiazine, mebendazole or thiabendazole for use as a broad-spectrum anthelmintic in horses, *Vet. Med./Small Anim. Clin., 70,* 1297, 1975.

61. **Drudge, J. H., Lyons, E. T., and Tolliver, S. C.,** Critical and controlled tests of the antilparasitic activity of liquid and paste formulations of trichlorfon in the horse, *Vet. Med./Small Anim. Clin., 70,* 975, 1975.

62. **Drudge, J. H., Lyons, E. T., and Taylor, E. L.,** Critical tests and safety studies on trichlorfon as an antiparasitic agent in the horse, *Am. J. Vet. Res., 37,* 139, 1976.

63. **Lyons, E. T., Drudge, J. H., and Tolliver, S. C.,** Critical tests of the antiparasitic activity of thiabendazole and trichlorfon sequentially administered to horses via stomach tube, *Am. J. Vet. Res., 38,* 721, 1977.

64. **McCurdy, H. D., Sharp, M. L., and Kruchkenberg, S. M.,** Critical and clinical trials of mebendazole and trichlorfon in the horse, *Vet. Med./Small Anim. Clin., 72,* 245, 1977.

65. **Drudge, J. H., Lyons, E. T., and Tolliver, S. C.,** Critical tests of the anthelmintic febantel in the horse: activity of a paste formulation alone or with a trichlorfon paste, *Am. J. Vet. Res., 39,* 1419, 1978.

66. **Drudge, J. H., Lyons, E. T., and Tolliver, S. C.,** Critical tests of febantel in the horse: antiparasitic activity of a suspension alone or with liquid trichlorfon, *J. Equine Med. Surg., 3,* 135, 1979.

67. **Asquith, R. L. and Kulwich, R.,** Concomitant use of oxfendazole & trichlorfon as an equine anthelmintic in mares, *Vet. Med./Small Anim. Clin., 75,* 682, 1980.

68. **DiPietro, J. A., Lock, T. F., Todd, K. S., Ewert, K., and Cole, N.,** Clinical trials with oxfendazole and commonly used boticides in horses, *Equine Pract., 3,* 16, 1981.

69. **Lyons, E. T., Drudge, J. H., and Tolliver, S. C.,** Haloxon: critical tests of antiparasitic activity in equids, *Am. J. Vet. Res., 42,* 1043, 1981.

70. **Drudge, J. H., Lyons, E. T., and Tolliver, S. C.,** Critical tests of morantel — trichlorfon paste formulation against internal parasites of the horse, *Vet. Parasitol., 14,* 55, 1984.

71. **Presson, B. L., Hamm, D., Yazwinski, T. A., and Pote, L. M.,** Critical test evaluation of oxfendazole and trichlorfon: effectiveness of a paste formulation in the horse, *Am. J. Vet. Res., 45,* 1203, 1984.

72. **Bello, T. R., Gaunt, S. D., and Torbert, B. J.,** Critical evaluation of environmental control of bots *(Gasterophilus intestinalis)* in horses, *J. Equine Med. Surg., 1,* 126, 1977.

73. **Sharp, A. J., Pennington, R. G., Scroggs, M. G., and Miller, W. V.,** Efficacy of an oral larvicide in controlling horse bots, *Vet. Med./Small Anim. Clin., 76,* 1207, 1981.

74. **Drudge, J. H., Lyons, E. T., and Tolliver, S.C.,** Parasite control in horses: a summary of contemporary drugs, *Vet. Med./Small Anim. Clin., 76,* 1479, 1981.

75. **Lyons, E. T., Drudge, J. H., and Tolliver, S. C.,** Antiparasitic activity of Ivermectin in critical tests in equids, *Am. J. Vet. Res., 41,* 2069, 1980.

76. **Bello, T. R. and Norfleet, C. M.,** Critical antiparasitic efficacy of Ivermectin against equine parasites, *J. Equine Vet. Sci., 1,* 14, 1981.

77. **Craig, T. M. and Kunde, J. M.,** Controlled evaluation of Ivermectin in Shetland ponies, *Am. J. Vet. Res., 42,* 1422, 1981.

78. **Bello, T. R.,** Ivermectin: a potential injectable equine anthelmintic, *Proc. Am. Soc. Equine Pract., 27,* 485, 1982.

79. **DiPietro, J. A., Todd, K. S., Lock, T. F., and McPherron, T. A.,** Anthelmintic efficacy of Ivermectin given intramuscularly in horses, *Am. J. Vet. Res., 43,* 145, 1982.

80. **Drudge, J. H., Lyons, E. T., and Tolliver, S. C.,** Controlled tests of activity of Ivermectin against natural infestions of migratory large strongyles and other internal parasites of equids, *Am. J. Vet. Res., 45,* 2267, 1984.

81. **Egerton, J. R., Brokken, E. S., Suhayda, D., Eary, C. H., Wooden, J. W., and Kilgore, R. L.,** The antiparasitic activity of Ivermectin in horses, *Vet. Parasitol., 8,* 83, 1981.

82. **Torbert, B. J., Kramer, B. S., and Klei, T. R.,** Efficacy of injectable and oral paste formulations of Ivermectin against gastrointestinal parasites in ponies, *Am. J. Vet. Res., 43,* 1451, 1982.

83. **Yazwinski, T. A., Hamm, D., Greenway, T., and Tilley, W.,** Antiparasitic effectiveness of Ivermectin in the horse, *Am. J. Vet. Res.,* 43, 1092, 1982.
84. **Guerrero, J., Michael, B. F., Rohovsky, M. W., and Campbell, B. P.,** The activity of Closantel as an equine antiparasitic agent, *Vet. Parasitol.,* 12, 71, 1983.
85. **Guerrero, J., Newcomb, K., Seibert, B. P., and Michael, B. F.,** Activity of Closantel in the prevention of *Gasterophilus* and *Strongylus vulgaris* larval infections in equine foals and yearlings, *Am. J. Vet. Res.,* 46, 16, 1985.

Chapter 13

CONTROL OF ARTHROPOD PESTS OF SHEEP AND GOATS*

I. INTRODUCTION

Sheep and goats are parasitized by a variety of arthropod pests. These pests can be grouped according to their relationship to sheep and goats as follows: those found (1) continuously in or on the skin — lice, keds, scab, itch or mange mites, and other parasitic mites; (2) in wounds or in soiled wool or mohair — screwworms, fleece worms, and larvae of other myiasis-producing flies; (3) in the nasal passages and sinuses — sheep bot fly larvae, and (4) intermittently sucking blood from or annoying sheep and goats — biting gnats, black flies, and other biting and nuisance flies. Because of these different relationships, different technologies have been and are being used to control these arthropods. Thus, this chapter is divided into six sections that present treatment technologies used to control specific groups of pests dependent upon these relationships. General information on the biology and control of the arthropod pests of sheep was recently presented in a chapter in *Livestock Entomology*.[1]

II. CONTROL OF LICE AND KEDS

Sheep are infested with the sheep biting louse*, *Bovicola ovis* (Schrank), and two species of sucking lice, *Linognathus ovillus* (Neumann) and *L. pedalis* (Osborn). Meat, dairy, and Angora goats are infested with two species of sucking lice (the goat sucking louse*, *L. stenopsis* [Burmeister], and *L. africanus* Kellogg and Paine) and three species of biting lice (the goat biting louse*, *Bovicola caprae* [Gurlt], the Angora goat biting louse*, *B. crassipes* [Rudow], and *B. limbatus* [Gervais]). Sheep and, to a lesser extent, goats are also infested with a wingless fly, the sheep ked*, *Melophagus ovinus* (Linnaeus), often called the sheep "tick" although it is a fly. Each of these species spends its life cycle on the host, and thus is generally controlled by the application of insecticides to the hosts. Treatments effective against lice are usually effective against keds and vice versa.

A. Early Treatment Technology

Osborn, in 1896,[2] described *L. pedalis* as a new species and listed treatments to control lice as spraying animals with pyrethrins or dipping them in standard dips, such as tobacco, tobacco-sulfur, or lime-sulfur. He also discussed the sheep "tick" and listed pyrethrins sprays or dipping in kerosene emulsion, tobacco, and other dips as effective treatments. The original issue of *U.S. Dep. Agric. Farmers' Bulletin* No. 798[3] in 1917 listed dipping of sheep in coal-tar creosote, cresol, nicotine, or lime-sulfur-arsenic as the only practical method known for eradicating sheep keds. One dipping controlled keds, but two dippings were generally necessary for eradication. U.S. Dep. Agric. Leaflet No. 13 in 1928[4] listed a variety of methods and materials to control lice on sheep and goats: (1) hand application of dusts of naphthalene or pyrethrins or washes of sodium fluoride, which controlled biting lice only, (2) fumigation with sulfur dioxide, which killed lice, but not their eggs, and, since the eyes and nostrils of the treated animals must be protected from the fumes, the method was not recommended, (3) spraying of the chemicals used in dipping vats, but sprays did not fully penetrate wool or mohair, and (4) dipping in arsenic, coal-tar creosote, or nicotine. One dipping controlled lice, but two dippings were necessary to eradicate lice, especially sucking lice.

* Common names of insects and acarines, as listed in *Common Names of Insects and Related Organisms* (published by the Entomological Society of America), are marked with a * the first time they are cited preceding the scientific name.

Treatments for keds changed little, for the 1939[5] and 1940[6] editions of Bulletin No. 798 still listed nicotine, coal-tar creosote, and cresol dips and added that one dipping in a fused bentonite sulfur dip usually eradicated keds. Sheep keds were found on ca.80% of the flocks in Illinois, and a newly designed, portable dipping vat, charged with standard dips, provided excellent control of lice and keds.[7] In the 1942 *U.S. Dep. Agric. Yearbook of Agriculture,*[8] dipping goats in wettable sulfur, wettable sulfur plus rotenone, or arsenic controlled both sucking and biting lice. A single dipping in rotenone eradicated keds.[9] Dipping sheep in rotenone-sulfur eliminated keds, but dips of fixed nicotine with or without sulfur were not completely effective.[10,11]

The daily oral administration of sulfur in capsules or in feed to Angora goats had no effect on the populations of biting or sucking lice.[12]

B. Organochlorine Treatments

At the end of World War II, DDT dip controlled keds on sheep[13,14] and biting and sucking lice on sheep and goats.[15-19] Schwardt and Matthysse[20] briefly reviewed the literature on the biology and control of keds and presented a considerable amount of information on current treatment materials, especially rotenone, and methods, especially a power duster and a portable dipping vat. The 1948 revision of Bulletin No. 798[21] listed dips of DDT and rotenone as the most effective treatments for keds but also presented information on the older dip materials as well. Benzene hexachloride (BHC), lindane, chlordane, toxaphene, methoxychlor, and TDE controlled keds and lice.[22-26] *U.S. Dep. Agric. Farmers' Bulletin* No. 2057,[27] which superseded Bulletin No. 798 in 1953, listed all previous dip materials and added seven new chlorinated hydrocarbon insecticides as dip treatments to control keds.

Power dusting equipment was used[28] on a large scale to apply rotenone to control keds on lambs in cold weather. DDT dusts were not effective and dieldrin dusts were more effective than dusts of chlordane, heptachlor, lindane, or toxaphene when applied in the spring after shearing or in the fall when sheep had fleece.[29-32] Dipping lambs in DDT-sulfur or dusting them with rotenone-sulfur gave better control of keds than pen spraying or spraying only along the top line, called "ribbon spraying", with DDT, rotenone, or sulfur.[33]

C. Organophosphorus Treatments

Dips of diazinon, chlorthion, trichlorfon, and coumaphos controlled biting lice on goats.[34] Sprays of ronnel, dioxathion, coumaphos, dicapthon, malathion, and trichlorfon controlled keds on sheep.[35,36]

The resistance of biting lice, *B. caprae* and *B. limbatus,* on Angora goats in central Texas to toxaphene was reported by Moore et al.,[37] but sprays of ronnel, malathion, coumaphos, trichlorfon, dioxathion, and a carbamate, carbaryl, provided complete control of biting and sucking lice. Of a variety of insecticides sprayed onto Angora goats for the control of biting and sucking lice and onto sheep for control of biting lice, the most effective were crufomate, chlorfenvinphos, and dichlofenthion.[38]

Dusts of coumaphos, diazinon, ronnel, malathion, and carbaryl were more effective in the spring with sheared sheep than in the fall with sheep in fleece for the control of keds.[39,40] Power dusting of shorn sheep with crotoxyphos, stirofos, and phosmet reduced ked populations but did not eradicate keds as did dusts of coumaphos and ronnel.[41]

Diazinon, ronnel, coumaphos, and malathion were effective against biting lice and keds on sheep when applied as high-volume, high-pressure sprays, but only diazinon and ronnel were effective as low-volume, low-pressure sprays and by the "sprinkler-can" application technique.[42]

D. Other Treatment Technologies

Recent research has shown that applications of low volumes of higher concentrations of insecticides were as effective as conventional power dusting, dip, or spray treatments.

Spraying of 4.8 to 9 mℓ per sheep of concentrated diazinon or ronnel controlled keds.[43] Pouron treatments of 0.01 to 0.6 mℓ of coumaphos, diazinon, ronnel, or crufomate per kilogram of body weight applied to one spot on or along the backline of sheared sheep controlled keds.[44] Spoton treatments of 4 mℓ per sheep of fenthion or 2 mℓ per sheep of chlorpyrifos lowered, but did not eliminate, populations of keds.[45,46]

Two spray treatments of the synthetic juvenile hormone, methyl 10, 11-epoxy-7-ethyl-3,11 demethyl-2,6-tridecadienoate, controlled biting lice on Angora goats.[47] Several insect growth regulators, hydroprene, triprene, Ciba-Geigy® CGA-13353, and Stauffer® HS-103, caused a slow decline in louse populations, and diflubenzuron, a chitin inhibitor, caused a rapid decline in populations of biting lice on Angora goats.[48]

Dichlorvos-impregnated resin collars placed around the necks of goats controlled biting lice.[49] Small ear tags impregnated with amitraz, flucythrinate, or fenvalerate, applied to sheared sheep, controlled keds.[50]

Recently, biting lice on Angora goats with 3 months of mohair growth were controlled with pourons, spotons, and sprays of several pyrethroids and organophosphorus insecticides.[51] Pourons of diflubenzuron, fenvalerate, and phenthoate, a fenvalerate-impregnated plastic neck band, and fenthion spoton controlled *B. limbatus* on Angora goats, but an ivermectin injection failed to control lice systemically.[52]

III. CONTROL OF *PSOROPTES OVIS*

A historically important ectoparasite of sheep throughout the world, the sheep scab mite◆, *Psoroptes ovis* (Hering), has been eradicated from sheep in the U.S. Details of the eradication program are presented by Graham and Hourrigan.[53] Here we shall discuss chemical control technology only.

A. Early Treatment Technology

U.S. Dep. Agric. Bureau of Animal Industry Bulletin No. 21[54] in 1898 presented a historical review of investigations on the biology of *P. ovis*, listed detailed procedures for preparation of dips of sulfur plus tobacco or lime, tobacco, arsenicals, or carbolic acid, and gave instructions for dipping sheep and for construction of dipping vats, including circular vats. This bulletin was condensed into *U.S. Dep. Agric. Farmers' Bulletin* No. 159 in 1903.[55] This bulletin was superseded by *U.S. Dep. Agric. Farmers' Bulletin* No. 713[56] in 1916 which described the problems associated with sheep scab, noted progress in scab eradication, listed only lime-sulfur or nicotine-sulfur as official dips, and stated that neither feeding sulfur, salt, or various other preparations to sheep nor hand dressing or "spot doctoring" of only affected areas were effective treatments. The 1923 edition of this bulletin[57] contained no major changes in control recommendations. However, in the 1935 edition,[58] the nicotine-sulfur dip was replaced by nicotine alone. The only official dips listed in *U.S. Dep. Agric. Yearbook of Agriculture* in 1942[59] were nicotine and heated lime-sulfur.

B. Benzene Hexachloride and Lindane

After World War II, the fact that a single dipping in BHC eradicated *P. ovis* from sheep[60-62] was hailed by Kemper and Roberts[63] as a "splendid weapon against an ancient enemy". The 1952 revision of Bulletin No. 713[64] added BHC and lindane (wettable powder) as very effective dips for the eradication of sheep scabies.

C. Organophosphorus Treatments

Of the many organophosphorus insecticides used to control arthropod pests of livestock, only a very few eradicated *P. ovis* on sheep with a single treatment. Coumaphos[65] and diazinon eradicated mites, while ronnel, crotoxyphos, chlorfenvinphos, and fenthion controlled mites.[66] Chlorpyrifos as a dip eliminated severe infestations of *P. ovis*.[67] Dips of crotoxyphos, ronnel, and diazinon provided protection against infestation by mites from infested sheep for periods as long as those provided by the standard treatments of lindane and toxaphene.[68] Two dips of coumaphos, chlorpyrifos, phosmet, and carbophenothion eliminated mites.[69] Daily oral treatment with famphur, an animal systemic insecticide, did not eliminate *P. ovis* from sheep.[70]

The eradication of *P. ovis* from sheep in the U.S. in 1973 precluded additional research on control of this pest on sheep in the U.S. Meleney[71] reviewed current information on the biology and control of *P. ovis*.

IV. CONTROL OF OTHER MITE PESTS

In addition to *P. ovis*, sheep may be infested with other mite pests, the itch mite♦, *Sarcoptes scabiei* (De Geer), *Chorioptes bovis* (Hering), *Psorergates ovis* Womersley, and the sheep follicle mite♦, *Demodex ovis* Railliet. Goats are infested with *S. scabiei* (De Geer), *C. texanus* Hirst, *Psoroptes cuniculi* (Delafond), and the goat follicle mite♦, *D. caprae* Railliet. Practical information on the biology and control of these species was presented by Lofstedt.[72] Meleney[71] presented a current, broad overview of the biology and control of these species.

Generally considered nonpathogenic, *Chorioptes bovis* is usually found around the lower legs and feet of sheep and is the cause of "foot scab". In the early USDA publications, the treatments listed for control of *P. ovis* were generally recognized as effective against the other mite pests, except *Demodex* spp., of sheep and goats. Infestations apparently cause little damage to fleece and have no effect on the growth of lambs.[73] Sweatman and Pullin[74] reviewed the literature on control of *C. bovis* and found that none of a variety of acaricides killed eggs, but dieldrin, lindane, ronnel, endosulfan, and carbophenothion controlled newly hatched mites. *C. bovis* was found on the feet and scrotum of almost every sheep examined,[75] and crotoxyphos was the most promising of a large number of insecticides tested.

Chorioptes texanus, which rarely occurs in the U.S., but can cause extensive lesions on Angora goats, was controlled by dipping goats twice in heated sulfur.[76] A single dipping of Angora goats in BHC eradicated *C. texanus*.[77] Chorioptic mange in goats was controlled by the same lime-sulfur wash that controlled sarcoptic mange; also, a coumaphos treatment was reported as effective.[78]

Psorergates ovis was discovered on sheep in the U.S. in Ohio in 1951[79] and subsequently in California and New Mexico.[80] In Australia, dips of arsenic-sulfur-rotenone, lime-sulfur, lime-sulfur-diazinon, phoxim, BHC, arsenic, dioxathion, malathion, coumaphos, and trichlorfon and injections of dimethoate controlled but failed to eradicate *P. ovis*.[81-83] There is no information on the control of this species in the U.S.

Sarcoptes scabiei infestations, often called "head scab", are generally found around the eyes of sheep and are of little consequence in the U.S. In India, sarcoptic mange in goats has been controlled with multiple sprays of malathion,[84] or in the Sudan with a single spray of chlorfenvinphos.[85]

Demodectic mange, generally found in the eyelids of sheep,[86] is also of little importance in sheep. In contrast, demodectic mange in goats may become a serious problem. *D. caprae* form nodules on the skin of goats, and treatment of the nodules with various ointments appeared to have little effect on the infestation.[87] Opening and injecting a few drops of carbolic acid into each nodule controlled infestations.[88,89] Another treatment consisted of opening the nodules, removing contents and injecting the nodules with coal-tar creosote dip.[90] Treatment of goats weekly for 3 weeks with rotenone in cottonseed oil apparently controlled mites and eliminated the lesions.[91] In India, cure of demodectic mange in Beetal goats was obtained with multiple oral treatments of trichlorfon,[92] and dressings of malathion were more effective than those of trichlorfon or coumaphos.[93] Williams and Williams[94] reported on recent cases of demodicosis in dairy goats in the U.S. but listed only the use of the carbolic acid treatment to control the mites. In France, a trichlorfon pouron is reported[95] to control this species.

Goats may be infested, primarily in the ears, with *Psoroptes cuniculi*, which may need to be treated when an infestation becomes extensive. In England, Littlejohn[96] reviewed the literature on *P. cuniculi* and reported the cure of psoroptic mange with washes of lindane. *P. cuniculi* infestations were common in dairy goats in Michigan, but clinical signs were limited to behavioral changes.[97] Treatment of ears with rotenone-containing ear drops gave good results in clinically affected goats.[98]

V. CONTROL OF MYIASIS-PRODUCING FLIES

In the U.S. and Canada, sheep, domestic and wild animals, and man are attacked by a variety of myiasis-producing flies whose larvae live in wounds or on the skin of animals. Osborn[2] described the screwworm♦, *Cochliomyia hominivorax* (Coquerel), which was then named *Compsomyia macellaria* Fabricius, as "unquestionably one of the most important of all the insects that affect domestic animals". Technologies used to control screwworms are discussed in Chapter 7, and the sterile insect technique that has been used to eradicate screwworms from the U.S. and most of Mexico is discussed in Chapter 20. Here, we will limit ourselves to the materials and methods used to control "secondary" myiasis-producing flies, including the black blow fly♦, *Phormia regina* (Meigen), the secondary screwworm♦, *Cocliomyia macellaria* (Fabricius), *Lucilia sericata* (Meigen), *Protophormia terrae-novae* (Robineau-Desvoidy), and several other species. There are a number of species of "fleece worms" and "wool maggots" in the U.S. and, although infestations can be found in sheep and goats, the magnitude and the economic importance of such infestations do not approach those for infestations of *Lucilia cuprina* (Wiedemann) in sheep-producing areas of Africa, Australia, and Europe. There the sheep blow fly problem, or cutaneous myiasis as a result of blow fly strike, is a major economic concern of sheep producers.

A. Early Treatment Technology

Osborn[2] listed that control of fly larvae on livestock was obtained with a wash of carbolic acid or creoline to kill larvae, followed by a final dressing of pine oil to repel flies. Bishopp and Laake[99] reported that various wool maggots were found in the U.S., but had received little attention. They described the life cycles of *P. regina* and *L. sericata* and briefly listed control measures which included burning or burying carcasses, breeding of ewes so that lambing was done in the winter when flies were not active, development of breeds of hornless sheep, treating infested areas with concoctions containing chloroform, and the trimming of soiled wool away from the perianal area and rear legs, which is called "tagging".

A critical point to be made with respect to the early literature on myiasis in sheep and other livestock in the U.S. is the fact that myiasis by the screwworm, *Cochliomyia hominivorax*, was not differentiated from that of the secondary screwworm, *C. macellaria* and other blow flies. This fact is illustrated by Bishopp[100] who stated "The screwworm, *C. macellaria*, has developed a very marked tendency to attack living animals, although it breeds in greatest numbers in carcasses", and observed that screwworms in wounds were controlled with chloroform, creosote products, pine tar, and other remedies. The initial issue of *U.S. Dep. Agric. Farmers' Bulletin* No. 734 in 1916[101] described a conical hoop fly trap, that, if baited with the mucous membrane from the lining of the intestine of hogs, called "gut slime", would attract and capture blow flies. The initial issue of *U.S. Dep. Agric. Farmers' Bulletin* No. 857 in 1917[102] described the life history and biology of wool maggots. Control measures included destruction of carcasses, treatment of maggots in wounds with chloroform, turpentine, or tar, and the use of lime dust to dry and deodorize infested areas. Also, the scheduling of lambing, castration, shearing, tail docking, dehorning, and tagging minimized wounds or exposure to flies.

Early research on repellents, attractants, and larvicides for screwworms and other flies[103] showed that pine tar oils and other oils were repellent, moistened dried whole egg or egg yolk was a good bait, and benzol was the best larvicide for wounds. Benzol was the most effective of a variety of chemicals applied to wounds to control screwworms.[104] Of many materials tested as repellents for screwworms and blow flies, chloropicrin, a tear gas, was highly repellent, but difficult to use.[105] The 1926 revision of Bulletin No. 857[106] stated that benzol controlled larvae in wounds and that pine tar oil repelled flies. Further tests with baits and repellents[107] found that beef or hog liver and rabbit meat were attractive baits for fly traps and that, although pine tar was an effective repellent, the search for other repellents lies in finding chemicals that absorb, adsorb, alter, or prevent formation of attractive volatile compounds from wounds, rather than in finding chemicals with masking odors, such as tear gases. The 1930 revision of Bulletin No. 734[108] included an expanded section on the selection of baits to attract screwworms and other blow flies to traps on the range.

In 1933, Cushing and Patton[109] determined that in the U.S. the true, primary screwworm, which they named *C. americana,* was the cause of initial wound myiasis of live animals and that the more numerous *C. macellaria* was an invader of dead and decaying flesh. Studies on the biology of the two species[110] revealed differences in life cycles, hosts, and abundance. Further research on the biology and control of the screwworm provided specific treatments (Chapter 7) and eventually led to the use of the sterile insect technique to eradicate this species from most of the North American continent (Chapter 20).

B. Blow Fly and Fleece Worm Larvae

Research on control of larvae of the "secondary" myiasis-producing flies showed that several organic compounds were highly active as larvicides.[111] In field tests, smears or ointments containing benzol, as a toxicant, and diphenylamine, as a wound protection agent, controlled fleece worms and prevented reinfestation.[112] After World War II, of several chlorinated hydrocarbon insecticides applied as sprays to sheep infested with *C. macellaria* and *P. regina,* toxaphene was the most effective in preventing reinfestation, less effective were chlordane and lindane, and least effective were DDT and BHC.[113] The 1956 *U.S. Dep. Agric. Yearbook of Agriculture*[114] reviewed the biology of fleece worms and listed the use of preventive ranching practices, spraying of the perianal region and tail with toxaphene, chlordane, or BHC to prevent fly attack, and treating larval infestations with 1 part of smear EQ-335 (3% lindane, 35% pine-tar oil plus inert ingredients) diluted with 9 parts of water as an excellent toxicant and protectant against reinfestation.

A systemic insecticide, ronnel, administered orally to sheep, afforded prompt kill of blow fly larvae; however, the treatment was considered practical for only deep, percutaneous infestations and did not prevent reinfestation.[115] Ronnel applied as a spray or dip was highly effective against screwworm larvae, fleece worm larvae, and wool maggots.[116] Coumaphos spray was also highly toxic to fleece worm larvae.[117]

Although the international literature on research on sheep strike or wool maggots since 1960 continues to contain large numbers of articles, there are none found in the literature for the U.S. Two recent general papers on parasites of sheep and goats in the U.S.[118,72] still list cutaneous myiasis as an ever-present problem that can be lessened or prevented by tagging sheep or preventing diarrhea of sheep and goats. Animals may be treated with insecticides to prevent infestation, or infested areas may be treated with smears, aerosols, or sprays of insecticides to kill larvae and prevent reinfestation.

VI. CONTROL OF *OESTRUS OVIS*

A. Early Treatment Technology

A review of the early literature indicates that larvae of the sheep bot fly[*], *Oestrus ovis* Linnaeus, called "grub in the head", have been observed in sheep since ancient times. Osborn[2] lists a variety of control measures to dislodge larvae from the nassal passages or prevent flies from larvipositing. Early technologies used to control *O. ovis* larvae in the nasal chambers of sheep were injecting materials into the frontal sinuses through openings made with a needle or trephine in the frontal bones;[119] injecting materials, especially carbon disulfide in mineral oil, into the nasal passages through the nostrils,[120] and introducing irritants into the nasal passages to cause the sheep to sneeze and expel larvae. Placing repellents, especially pine tar, around the nasal openings prevented flies from depositing larvae into the nares.[121] Saponified cresol (lysol) injected into the nasal passages through the nostrils[122] killed larvae on the nasal mucosa of sheep and was used to treat thousands of sheep with satisfactory results.[123]

B. Systemic Insecticides

Technologies used to control sheep bot larvae were basically unchanged until the advent of animal systemic insecticides in the 1950s. The first practical animal systemic insecticide, ronnel, as an oral drench, controlled first instar larvae, but not second and third instar larvae.[124] Soon other systemics were found to be effective against sheep bot larvae in sheep: dimethoate orally or as an intramuscular injection;[125] coumaphos as a dip, crufomate, Dowco®-109, and dimethoate orally;[126] trichlorfon orally;[127] and crufomate orally.[128] In preliminary tests, 13 of 20 systemics were effective orally, in feed or as intramuscular injections against one or more instars.[129] Bayer B-9017, Bayer B-9018, famphur, trichlorfon, fenthion, a coumaphos-trichlorfon mixture administered orally, and dimethoate and trichlorfon administered as intramuscular injections controlled first instar larvae.[130] Oral treatments of B-9017, B-9018, crufomate, famphur, and Stauffer R-3828 and a pouron treatment of crufomate controlled all three instars.[131] Fenthion, Bayer B-9017, and Bayer B-9018 were effective when administered orally or as sprays or pourons.[132,133] Spoton treatments of crufomate and pouron treatments of famphur, fenthion, and phosmet, but not permethrin, controlled first instar larvae.[134]

Injecting dimethoate into almost all of an isolated flock of sheep consecutively for 4 years caused a 83% reduction in the average number of larvae, but the treatment did not eradicate *O. ovis*.[135]

A subcutaneous treatment of trichlorfon or oral treatments of thiabendozole or Maretin® were effective anthelmintics but did not control *O. ovis* larvae.[136,137] A commercially available drench that contained crufomate controlled all three instars.[138] Although not tested in the U.S., an anthelmintic, rafoxanide, given orally to sheep controlled all larval instars of *O. ovis*.[139-141] Another anthelmintic, nitroxynil, given subcutaneously to sheep, also controlled *O. ovis* larvae.[142] Most recently, a single oral treatment of ivermectin, a highly effective, broad-spectrum anthelmintic and systemic insecticide, was systemically active against all instars of *O. ovis*.[143-145]

C. Nasal Treatments

Dichlorvos, applied into nostrils of sheep in petroleum jelly[146] or as a nasal spray,[132,133] controlled first instar larvae, although high dosages poisoned some of the sheep. Nasal sprays of a trichlorfon-coumaphos mixture and Bayer 9017 were also effective. Irrigation of nasal passages with methoprene significantly reduced pupation and emergence of adult flies but did not affect larval development.[147]

VII. CONTROL OF BITING AND NUISANCE FLIES

Sheep, especially recently shorn animals, are often attached by a variety of biting flies, including the horn fly*, *Haematobia irritans* (Linnaeus), and small biting flies, such as *Culicoides* spp., *Leptoconops* spp., *Simulium* spp., and mosquitoes.[148] Control of horn flies has been accomplished by spraying sheep with ronnel.[116] The house fly*, *Musca domestica* Linnaeus, the stable fly*, *Stomoxys calcitrans* (Linnaeus), and other flies were controlled by sprays of ronnel, a mixture of stirofos, plus dichlorvos and dioxathion, but forced use of crotoxyphos dust bags was less effective.[149]

VIII. OVERVIEW AND CURRENT TECHNOLOGY

Historically, the control of lice and keds on sheep and goats was accomplished by treating animals with insecticides applied as dips or sprays. More modern technology involves treatment of sheep and goats with power dusters, low-volume sprays, pouron, or spoton treatments.

The most important mite pest of sheep and goats, the sheep scab mite, has been eradicated from the U.S. The remaining mite pests are of much less economic significance. Infestations of most species can be controlled, if warranted, with currently available treatment technology.

Screwworms have also been eradicated from the U.S., and infestations of fleece worms or wool maggots can be lessened by appropriate sheep and goat production and management operations. Occasional infestations of these species can be controlled by treating infested individuals with smears, aerosols, or other dermal treatments of effective insecticides.

A variety of systemic insecticides is effective against larvae of the sheep bot fly, but, as of this writing, there are no commercially available treatments for this species. The effectiveness of ivermectin as both an anthelmintic and a systemic insecticide make it an excellent candidate for a practical, commercially available treatment.

With the eradication of the sheep scab mite and the screwworm, two major pests of sheep and goats, there has been a decrease in need to develop new technologies for the control of the other arthropod pests of sheep and goats. In addition, the sheep and goat production is of lesser economic importance and thus has limited resources to devote to research on the control of arthropod pests.

REFERENCES

1. **Lloyd, J. E.**, Arthropod pests of sheep, in *Livestock Entomology*, Williams, R. E., Hall, R. D., Broce, A. B., and Scholl, P. J., Eds., John Wiley & Sons, New York, 1985, 253.
2. **Osborn, H.**, Insects affecting domestic animals: an account of the species of importance in North America with mention of related forms occurring on other animals, *U.S. Dep. Agric. Bull.*, 5, 1896.
3. **Imes, M.**, The sheep tick and its eradication by dipping, *U.S. Dep. Agric. Farmers' Bull.*, 798, 1917.
4. **Imes, M.**, Sheep and goat lice and methods of control and eradication, *U.S. Department of Agriculture*, Leaflet Number 13, 1928.
5. **Imes, M.**, The sheep tick and its eradication by dipping, *U.S. Dep. Agric. Farmers' Bull.*, 798, 1939.
6. **Imes, M.**, The sheep tick and its eradication by dipping, *U.S. Dep. Agric. Farmers' Bull.*, 798, 1940.
7. **McCauley, W. E. and Russell, H. G.**, External parasites of sheep in Illinois: a portable dipping vat, *J. Econ. Entomol.*, 33, 547, 1940.
8. **Babcock, O. G. and Cushing, E. C.**, Goat lice, *U.S. Dep. Agric. Yearb. Agric.*, 917, 1942.
9. **Cobbett, N. G. and Smith, C. E.**, The eradication of sheep ticks, *Melophagus ovinus*, by one dipping in dilute derris-water or cube-water dips, *J. Am. Vet. Med. Assoc.*, 103, 6, 1943.
10. **Schwardt, H. H. and Matthysse, J. G.**, New recommendations for large scale control of the sheep tick in the northeast, *J. Econ. Entomol.*, 36, 105, 1943.

11. **Cobbett, N. G. and Smith, C. E.,** Field tests with fixed nicotine for the control of "sheep ticks", *Melophagus ovinus, N. Am. Vet.,* 25, 536, 1944.

12. **Babcock, O. G. and Boughton, I. B.,** Sulfur-feeding tests for the control of ectoparasites of animals, *J. Am. Vet. Med. Assoc.,* 103, 209, 1943.

13. **Cobbett, N. G. and Smith, C. E.,** DDT has possibilities of becoming a remedy for sheep ticks, *J. Am. Vet. Med. Assoc.,* 107, 147, 1945.

14. **Kemper, H. E., Roberts, I. H., Smith, C. E., and Cobbett, N. G.,** DDT dips for the control of sheep ticks, *Melophagus ovinus, J. Am. Vet. Med. Assoc.,* 111, 196, 1947.

15. **Babcock, O. G.,** DDT for control of goat lice, *J. Econ. Entomol.,* 37, 138, 1944.

16. **Parish, H. E. and Rude, C. S.,** DDT for the control of goat lice, *J. Econ. Entomol.,* 38, 612, 1945.

17. **Parish, H. E. and Rude, C. S.,** DDT control of the biting sheep louse, *J. Econ. Entomol.,* 39, 546, 1946.

18. **Brown, A. W. A.,** A DDT emulsion dip to control goat lice, *J. Econ. Entomol.,* 40, 605, 1947.

19. **Kemper, H. E., Cobbett, N. G., Roberts, I. H., and Peterson, H. O.,** DDT emulsions for the destruction of lice on cattle, sheep, and goats, *Am. J. Vet. Res.,* 9, 373, 1948.

20. **Schwardt, H. H. and Matthysse, J. G.,** The sheep tick *(Melophagus ovinus* L.) materials and equipment for its control, *Cornell Univ. Agric. Exp. Stat. Bull. No. 844,* 1948.

21. **Imes, M.,** The sheep tick and its eradication by dipping, *U.S. Dep. Agric. Farmers' Bull.,* 798, 1948.

22. **Telford, H. S.,** Benzene hexachloride to control certain insects affecting domestic animals, *J. Econ. Entomol.,* 40, 918, 1947.

23. **Kemper, H. E., Cobbett, N. G., and Roberts, I. H.,** Tests with benzene hexachloride for the destruction of coexistent infestations of the foot louse and keds on sheep, *N. Am. Vet.,* 29, 422, 1948.

24. **Fairchild, H. E., Hoffman, R. A., and Lindquist, A. W.,** A comparison of the chlorinated hydrocarbon insecticides for control of the sheep tick, *J. Econ. Entomol.,* 42, 410, 1949.

25. **Dicke, R. J., Pope, A. L., Bray, R. W., and Hanning, F.,** Investigation of rotenone and benzene hexachloride dusts for the control of insect ectoparasites on sheep, *J. Agric. Res.,* 78, 565, 1949.

26. **Kemper, H. E. and Hindman, W. M.,** Occurrence of and treatment for the destruction of the African blue louse on sheep in northern Arizona, *Vet. Med.,* 45, 39, 1950.

27. **Kemper, H. E. and Peterson, H. O.,** The sheep tick and its eradication, *U.S. Dep. Agric. Farmers' Bull.,* 2057, 1953.

28. **Matthysse, J. G.,** Large scale power dusting of feeder lambs for winter control of the sheep tick, *J. Econ. Entomol.,* 38, 285, 1945.

29. **Denning, D. G.,** Dusting for sheep tick control, *J. Econ. Entomol.,* 42, 852, 1949.

30. **Pfadt, R. E. and Ryff, J. F.,** Safe use of dieldrin dust for sheep ked control, *J. Econ. Entomol.,* 48, 195, 1955.

31. **Pfadt, R. E. and DeFoliart, G. R.,** Power dusting to control the sheep ked, *J. Econ. Entomol.,* 50, 190, 1957.

32. **Goulding, R. L.,** Sheep ked control in Oregon farm flocks, *J. Econ. Entomol.,* 51, 585, 1958.

33. **Muma, M. H., Hill, R. E., Hixson, E., and Harris, L.,** Control of sheep-ticks on feeder lambs, *J. Econ. Entomol.,* 45, 833, 1952.

34. **Smith, C. L. and Richards, R.,** Evaluations of some new insecticides against lice on livestock and poultry, *J. Econ. Entomol.,* 48, 566, 1955.

35. **Roth, A. R. and Bigley, W. S.,** Sheep ked control with organic phosphorus compounds, *J. Econ. Entomol.,* 52, 539, 1959.

36. **McGregor, W. S. and Miller, W. O.,** Trolene and korlan show promise for parasite control in sheep, *Down Earth,* 14, 7, 1958.

37. **Moore, B., Drummond, R. O., and Brundrett, H. M.,** Tests of insecticides for the control of goat lice in 1957 and 1958, *J. Econ. Entomol.,* 52, 980, 1959.

38. **Medley, J. G. and Drummond, R. O.,** Tests with insecticides for control of lice on goats and sheep, *J. Econ. Entomol.,* 56, 658, 1963.

39. **Pfadt, R. E.,** Fall dusting to control the sheep ked, *J. Econ. Entomol.,* 52, 380, 1959.

40. **Pfadt, R. E. and Lavigne, R. J.,** Further tests with power dusting to control the sheep ked, *J. Econ. Entomol.,* 58, 37, 1965.

41. **Pfadt, R. E., Lloyd, J. E., and Spackman, E. W.,** Power dusting with organophosphorus insecticides to control the sheep ked, *J. Econ. Entomol.,* 68, 468, 1975.

42. **Matthysse, J. G.,** Sheep ectoparasite control. I. Insecticides and application methods for keds and biting lice, *J. Econ. Entomol.,* 60, 1645, 1967.

43. **Lloyd, J. E., Olson, E. J., and Pfadt, R. E.,** Low volume spraying of sheep to control the sheep ked, *J. Econ. Entomol.,* 71, 548, 1978.

44. **Lloyd, J. E., Pfadt, R. E., and Kumar, R.,** Sheep ked control with pour-on applications of organophosphorus insecticides, *J. Econ. Entomol.,* 75, 5, 1982.

45. **Surgeoner, G. A., Ralley, W. E., Madder, D. J., Beattle, B., and Westwood, R.,** Efficacy of fenthion Spotton® for control of the sheep ked, *Melophagus ovinus, Agric. Can. Pestic. Res. Rep.,* 185, 1983.

46. **Surgeoner, G. A., Ralley, W. E., Madder, D. J., Beattle, B., and Westwood, R.,** Efficacy of chlorpyrifos Dursban-44® for control of the sheep ked, *Melophagus ovinus* (L.), *Pestic. Res. Rep.* (Agric. Can.), 186, 1983.

47. **Chamberlain, W. F. and Hopkins, D. E.,** The synthetic juvenile hormone for control of *Bovicola limbata* on Angora goats, *J. Econ. Entomol.,* 64, 1198, 1971.

48. **Chamberlain, W. F., Hopkins, D. E., and Gingrich, A. R.,** Applications of insect growth regulators for control of Angora goat biting lice, *Southwest. Entomol.,* 1, 1, 1976.

49. **Darrow, D. I.,** Biting lice of goats: control with dichlorvos-impregnated resin neck collars, *J. Econ. Entomol.,* 66, 133, 1973.

50. **Lloyd, J. E., Kumar, R., Pfadt, R. E., Watson, D. W., and LeaMasters, B. R.,** Sheep ked control with insecticide ear tags, 1984, *Insectic. Acaric. Tests,* 10, 353, 1985.

51. **Fuchs, T. W., and Shelton, M.,** Effectiveness of new methods of biting lice control on Angora goats, *Southwest. Entomol.,* 10, 15, 1985.

52. **Miller, J. A., Chamberlain, W. F., and Oehler, D. D.,** Methods for control of the Angora goat biting louse, *Southwest. Entomol.,* 10, 181, 1985.

53. **Graham, O. H. and Hourrigan, J. L.,** Eradication programs for the arthropod parasites of livestock, *J. Med. Entomol.,* 13, 629, 1977.

54. **Salmon, D. E. and Stiles, C. W.,** Sheep scab: its nature and treatment, *U.S. Dep. Agric. Bur. Anim. Ind. Bull.,* 21, 1898.

55. **Salmon, D. E. and Stiles, C. W.,** Scab in sheep, *U.S. Dep. Agric. Farmers' Bull.,* 159, 1903.

56. **Imes, M.,** Sheep scab, *U.S. Dep. Agric. Farmers' Bull.,* 713, 1916.

57. **Imes, M.,** Sheep scab, *U.S. Dep. Agric. Farmers' Bull.,* 713, 1923.

58. **Imes, M.,** Sheep scab, *U.S. Dep. Agric. Farmers' Bull.,* 713, 1935.

59. **Miller, A. W.,** Sheep scab and its control, *U.S. Dep. Agric. Yearb. Agric.,* 904, 1942.

60. **Kemper, H. E.,** Progress report on benzene hexachloride for the destruction of sheep scab mites, *Vet. Med.,* 43, 76, 1948.

61. **Kemper, H. E. and Roberts, I. H.,** Benzene hexachloride dip to destroy scab mites on unborn *(sic)* sheep, *Vet. Med.,* 44, 163, 1949.

62. **Roberts, I. H.,** Benzene hexachloride dips for the destruction of psoroptic scabies mites on shorn sheep, *Vet. Med.,* 44, 471, 1949.

63. **Kemper, H. E. and Roberts, I. H.,** Eradication of sheep scabies, *Proc. U.S. Livestock Sanit. Assoc.,* 247, 1950.

64. **Kemper, H. E.,** Sheep scab, *U.S. Dep. Agric. Farmers' Bull.,* 713, 1952.

65. **Strickland, R. K. and Gerrish, R. R.,** Efficacy of coumaphos against *Psoroptes ovis, J. Am. Vet. Med. Assoc.,* 148, 553, 1966.

66. **Meleney, W. P. and Roberts, I. H.,** Evaluation of acaricidal dips for control of *Psoroptes ovis* on sheep, *J. Am. Vet. Med. Assoc.,* 151, 725, 1967.

67. **Strickland, R. K., Gerrish, R. R., Hourrigan, J. L., and Czech, F. P.,** Chloropyridyl phosphorothioate insecticide as dip and spray: efficacy against *Psoroptes ovis,* dermal toxicity for domesticated animals, selective carryout, and stability in the dipping vat, *Am. J. Vet. Res.,* 31, 2135, 1970.

68. **Roberts, I. H. and Meleney, W. P.,** Acaricidal treatments for protection of sheep against *Psoroptes ovis, J. Am. Vet. Med. Assoc.,* 158, 372, 1971.

69. **Meleney, W. P. and Roberts, I. H.,** Trials with eight acaricides against *Psoroptes ovis* the sheep scabies mite, in *Recent Advances in Acarology,* Vol. 2, Rodriguez, J. G., Ed., Academic Press, New York, 1979, 95.

70. **Roberts, I. H., Meleney, W. P., and Apodaca, S. A.,** Oral famphur for treatment of cattle lice, and against scabies mites and ear ticks of cattle and sheep, *J. Am. Vet. Med. Assoc.,* 155, 504, 1969.

71. **Meleney, W. P.,** Mange mites and other parasitic mites, in *Parasites, Pests and Predators,* Gaafar, S. M., Howard, W. E., and Marsh, R. E., Eds., Elsevier, Amsterdam, 1985, 317.

72. **Lofstedt, J.,** Dermatologic diseases of sheep, *Vet. Clin. N. Am. Large Anim. Pract.,* 5, 427, 1983.

73. **Roberts, I. H., Hanosh, G. J., and Apodaca, S. A.,** Observations on the incidence of chorioptic acariasis of sheep in the United States, *Am. J. Vet. Res.,* 25, 478, 1964.

74. **Sweatman, G. K. and Pullin, J. W.,** Toxicity of lindane and other acaricides to the eggs of the mange mite *Chorioptes bovis, Can. J. Comp. Med.,* 22, 409, 1958.

75. **Matthysse, J. G. and Marshall, J.,** The importance, relation to foot rot, and control of *Chorioptes bovis* on cattle and sheep, in *Advances in Acarology,* Vol. 1, Naegele, J. A., Ed., Cornell University Press, Ithaca, N.Y., 1963, 39.

76. **Babcock, O. G. and Hardy, W. T.,** The goat scab mite *Chorioptes caprae, Sheep Goat Raiser,* 40, 44, 1960.

77. **Kemper, H. E., Roberts, I. H., and Peterson, H. O.,** Tests with benzene hexachloride on chorioptic scab mites, *Sheep Goat Raiser,* 32, 56, 1952.

78. **Smith, M. C.,** Caprine dermatologic problems: a review, *J. Am. Vet. Med. Assoc.,* 178, 724, 1981.

79. **Bell, D. S., Pounden, W. D., Edgington, B. H., and Bentley, O. G.,** *Psorergates ovis*— a cause of itchiness in sheep, *J. Am. Vet. Med. Assoc.,* 120, 117, 1952.

80. **Roberts, I. H., Meleney, W. P., and Colbenson, H. P.,** Psorergatic acariasis on a New Mexico range ewe, *J. Am. Vet. Med. Assoc.,* 146, 24, 1965.

81. **Downing, W. and Mort, P.,** Experiments in the control of the itch mite, *Psorergates ovis,* Womersley, 1941, *Aust. Vet. J.,* 38, 269, 1962.

82. **Sinclair, A. N.,** Fleece derangement of Merino sheep infested by the itch mite *Psorergates ovis, N.Z. Vet. J.,* 24, 149, 1976.

83. **Hopkins, T. J.,** A new method for evaluating chemicals to control *Psorergates ovis* on sheep, *Vet. Med. Rev.,* 1981, 122, 1981.

84. **Swarup, D., Parai, T. P., and Lai, M.,** A report on clinical trial with malathion against sarcoptic mange in pashmina bearing goats, *Ind. Vet. J.,* 60, 399, 1983.

85. **Osman, O. M.,** A note on supatox against *Sarcoptes scabiei, Sudan J. Vet. Res.,* 1, 53, 1979.

86. **Baker, D. W. and Nutting, W. B.,** Demodectic mange in New York State sheep, *Cornell Vet.,* 40, 140, 1950.

87. **Cram, E. B.,** Demodectic mange of the goat in the United States, *J. Am. Vet. Med. Assoc.,* 66, 475, 1925.

88. **Hardenbergh, J. G. and Schlotthauer, C. F.,** Demodectic mange of the goat and its treatment, *J. Am. Vet. Med. Assoc.,* 67, 486, 1925.

89. **Durant, A. J.,** Demodectic mange of the milk goat, *Vet. Med.,* 39, 268, 1944.

90. **Miller, A. W.,** Sheep scab and its control, *U.S. Dep. Agric. Yearb. Agric.,* 904, 1942.

91. **Griffin, C. A. and Dean, D. J.,** Demodectic mange in goats, *Cornell Vet.,* 34, 308, 1944.

92. **Misra, A.,** Neguvon on demodectic mange in Beetal goats, *Ind. Vet. J.,* 41, 435, 1964.

93. **Das, D. N. and Misra, S. C.,** Studies on caprine demodectic mange with institution of effective therapeutic measures, *Ind. Vet. J.,* 49, 96, 1972.

94. **Williams, J. F. and Williams, C. S. F.,** Demodicosis in dairy goats, *J. Am. Vet. Med. Assoc.,* 180, 168, 1982.

95. **Euzeby, J., Chermiette, R., and Gevry, J.,** La demodecie de la chevre en France, *Inst. Nat. Rech. Agron. Publ. Les Maladus de la Chevre,* 28, 573, 1984.

96. **Littlejohn, A. I.,** Psoroptic mange in the goat, *Vet. Rec.,* 82, 148, 1968.

97. **Williams, J. F. and Williams, C. S. F.,** Psoroptic ear mites in dairy goats, *J. Am. Vet. Med. Assoc.,* 173, 1582, 1978.

98. **Schillhorn van Veen, T. W. and Williams, J. F.,** Some typical parasitic diseases of the goat, *Mod. Vet. Pract.,* 61, 847, 1980.

99. **Bishopp, F. C. and Laake, E. W.,** A preliminary statement regarding wool maggots of sheep in the United States, *J. Econ. Entomol.,* 8, 466, 1915.

100. **Bishopp, F. C.,** Flies which cause myiasis in man and animals—some aspects of the problem, *J. Econ. Entomol.,* 8, 317, 1915.

101. **Bishopp, F. C.,** Flytraps and their operation, *U.S. Dep. Agric. Farmers' Bull.,* 734, 1916.

102. **Bishopp, F. C., Mitchell, J. D., and Parman,, D. C.,** Screw-worms and other maggots affecting animals, *U.S. Dep. Agric. Farmers' Bull.,* 857, 1917.

103. **Bishopp, F. C., Cook, F. C., Parman, D. C., and Laake, E. W.,** Progress report of investigations relating to repellents, attractants and larvicides for the screw-worm and other flies, *J. Econ. Entomol.,* 16, 222, 1923.

104. **Parman, D. C.,** Benzene as a larvicide for screw worms, *J. Agric. Res.,* 31, 885, 1925.

105. **Bishopp, F. C., Roark, R. C., Parman, D. C., and Laake, E. W.,** Repellents and larvicides for the screw worm and other flies, *J. Econ. Entomol.,* 18, 776, 1925.

106. **Bishopp, F. C., Laake, E. W., and Parman D. C.,** Screw worms and other maggots affecting animals, *U.S. Dep. Agric. Farmers' Bull.,* 857, 1926.

107. **Parman, D. C., Laake, E. W., Bishopp, F. C., and Roark, R. C.,** Tests of blowfly baits and repellents during 1926, *U.S. Dep. Agric. Tech. Bull.,* 80, 1928.

108. **Bishopp, F. C.,** Flytraps and their operation, *U.S. Dep. Agric. Farmers' Bull.* 734, 1930.

109. **Cushing, E. C., and Patton, W. S.,** Studies on the higher Diptera of medical and veterinary importance, *Cochliomyia americana* sp.nov., the screw-worm fly of the new world, *Ann. Trop. Med. Parasitol.,* 27, 539, 1933.

110. **Laake, E. W., Cushing, E. C., and Parish, H. E.,** Biology of the primary screw worm fly, *Cochliomyia americana,* and a comparison of its stages with those of *C. macellaria, U.S. Dep. Agric. Tech. Bull.,* 500, 1936.

111. **Knipling, E. F.,** Toxicity of certain chemicals to the fleece worms *Phormia regina* (Meig.), *Cochliomyia macellaria* (F.) and *Lucillia sericata* (Meig.), *J. Econ. Entomol.,* 34, 314, 1941.

112. **Knipling, E. F.,** A preliminary report on a treatment for fleece-worm infestations in sheep, *J. Econ. Entomol.,* 35, 896, 1942.

113. **Graham, O. H. and Eddy, G. W.**, Persistence of chlorinated camphene as a fleece worm larvicide, *J. Econ. Entomol.*, 41, 521, 1948.

114. **Eddy, G. W. And Bushland, R. C.,**, Fleeceworms, *U.S. Dep. Agric. Yearb. Agric.*, 175, 1956.

115. **Marquardt, W. C. and Hawkins, W. W., Jr.**, Experimental therapy of fly strike in sheep, using a systemic insecticide, *J. Am. Vet. Med. Assoc.*, 132, 429, 1958.

116. **McGregor, W. S. and Miller, W. O.**, Trolene and Korlan show promise for parasite control in sheep, *Down Earth*, 14, 7, 1958.

117. **Brundrett, H. M. and Graham, O. H.**, Bayer 21/199 as a deterrent to screw-worm attack in sheep, *J. Econ. Entomol.*, 51, 407, 1958.

118. **Fuchs, T. W.**, External parasites of sheep and goats, *Proc. Int. Ranchers Roundup*, 313, 1983.

119. **Stewart, J. R.**, Treatment for *Oestrus ovis*, *J. Am. Vet. Med. Assoc.*, 80, 108, 1932.

120. **Gildow, E. M. and Hickman, C. W.**, A new treatment for *Oestrus ovis*, larvae in the head of sheep, *J. Am. Vet. Med. Assoc.*, 79, 210, 1931.

121. **Mitchell, W. C. and Cobbett, N. G.**, Field investigations relative to control of *Oestrus ovis*, *J. Am. Vet. Med. Assoc.*, 83, 247, 1933.

122. **Cobbett, N. G.**, An effective treatment for the control of the sheep head grub, *Oestrus ovis*, in areas where the winters are cold, *J. Am. Vet. Med. Assoc.*, 97, 565, 1940.

123. **Cobbett, N. G.**, A method of large-scale treatment of sheep for the destruction of head grubs ($=$ *Oestrus ovis*), *J. Am. Vet. Med. Assoc.*, 97, 571, 1940.

124. **Peterson, H. O., Jones, E. M., and Cobbett, N. G.**, Effectiveness of Dow ET-57 (Trolene) against the nasal botfly of sheep, *Am. J. Vet. Res.*, 19, 129, 1958.

125. **Peterson, H. O., Cobbett, N. G., and Meleney, W. P.**, Treatment of *Oestrus ovis* with dimethoate, *Vet. Med.*, 54, 377, 1959.

126. **Peterson, H. O., Meleney, W. P., and Cobbett, N. G.**, The use of organic phosphorus compounds in destroying *Oestrus ovis* larvae, *Proc. U.S. Livestock Sanit. Assoc.*, 178, 1960.

127. **Chavarria, M. and Carrillo, R. A.**, A new and effective treatment for nasal myiasis caused by *Oestrus ovis* Linn., *Zentralbl. Veterinaermed.*, 6, 816, 1959.

128. **Miller, J. H., Johnson, H. E., and Stout, A. L.**, Control of nasal botfly in sheep, *J. Am. Vet. Med. Assoc.*, 138, 431, 1961.

129. **Drummond, R. O.**, Control of larvae of *Oestrus ovis* in sheep with systemic insecticides, *J. Parasitol.*, 48, 211, 1962.

130. **Knapp, F. W. and Drudge, J. H.**, Efficacy of several organic phosphates against the botfly of sheep, *Am. J. Vet. Res.*, 25, 1686, 1964.

131. **Drummond, R. O.**, Systemic insecticides to control larvae of *Oestrus ovis* in sheep, *J. Parasitol.*, 52, 192, 1966.

132. **Pfadt, R. E.**, Sheep bot fly control tests, *J. Econ. Entomol.*, 57, 928, 1964.

133. **Pfadt, R. E.**, Mortality of nasal bots in sheep treated with systemic insecticides, *J. Econ. Entomol.*, 60, 1420, 1967.

134. **Pfadt, R. E., Lloyd, J. E., and Spackman, E.**, Sheep, mortality of nasal bots in sheep treated with systemic insecticides, 1977. *Insectic. Acaric. Tests*, 3, 189, 1978.

135. **Meleney, W. P., Cobbett, N. G., and Peterson, H. O.**, Control of *Oestrus ovis* in sheep on an isolated range, *J. Am. Vet. Med. Assoc.*, 143, 986, 1963.

136. **Lyons, E. T., Drudge, J. H., and Knapp, F. W.**, Controlled test of anthelmintic activity of trichlorfon and thiabendazole in lambs, with observations on *Oestrus ovis*, *Am. J. Vet. Res.*, 28, 111, 1967.

137. **Partosoedjono, S., Drudge, J. H., Lyons, E. T., and Knapp, F. W.**, Evaluation of naphthalophos against *Oestrus ovis* and a thiabendazole-tolerant strain of *Haemonchus contortus* in lambs, *Am. J. Vet. Res.*, 30, 81, 1969.

138. **Buchanan, R. S., Dewhirst, L. W., and Ware, G. W.**, The importance of sheep bot fly larvae and their control with systemic insecticides in Arizona, *J. Econ. Entomol.*, 62, 675, 1969.

139. **Roncalli, R. A., Barbosa, A., and Fernandez, J. F.**, The efficacy of rafoxanide against the larval stages of *Oestrus ovis* in sheep, *Vet. Rec.*, 289, 1971.

140. **Horak, I. G., Louw, J. P., and Raymond, S. M.**, Trials with rafoxanide, 3. Efficacy of rafoxanide against the larvae of the sheep nasal bot fly *Oestrus ovis*, Linne, 1761, *J. S. Afr. Vet. Med. Assoc.*, 42, 337, 1971.

141. **Snijders, A. J., Horak, I. G., and Louw, J. P.**, Trails with rafoxanide, 6. The effect of repeated and single treatments with rafoxanide against *Haemonchus contortus* and *Oestrus ovis* in sheep, *J. S. Afr. Vet. Med. Assoc.*, 44, 251, 1973.

142. **Wellington, A. C.**, Efficacy of nitroxynil against *Oestrus ovis* in sheep, *Vet. Rec.*, 116, 322, 1985.

143. **Yawzinski, T. A., Greenway, T., Presson, B. L., Pote, L. M., Featherstone, H., and Williams, M.**, Antiparasitic efficacy of Ivermectin in naturally parasitized sheep, *Am. J. Vet. Res.*, 44, 2186, 1983.

144. **Preston, J. M.**, Ivermectin and the control of nematodiasis in sheep, *Prev. Vet. Med.*, 2, 309, 1984.

145. **Roncalli, R. A.**, Efficacy of Ivermectin against *Oestrus ovis* in sheep, *Vet. Med.*, 79, 1095, 1984.

146. **Pfadt, R. E. and Campbell, J.,** Sheep bot fly control tests with DDVP, *J. Econ. Entomol.,* 56, 530, 1963.
147. **Prasert, V., Knapp, F. W., Lyons, E. T., and Drudge, J. H.,** Biological effects of methroprene on the sheep bot fly, *J. Econ. Entomol.,* 68, 639, 1975.
148. **Jones, R. H.,** Some observations on biting flies attacking sheep, *Mosq. News,* 21, 113, 1961.
149. **Campbell, J. B. and Doane, T. H.,** Weight gain response and efficacy of washing and various insecticide treatments for prevention of flies feeding on shear wounds of summer shorn lambs, *J. Econ. Entomol.,* 70, 132, 1977.

Chapter 14

CONTROL OF ARTHROPOD PESTS OF SWINE*

I. INTRODUCTION

In the U.S. and Canada, the two major arthropod pests of swine are a blood-sucking louse, the hog louse[*], *Haematopinus suis* (Linnaeus), and the itch mite[*], *Sarcoptes scabiei* (DeGeer). Also, swine may be infested with the hog follicle mite[*], *Demodex phylloides* Csokor, the cause of demodectic mange, and, in some locations, fleas and ticks. In addition, swine may be hosts for biting flies, such as the stable fly[*], *Stomoxys calcitrans* (Linnaeus), mosquitoes, horse and deer flies, and biting gnats. A variety of nonbiting flies, such as the house fly[*], *Musca domestica* Linnaeus, *Fannia* spp., *Ophyra* spp., and other species, may be found associated with swine and swine-rearing areas, which can vary from very intensive, highly cleaned, and environmentally controlled facilities to open, unmanaged extensive lots. Technologies used to control flies that breed in manure and are found around structures are presented in Chapter 18. Therefore, this chapter will concentrate only on technologies used to control arthropod pests that directly parasitize swine.

A comprehensive, practical review of the current technologies used in the U.S. to control lice and mites of swine was presented by Williams.[1] Some general control measures were also presented in a chapter in *Livestock Entomology*.[2] Sarcoptic mange in swine was reviewed by Yeoman,[3,4] who described the problems associated with *S. scabiei*, listed shortcomings of present treatment materials, and was encouraged by activity of systemic acaricides that may allow for the eradication of the mite from swine. Recently, Meleney[5] included biology and control of *S. scabiei* on swine in his broad review of parasitic mites of livestock.

II. CONTROL OF THE HOG LOUSE AND ITCH MITE

A. Early Treatment Technology

In 1896, Osborn[6] described the pest aspects of the hog louse (then called *H. urius* Nitzsch) and listed the following control technologies: washes or sprays of tobacco water, carbolic acid, or kerosene emulsion; ointments of sulfur or kerosene in lard; and dusting with ashes, charcoal, or road dust. *S. scabiei* was not listed as an important pest. The first issue of *U.S. Dep. Agric. Farmers' Bulletin* No. 1085 in 1920[7] listed five methods of applying treatments to swine to control lice and itch mites: hand application of liquids, spraying, hog oilers, medicated hog wallows, and dipping vats. There were no effective treatments for demodectic mange. Hand-applied materials, which included crude petroleum, a mixture of cottonseed oil and kerosene, or a mixture of kerosene and lard, were to be liberally applied to each animal with a brush, mop, or cloth. Sprayers could be used to apply the chemicals used as dips. Hog oilers consisted of a post or rod on which was placed a sack, rope, or other absorbent material that was saturated with oil which was transferred to the swine when they rubbed the device. Coverage was limited, treatment erratic, and oilers tended to become dry and caked with mud. Swine instinctively wallow in shallow water in warm weather to cool themselves. Medicated wallows consisted of man-made shallow troughs usually charged with water, but intermittently charged with chemicals in order to treat swine; crude petroleum that floated on the surface of water in the wallow was suggested as the most effective

---

* Common names of insects and acarines, as listed in *Common Names of Insects and Related Organisms* (published by the Entomological Society of America), are marked with a [*] the first time they are cited preceding the scientific name.

material. The dipping of swine in a small dipping vat was considered the most effective method of treatment. Dip materials included crude petroleum, lime-sulfur, coal-tar creosote, and the arsenical dip used to control cattle ticks. The treatment methods and materials listed in the original issue of this bulletin were only slightly changed in the 1923,[8] 1924,[9] 1933,[10] and 1937[11] issues of the bulletin.

Sprays of an emulsion of a white oil, called Volck oil, killed adult and nymphal lice but had no effect on louse eggs or itch mites.[12] In the 1942 *U.S. Dep. Agric. Yearbook of Agriculture,* the most practical treatments listed for louse control were dipping swine in crude petroleium and applying kerosene emulsion by hand.[13] Mange control consisted of two or more dippings in crude petroleum or four or more dippings in lime sulfur.[14] Pyrethrins synergized with piperonyl butoxide in "hog oil" sprayed onto swine or onto burlap attached to a rubbing post controlled hog lice.[15]

B. Organochlorine Treatments

The materials used to control mites and lice on swine were relatively unchanged until the appearance of the organochlorine insecticides after World War II. Because a single spray or dip treatment DDT, TDE, or chlordane killed nymphs and adults and had sufficient residual activity to kill newly hatched nymphs, usually one treatment eradicated lice.[16,17] Sarcoptic mange was eradicated with a single spray of benzene hexachloride (BHC), lindane, or chlordane, but benzyl benzoate, DDT, and rotenone were not completely effective.[18-21] Single sprays of lindane or chlordane generally eradicated itch mites, and toxaphene was highly effective.[22] The 1952 issue of Bulletin No. 1085[23] still listed the treatment methods and materials presented in the earlier editions of the bulletin and also noted that lindane, BHC, chlordane, and toxaphene dips were replacing earlier treatments for both pests. DDT controlled lice but not mites.

The 1956 *U.S. Dep. Agric. Yearbook of Agriculture* noted that the older preparations for louse control had been replaced by BHC, lindane, DDT, chlordane, and toxaphene, which should be applied twice as dips or sprays with a 10 to 14-day interval to eliminate lice.[24] BHC, lindane, and chlordane replaced the older remedies for sarcoptic mange and, although no specific cure for demodectic mange was known, frequent treatment in crude petroleum, lindane, or BHC may control the disease.[25]

C. Organophosphorus Treatments

Starting in the late 1950s, malathion,[26] coumaphos, and trichlorfon,[27] chlorfenvinphos, crotoxyphos, carbaryl (a carbamate), methoxychlor and Dilan,®[28] and stirofos[29] controlled lice as sprays. Itch mites were controlled with a single spray of malathion.[30]

In a unique treatment technique in which organophosphorus granules were placed in dry hog wallows so that the swine would treat themselves, ronnel killed both lice and eggs, but dimethoate was ineffective.[31,32] Dusts of crotoxyphos, coumaphos, and stirofos applied to bedding areas also controlled lice.[33] However, sprays of ronnel or a combination of crotoxyphos and dichlorvos or a dust of crotoxyphos did not control itch mites.[34] Ronnel controlled lice when applied to swine as a cold fog mist in mineral oil.[35] Phosmet spray provided poor to fair control of itch mites.[36]

The pouron treatment method, in which ca. 15 to 30 cm^3 of concentrated insecticide per 45 kg of body weight was applied along the backline of swine, was used[37] for lice control; two treatments of fenthion pouron at a 3-week interval were necessary to control lice. The spoton treatment method, in which 2 cm^3 of concentrated insecticide per 45 kg of body weight was applied to a single spot on the backline, was also used for lice control; a single treatment of fenthion spoton controlled lice.[38] A similar spoton treatment of chlorpyrifos killed all lice and their eggs apparently by both contact and fumigant action.[39] A pouron treatment of 30 cm^3 of phosmet per 45 kg provided excellent control of lice.[40] In England, phosmet applied as a pouron at the rate of 1 cm³/10 kg to the backline (and to the ears) controlled itch mites by both contact and systemic activity.[41]

D. Newer Treatment Technology

In tests in England, sarcoptic mange in pigs was controlled by one or two applications of a spray of amitraz.[42]

Permethrin dust or spray killed nymphal and adult lice, but a second treatment was necessary to provide complete control of lice.[43] Two sprays of permethrin were ineffective against itch mites.[44]

A unique method of treatment for the control of lice was the application of fenvalerate-impregnated ear tags (one per year) to swine.[45] Lice were eliminated in three of four tests and there were no adverse reactions in the animals.

Issues of *Insecticides and Acaricide Tests* since 1979 have contained data on the control of lice and mites on swine: a single spray of fenvalerate eliminated lice, but two sprays were necessary to eliminate mites; phosmet spray did not control itch mites, but a pouron was effective against lice; two treatments with permethrin spray or dust eliminated lice; fenvalerate-impregnated ear tags eliminated lice, while permethrin- or flucythrinate-impregnated ear tags were only slightly less effective; a single spray of permethrin eliminated lice while a phosmet spray was slightly less effective.

E. Systemic Insecticides

The use of systemic insecticides has been investigated for the control of lice and mites on swine. Coumaphos given orally was ineffective, but oral treatments of trichlorfon were systemically effective against nymphs but not adults.[27] In Germany, trichlorfon was administered orally for 3 consecutive days and the treatment repeated at 2 weeks controlled itch mites.[46] Famphur was ineffective orally against itch mites.[34]

The advent of ivermectin, a highly effective animal systemic insecticide that controls a variety of external and internal parasites of livestock, has the potential to revolutionize the control of lice and mites of swine. A single oral or subcutaneous treatment usually eliminated both species.[47-55]

III. CONTROL OF FLIES, FLEAS, AND OTHER PESTS

Although certain biting flies, nonbiting flies, fleas, and other arthropods are listed as pests of swine,[56,57] there are no reports in the literature on the use of specific methods or materials applied directly to swine for their control. In the original edition of *U.S. Dep. Agric. Farmers' Bulletin* No. 683[58] in 1915, control of the human flea♦, *Pulex irritans* (Linnaeus), or the sticktight flea♦, *Echidnophaga gallinacea* (Westwood), on swine was accomplished by dipping swine in creosote dips or sprinkling crude petroleum on them. Some of the insecticides and acaricides that were labeled for application directly to swine for the control of lice and mites were also listed as treatments that will control house flies, fleas, the horn fly♦, *Haematobia irritans* (Linnaeus), stable flies, and ticks.[59]

IV. OVERVIEW AND CURRENT TECHNOLOGY

The changes in swine production systems, in that more and more swine are being raised in confinement and under strict management practices, have not lessened the parasitism by external pests. Although fleas are seldom seen in modern systems, swine can be infested with lice and mites. These confinement systems have increased the problems of flies and other pests that breed in the manure from these facilities. The stresses of confinement and demands of modern swine production make it more important than ever that the external parasites of swine be controlled or eliminated, for their presence can cause serious production losses.

The treatment methodology used to control the hog louse and the itch mite, which are the major arthropod pests of swine, has changed litttle since the 1900s. Swine have been and can be sprayed or dipped in a variety of insecticides. Pouron or spoton treatments are relatively easy to apply to swine and dusts or granules can be used to treat bedding areas.

Although not a part of current technology, the use of ivermectin, an extremely effective animal systemic insecticide, has the potential to change treatment methodology. A single oral or subcutaneous treatment essentially eliminates lice and mites. However, if such a systemic treatment is used to treat swine, then a concurrent treatment of the swine holding facilities is needed in order to control those mites and lice that are not on the swine when they are treated.

REFERENCES

1. **Williams, R. E.**, External swine parasites lice and mite infestations still a common problem, *Anim. Nutr. Health*, 36, 16, 1981.
2. **Williams, R. E.**, Arthropod pests of swine, in *Livestock Entomology*, Williams, R. E., Hall, R. D., Broce, A. B., and Scholl, P. J., Eds., John Wiley & Sons, New York, 1985, 239.
3. **Yeoman, G. H.**, Pig mange. I. A management problem of modern systems, *Livestock Int.*, 11, 116, 1983.
4. **Yeoman, G. H.**, Pig mange. II. Control by modern methods, *Livestock Int.*, 11, 146, 1983.
5. **Meleney, W. P.**, Mange mites and other parasitic mites, in *Parasites, Pests and Predators*, Gaafar, S. M., Howard, W. E., and Marsh, R. E., Eds., Elsevier, Amsterdam, 1985, 317.
6. **Osborn, H.**, Insects affecting domestic animals: an account of the species of importance in North America, with mention of related forms occurring on other animals, *U.S. Dep. Agric. Bull.*, 5, 1896.
7. **Imes, M.**, Hog lice and hog mange methods of control and eradication, *U.S. Dep. Agric. Farmers' Bull.*, 1085, 1920.
8. **Imes, M.**, Hog lice and hog mange methods of control and eradication, *U.S. Dep. Agric. Farmers' Bull.*, 1085, 1923.
9. **Imes, M.**, Hog lice and hog mange methods of control and eradication, *U.S. Dep. Agric. Farmers' Bull.*, 1085, 1924.
10. **Imes, M.**, Hog lice and hog mange methods of control and eradication, *U.S. Dep. Agric. Farmers' Bull.*, 1085, 1933.
11. **Imes, M.**, Hog lice and hog mange methods of control and eradication, *U.S. Dep. Agric. Farmers' Bull.*, 1085, 1937.
12. **Hall, D. G.**, Volck oil, special emulsion number two, as an animal insecticide, *J. Kans. Entomol. Soc.*, 2, 74, 1929.
13. **Babcock, O. G. and Cushing, E. C.**, Hog lice, *U.S. Dep. Agric. Yearb. Agric.*, 741, 1942.
14. **Imes, M.**, Mange of swine, *U.S. Dep. Agric. Yearb. Agric.*, 734, 1942.
15. **Moore, D. H.**, Effectiveness of piperonyl butoxide and pyrethrum as a practical treatment for hog lice, *J. Parasitol.*, 33, 439, 1947.
16. **Kemper, H. E. and Roberts, I. H.**, Preliminary tests with DDT for single-treatment eradication of the swine louse, *Haematopinus suis*, *J. Am. Vet. Med. Assoc.*, 109, 252, 1946.
17. **Sweetman, H. L.**, New organic insecticides to control hog lice, *J. Econ. Entomol.*, 40, 454, 1947.
18. **Hixson, E. and Muma, M. H.**, Hog mange control tests, *J. Econ. Entomol.*, 40, 451, 1947.
19. **Spencer, W. T.**, Sarcoptic swine mange control tests with chlordane, *J. Am. Vet. Med. Assoc.*, 113, 153, 1948.
20. **Cobbett, N. G., Peterman, J. E., and Beagle, A. G.**, Eradication of sarcoptic mange of hogs by a single treatment of benzene hexachloride sprays, *Vet. Med.*, 43, 407, 1948.
21. **Sweetman, H. L., Wells, L. F., Jr., Toczydlowski, A. H., and Moore, S., III**, Mange and fly control with lindane in a piggery, *J. Econ. Entomol.*, 44, 112, 1951.
22. **Roberts, I. H. and Rogoff, W. M.**, Organic insecticides for the control of swine mange, *J. Am. Vet. Med. Assoc.*, 123, 227, 1953.
23. **Kemper, H. E. and Peterson, H. O.**, Hog lice and hog mange methods of control and eradication, *U. S. Dep. Agric. Farmers' Bull.*, 1085, 1952.

24. **Cobbett, N. G. and Bushland, R. C.,** The hog louse, *U.S. Dep. Agric. Yearb. Agric.*, 345, 1956.

25. **Cobbett, N. G.,** Hog mange, *U.S. Dep. Agric. Yearb. Agric.*, 347, 1956.

26. **Johnson, W. T.,** Tests with malathion for hog lice control, *J. Econ. Entomol.*, 51, 255, 1958.

27. **DeLeon, D. D., Turk, R. D., and Hale, F.,** Observations on the control of *Haematopinus suis* and *Ascaris lumbricoides* of swine, *J. Am. Vet. Med. Assoc.*, 138, 179, 1961.

28. **Roberts, R. H.,** Studies on the control of the hog louse, *Haematopinus suis, J. Econ. Entomol.*, 58, 378, 1965.

29. **Butler, J. F.,** Rabon for hog louse control in Florida, *Fla. Entomol.*, 56, 227, 1973.

30. **Raun, E. S. and Ahrens, R. H.,** A field test of malathion to control sarcoptic mange of hogs, *J. Econ. Entomol.*, 49, 140, 1956.

31. **Johnson, W. T.,** Hog louse control by ground treatment, *J. Econ. Entomol.*, 54, 821, 1961.

32. **McGregor, W. S. and Gray, H. E.,** Korlan insecticide granules for control of hog lice, *Down Earth*, 19, 1, 1963.

33. **Lancaster, J. L., Jr. and Simco, J. S.,** Applying dust to bedding to control hog louse, *Arkansas Farm Res.*, 17, 5, 1968.

34. **Magee, J. C.,** Studies on *Sarcoptes scabiei* on swine in Iowa, *Proc. North Cent. Branch Entomol. Soc. Am.*, 29, 125, 1974.

35. **DeWitt, J. R.,** A new technique provides control of lice on swine with korlan insecticide, *Pract. Nutr.*, 9, 1, 1975.

36. **Roberts, J. E., Sr. and Kondratieff, B. C.,** Swine, sarcoptic mange control, 1979, *Va. J. Sci.*, 31(Abstr.), 85, 1980.

37. **Buckman, A. F. and Roberts, J. E., Sr.,** Insecticidal control of lice on swine, *Va. J. Sci.*, 27 (Abstr.), 31, 1976.

38. **Knapp, F. W., Christensen, C. M., and Whiteker, M. D.,** Fenthion spot treatment for control of the hog louse, *J. Anim. Sci.*, 45, 216, 1977.

39. **Surgeoner, G. A.,** Evidence of ovicidal activity by fumigant action using chlorpyrifos for control *Haematopinus suis* (Anoplura: Haematopinidae), *Proc. Entomol. Soc. Ont.*, 110, 3, 1979.

40. **Roberts, J. E., Sr. and Kondratieff, B.,** Swine, control of hog lice on brood sows, 1978, *Va. J. Sci.*, 31 (Abstr.), 85, 1980.

41. **Hewett, G. R., and Heard, T. W.,** Phosmet for the systemic control of pig mange, *Vet. Rec.*, 111, 558, 1982.

42. **Griffiths, A. J.,** Amitraz — for the control of animal ectoparasites with particular reference to sheep tick *(Ixodes ricinus)* and pig mange *(Sarcoptes scabiei), Proc. 8th Br. Insect. Fungic. Conf.*, 2, 557, 1975.

43. **Roberts, J. E., Sr. and Kondratieff, B.,** Swine, hog louse control with Ectiban®, 1979, *Va. J. Sci.*, 31(Abstr.), 86, 1980.

44. **Galloway, T. D. and Giberson, D. J.,** Efficacy of permethrin as a whole body spray against hog mange mite, *Pestic. Res. Rep.* (Agric. Can.), 204, 1983.

45. **Roberts, J. E., Sr. and Saluta, M.,** Control of the hog louse, *Haematopinus suis* (Linnaeus) (Anoplura: Haematopinadae), on brood sows, *Sus scrofa* (Linnaeus), with Ectrin® 8% ear tags, *Va. J. Sci.*, 34(Abstr.), 107, 1983.

46. **Mauck, C. and Mickwitz, G.,** Combined mange and *Ascaris* treatment in weaned pigs with Neguvon®, *Dtsch. Tierarzt. Woschr.*, 72, 521, 1965.

47. **Barth, D. and Brokken, E. S.,** The activity of 22, 23-dihydroavermectin B_1 against the pig louse, *Haematopinus suis, Vet. Rec.*, 106, 388, 1980.

48. **Lee, R. P., Dooge, D. J. D., and Preston, J. M.,** Efficacy of Ivermectin against *Sarcoptes scabiei* in pigs, *Vet. Rec.*, 107, 503, 1980.

49. **Hogg, A.,** Treatment of sarcoptic mange in swine with Ivermectin: a pilot study, in *Proc. Annu. Meet. Livest. Conserv. Inst.*, 134, 1981.

50. **Stewart, T. B., Marti, O. G., and Hale, O. M.,** Efficacy of Ivermectin against five genera of swine nematodes and the hog louse, *Haematopinus suis, Am. J. Vet. Res.*, 42, 1425, 1981.

51. **Courtney, C. H., Ingalls, W. L., and Stitzlein, S. L.,** Ivermectin for the control of swine scabies: relative values of prefarrowing treatment of sows and weaning treatment of pigs, *Am. J. Vet. Res.*, 44, 1220, 1983.

52. **Martineau, G. P., Vaillancourt, J., and Frechette, J. L.,** Control of *Sarcoptes scabiei* infestation with Ivermectin in a large intensive breeding piggery, *Can. Vet. J.*, 25, 235, 1984.

53. **Alva-Valdes, R., Wallace, D. H., Benz, G. W., Foster, A. G., and Holste, J. E.,** Efficacy of Ivermectin against the mange mite *Sarcoptes scabiei var suis* in pigs, *Am. J. Vet. Res.*, 45, 2113, 1984.

54. **Brokken, E. S., Roncalli, R. A., Sutherland, I. H., and Leaning, W. H. D.,** Ivermectin, a new broad spectrum antiparastic agent for swine, *Int. Pig Vet. Soc. Proc. 8th Congr.*, 205, 1984.

55. **Hogg, A.,** Eradication of sarcoptic mange in swine with ivermectin, *Int. Pig Vet. Soc. Proc. 8th Congr.*, 206, 1984.

56. **Griffiths, H. J.,** External parasites, in *Diseases of Swine,* Dunne, H. W., Ed., Iowa State College Press, Ames, 1958, 405.

57. **Weiner, T. J. and Hansens, E. J.**, Species and numbers of bloodsucking flies feeding on hogs and other animals in southern New Jersey, *J. N. Y. Entomol. Soc.*, 83, 198, 1975.
58. **Bishopp, F. C.**, Fleas as pests to man and animals, with suggestions for their control, *U.S. Dep. Agric., Farmers' Bull. No. 683*, 1915.
59. **Hogg, A. and Swieczkowski, T.**, External parasites of swine, *Vet. Clin. N. Am. Large Anim. Pract.*, 4, 343, 1982.

Chapter 15

CONTROL OF ARTHROPOD PESTS OF POULTRY*

I. INTRODUCTION

Domesticated fowl, primarily chickens and turkeys, and, to a lesser extent, ducks, geese, pigeons, guinea fowl, quail, and pheasants are parasitized by a wide variety of arthropod pests. Certain pests, such as lice and several species of mites, all stages of which are found on the host, and fleas, which spend their adult stage on the host, are continuous parasites and are usually controlled by application of chemicals directly to the host. Other pests, such as other species of mites, bed bugs, chiggers, ticks, and biting flies (mosquitoes, gnats, etc.), found only on poultry while feeding, spend the remainder of their life cycles away from the hosts and are usually controlled by application of chemicals to the environment of poultry.

In addition to these external pests of poultry, the large amounts of poultry manure that accumulate beneath caged poultry in modern, large-scale poultry production systems can be the source of massive numbers of nuisance flies that can be a serious problem to poultry, poultry owners, and their often outraged neighbors. The technologies used to control flies and other pests that breed in poultry manure are reviewed in Chapter 16.

This chapter will focus on the technology used to control ectoparasitic arthropod pests. Loomis[1] presented a practical, comprehensive review of arthropod parasites of poultry and detailed a number of control technologies. General information on the biology and control of arthropod pests of poultry was presented in a chapter in *Livestock Entomology*.[2]

Currently, the most important and common arthropod pest of poultry, especially caged layers, in the U.S., is the northern fowl mite*, *Ornithonyssus sylviarum* (Canestrini and Fanzago). This mite spends its life cycle on the host, and the stresses induced by large populations of these mites can cause lowered egg production, reduced weight gains, increased feed consumption, and reduced production of seminal fluid. The crawling and biting of these mites also irritate persons who work with poultry or handle eggs. A closely related species, the tropical fowl mite*, *O. bursa* (Berlese), has been rarely reported in more tropical climates of the southern U.S.

Poultry are hosts for a variety of biting lice. The most important species, in terms of need for control, are the chicken body louse*, *Menacanthus stramineus* (Nitzsch), and the shaft louse*, *Menopon gallinae* (Linnaeus). Other biting lice found on domesticated poultry are the chicken head louse*, *Cuclotogaster heterographus* (Nitzsch), the fluff louse*, *Goniocotes gallinae* (DeGeer), the brown chicken louse *, *Goniodes dissimilis* Denny, the large chicken louse*, *G. gigas* (Taschenberg), the wing louse*, *Lipeurus caponis* (Linnaeus), the slender turkey louse*, *Oxylipeurus polytrapezius* (Burmeister), and the large turkey louse*, *Chelopistes meleagridis* (Linnaeus). In addition, other species of poultry — ducks, geese, pigeons, guinea fowl — have their own species of lice.

Because of modern methods of mass rearing poultry, infestations of the depluming mite*, *Knemidokoptes gallinae* (Railliet), or the scalyleg mite*, *K. mutans* (Robin & Lauguetin), are rare. These mites live at the base of the feathers or under scales on legs and can cause loss of feathers or severe crusts to form on legs. All stages are found on hosts. The feather mite*, *Megninia cubitalis* (Megnin), may rarely be found on feathers of fowl, but is not economically important.

---

* Common names of insects and acarines, as listed in *Common Names of Insects and Related Organisms* (published by the Entomological Society of America), are marked with a * the first time they are cited preceding the scientific name.

Poultry are parasitized by fleas, especially the sticktight flea♦, *Echidnophaga gallinacea* (Westwood). Other species of fleas that may be found on poultry include the European chicken flea♦, *Ceratophyllus gallinae* (Schrank); the western chicken flea♦, *C. niger* Fox; the dog flea♦, *Ctenocephalides canis* (Curtis); the cat flea♦, *C. felis* (Bouche); and the human flea♦, *Pulex irritans* Linnaeus. Adult fleas are highly mobile, except for the sticktight flea, which tends to permanently attach on the head of fowl and are found continually on the host. Females lay eggs that fall to the litter or bedding material where the nonparasitic larvae feed on organic matter. It is important to clean the premises so that there is little or no food available for flea larvae. Treatment of the premises also can control flea larvae.

Several other important pests spend some or most of their life cycle off of poultry. The chicken mite♦, *Dermanyssus gallinae* (DeGeer), lives on roosts and in cracks and crevices of poultry houses, and all feeding stages migrate to poultry to feed while the fowl roost or spend time in nests. Females lay eggs in the cracks and crevices of poultry structures. Nymphs and adults of the fowl tick♦, *Argas persicus* (Oken), or closely related species, *A. radiatus* Railliet, *A. sanchesi* Duges, and *A. miniatus* Koch, feed on poultry for short periods of time, from a few minutes to a few hours, but larvae may stay attached to poultry and feed for 1 week or so. Eggs are laid in cracks and crevices of buildings and other structures that house poultry. Nymphal and adult fowl ticks may live for several years without feeding.

Poultry may be infested with the bed bug♦, *Cimex lectularius* Linnaeus. The nymphal and adult stages feed on poultry for 5 to 30 min at night; the remainder of the time they stay hidden in cracks and crevices of structures. In modern, well-constructed caged layer, broiler, or breeder houses, infestations of the chicken mite, fowl ticks, and bed bugs are rarely encountered. However, infestations of these arthropods may still be encountered in older breeder houses and small "backyard" or homeowner flocks.

In certain areas of the southern U.S., turkeys confined to ranges with heavy clay soils may be attacked by larvae of the turkey chigger♦, *Neoschongastia americana* (Hirst). These larvae tend to feed in groups on turkeys and cause skin lesions at the feeding site. If turkeys are processed before the lesions heal, the lesions must be removed by trimming away the skin. Such trimming causes a downgrading of the carcass and an economic loss to the processor. Control of turkey chiggers consists of applying insecticides to the ranges to kill the chiggers before they can attach to turkeys.

Poultry can be hosts to a variety of mosquitoes, biting gnats, and black flies. Of special significance are black flies in the genus *Simulium* that are vectors of a protozoan, *Leucocytozoon smithi* (Lavern and Sucet), the agent of gnat fever or turkey malaria, an important disease of turkeys in South Carolina. Control of these arthropods is accomplished by treating streams with insecticides to kill the larval stages of the flies.

II. CONTROL OF LICE AND MITES

A. Early Treatment Technology

Early literature on the control of arthropod pests of poultry focused on the control of the chicken mite, lice, *Knemidokoptes* mites, ticks, and fleas. Poultry raising was generally limited to the keeping of "backyard" flocks and a few laying hens for eggs. In 1896, Osborn[3] described the pest aspects of many species of biting lice on domestic and wild fowl and listed treatment of poultry with washes of glycerin and carbolic acid in water, pyrethrins dust, and tobacco dust or dip, or allowing poultry access to road dust or ashes in self-treatment dust-bath boxes. To control the chicken mite, he suggested spraying poultry houses with kerosene, kerosene emulsion, benzene, or gasoline, dusting with carbolated lime, painting with lime whitewash, or sulfur fumigation. Banks[4] listed many of the same treatments plus the use of a mixture of sulfur and lime as a dust or naphthalene as a fumigant to control lice. *K. mutans* could be controlled with sulfur ointment or naphthalene in lard applied to the infested areas of the animal. He noted that a sure preventive for these mites and lice was to never allow them to enter the premises on infested poultry.

Other early authors emphasized the need for clean surroundings and light as a prerequisite for control of the chicken mite and fleas. Even burning down the building was suggested as a method to eliminate the chicken mite. A mixture of plaster of Paris and carbolic acid in self-treatment dust-bath boxes controlled lice. Lice were also controlled by putting a minute amount of mercurial ointment under the wing or around the vent. Sulfur ointment or a mixture of caraway oil and lard or vasoline applied to the legs controlled scalyleg mites; the chicken mite was controlled by treating roosts with a variety of materials including carbolenium, a mixture of coal tar and carbolic acid.[5,6] Fumigation of poultry with nitro-benzene controlled lice and scalyleg mites.[7]

The first issue of *U.S. Dep. Agric. Farmers' Bulletin* No. 801[8] in 1917 focused on control of the chicken mite by treating premises, nest boxes, and roosts with crude petroleum, anthracene oil, or even arsenic cattle dip. The scalyleg mite was controlled with crude petroleum and the depluming mite with sulfur ointment. Chiggers that infested chickens on summer range were controlled by treating limited areas of their range with sulfur or treating poultry with sulfur ointment or kerosene and lard. This bulletin described the "pinch method" used to apply dusts to fowl for louse control, and the most effective treatment was sodium fluoride dust or dip. Sanitary conditions were listed as a prerequisite to profitable poultry raising. Naphthalene dust controlled lice, but naphthalene-treated nest eggs were ineffective and injured hens.[9]

Dipping fowl in a mixture of sodium fluoride, sulfur, and soap eradicated lice and the depluming mite.[10] Of a number of materials applied as dusts, sprays, dips, vent treatments, fumigants, and premises treatments to control lice, the most effective were mercurial ointment, sodium fluoride dust or dip, and sulfur or pyrethrins dust.[11] Rotenone as a dust or dip controlled lice.[12] Fumigation, painting roosts, using treated nest eggs, treating nesting materials and hens topically were tested, but only spraying premises thoroughly with coal-tar oil, wood tar, or heavy mineral oil controlled the chicken mite.[13] Dipping of chickens in an emulsion of Volck® oil eliminated lice, and spraying of roosts and houses controlled the chicken mite.[14,15] Nicotine sulfate thoroughly applied to structures controlled the chicken mite, but the treatment of roosts only did not completely control chicken lice.[16]

The 1939 revision of Bulletin No. 801[17] listed control of the chicken mite with premises sprays of carbolineum or crude petroleum. Treating legs with crude petroleum controlled *K. mutans,* and dipping chickens in sulfur controlled *K. gallinae.* Lice were controlled by sodium fluoride dusts or dips. Roost paints of nicotine sulfate were also listed as a partially effective treatment for lice. Phenothiazine as a dust controlled chicken lice.[18] A mixture of nicotine sulfate, naphthalene, and oil of tar, contained in a "pack" on a metal band placed around the legs of chickens, did not control lice.[19]

The 1942 *Yearbook of Agriculture*[20] listed dusting or dipping in sodium fluoride as the most effective treatment for lice. The chicken mite could be controlled by treating premises with carbolineums, crude petroleum, or creosote oil.[21] Sodium fluosilicate dusts or dips were as effective as sodium fluoride, which was an essential defense material during World War II, for the control of poultry lice.[22]

B. Organochlorine Treatments

DDT controlled lice when applied to poultry as a dip or spray or when sprayed or dusted onto floors, roosts, and nests, but oral treatments of DDT in gelatin capsules were ineffective.[23,24] However, DDT dust was no more effective than the standard sodium fluoride treatment.[25] Telford[26] reviewed the history of insecticidal control of chicken lice, tested 37 louse powders applied with a salt-shaker-type applicator, and reported DDT, rotenone, and sulfur were fast-acting and provided residual activity against reinfestation. Dusts of DDT, sodium fluoride, sodium fluosilicate, and Lethane A-70® also controlled lice.[27] DDT dust controlled lice when applied directly to roosting hens.[28]

Benzene hexachloride (BHC) sprayed onto roosts and the floor controlled lice but was irritating to the spray operator and malodorous; however, gamma isomer extracts of BHC were also effective as roost paints and had none of the objectional properties of BHC.[29] BHC painted on roosts controlled lice by fumigant action.[30] Of several insecticides applied to poultry houses, DDT and pentachlorophenol were superior to carbolineum for control of the chicken mite.[31] Lice and *M. cubitalis* were controlled by spraying poultry with DDT plus Lethane B-72®.[32] Treating roosts or soil in poultry houses with chlordane, BHC, or DDT dust controlled lice.[33] The chicken mite was controlled with premises sprays of Lethane A-70®, BHC, and pentachlorophenyl.[34]

Edgar et al.[35] reviewed the history of technologies used to control poultry lice and reported that sodium fluoride dust applied to poultry was most effective and sulfur dust applied to litter was least expensive. Other effective treatments were spraying poultry with DDT and methoxychlor and applying chlordane dust to litter and nicotine to roosts. BHC was less effective than other materials. Body lice were controlled with lindane roost paint or DDT dust, and, although sprays of methoxychlor, chlordane, toxaphene, dieldrin, and aldrin were at times effective against the chicken mite, this species was difficult to control when poultry roosted in substandard houses or in trees which were impossible to treat adequately.[36] Lindane as a dust or a vapor provided by automatic, heat-generating vaporizers controlled lice.[37] Aldrin, chlordane, dieldrin, heptachlor, and lindane dusts applied to poultry controlled lice.[38]

C. Organophosphorus, Carbamate, and Other Treatments

Malathion was as effective as a variety of older treatments against lice and the chicken mite when applied as a spray to roosting areas.[39] With this report began the "malathion era" of poultry ectoparasite pest control. Both malathion and diazinon dusts applied by the shaker-can method controlled body lice.[40] Malathion roost sprays controlled body lice, and sprays applied to poultry house surfaces controlled the chicken mite.[41] Litter treatments also controlled lice.[42] Malathion, lindane, and chlorthion controlled lice when applied as dusts to poultry litter.[43] Sprays or dusts of malathion applied to walls, nests, roosts, and other areas controlled lice and the chicken mite.[44] The 1956 *Yearbook of Agriculture*[45] listed that treating roosts and other structures with DDT, lindane, or malathion controlled the chicken mite and crude oil and kerosene still controlled the scalyleg mite and depluming mite. Malathion dust placed in self-treatment dust-bath boxes or onto floor litter controlled lice.[46] Malathion sprayed onto the wooden frames of large community-type cages provided excellent control of the chicken mite.[47] Sprays of diazinon or dicapthon applied to roosts, nest boxes, and other structures controlled the chicken mite.[48] A dust of ronnel applied to litter controlled several species of biting lice.[49]

Of insecticides applied to range turkeys by a unique spraying system in which turkeys were driven through a curtain of spray, malathion was more effective than lindane and DDT failed to control body lice.[50] Trichlorfon, ronnel, and carbaryl sprays controlled lice.[51] Malathion dust in self-treatment dust-bath boxes was an efficient way to control lice[52] and, when applied to chickens in houses or cages, also controlled the chicken mite.[53] Treating litter with dusts of ronnel,[54] malathion, carbaryl, dioxathion, and coumaphos controlled poultry lice.[55,56] Body sprays of chlorfenvinphos[57] and coumaphos dust applied to nests and litter provided excellent control of lice.[58] Coumaphos or carbaryl dusts applied to litter controlled lice. Dichlorvos, which controlled lice as a spray, granules, or dust, but had short residual activity, was more effective when applied in resin strands to the floors of cages holding laying hens. Dimethoate sprays applied to structures controlled the chicken mite.[59] Dichlorvos controlled lice when applied in insecticide-impregnated resin strands attached to the legs of chickens or to the bottoms of wire layer cages.[60] Zytron® granules and dusts of phosmet and carbophenothion as litter treatments controlled lice, but a dust of Dowco® 175 and granules of Zytron® were never completely effective in self-treatment dust-bath boxes.[61] Chlorpyrifos sprays eliminated infestations of lice on chickens.[62]

Dusts containing *Bacillus thuringiensis* (BT) applied to hens controlled lice, but in self-treatment, dust-bath boxes were less effective.[63] Sprays of exotoxin, crystals, or spores of BT controlled lice[64] and the chicken mite.[65]

III. CONTROL OF FLEAS

The original issue of *U.S. Dep. Agric. Farmers' Bulletin* No. 683 in 1915[66] addressed the biology and control of fleas on man and animals. The section on sticktight fleas on poultry reported that control was accomplished by applying a mixture of kerosene and lard or carbolated vasoline to poultry, constructing chicken houses of metal instead of wood, removing manure and other larval breeding material, and applying crude petroleum or salt onto breeding places. Several of these same techniques were listed in *U.S. Dep. Agric. Bulletin* No. 248.[67] A revision of Bulletin No. 683, designated Farmers' Bulletin No. 897 in 1917,[68] contained no changes in control measures for fleas on poultry, but noted that fowl should not be allowed to eat the salt applied to breeding places for it is poisonous to them. The 1921 revision of this bulletin[69] also contained no changes in technologies to control sticktight fleas. Nicotine sulfate sprayed onto floors of poultry houses controlled sticktight fleas.[16]

Since 1940, very few articles have been published on control of the sticktight flea. Dusting of poultry houses with DDT controlled sticktight fleas, and treatment of chickens was not necessary.[70] Malathion dust applied to litter eliminated sticktight fleas.[49] Sticktight fleas were also controlled by malathion dust in natural soil wallows or in self-treatment dust-bath boxes.[71]

IV. CONTROL OF BED BUGS

In the first issue of *U.S. Dep. Agric. Farmers' Bulletin* No. 754 in 1916,[72] bed bugs were addressed as a problem for man and human dwellings, and control was obtained with fumigation of premises with hydrocyanic acid gas or burning sulfur. The 1942 *U.S. Dep. Agric. Yearbook of Agriculture*[73] suggested that bed bugs in poultry houses could be controlled by sulfur fumigation and spraying the premises with creosote oil or carbolineums.

DDT in kerosene also controlled bed bugs when applied to walls, roosts, dropping boards, and feed boxes.[74] An aqueous spray of DDT, applied to roosts, floors, walls, and other structures, controlled bed bugs.[28]

V. CONTROL OF FOWL TICKS

Osborn[3] listed spraying poultry houses with kerosene, kerosene emulsion, benzene, gasoline, dusting with carbolated lime, painting with lime whitewash or fumigation with sulfur to control fowl ticks. The original issue of *U.S. Dep. Agric. Farmers' Bulletin* No. 1070 in 1919[75] recommended control of the fowl tick, found principally in Florida and from Texas to California, by spraying the premises with crude petroleum or carbolineum and by construction of tick-proof poultry houses. A thorough spraying of poultry structures with nicotine sulfate controlled fowl ticks.[16]

The 1941 revision of Bulletin No. 1070[76] noted an increase in the distribution in the U.S. of the fowl tick but listed no changes in control techniques. The 1942 *U.S. Dep. Agric. Yearbook of Agriculture*[77] listed control measures as premises treatments with carbolineums, crude petroleum, and creosote oil. Proper house, roost, and nest construction were also stressed.

Aldrin was more effective than lindane or heptachlor as a thorough premises spray to control the fowl tick.[78] Sprays of lindane, chlordane, toxaphene, dieldrin, and aldrin provided some control of the fowl tick, but incomplete coverage of hiding places, because the fowl roosted and nested in trees and substandard houses, made results questionable.[36]

A malathion surface spray was not as effective as an aldrin spray for the control of the fowl tick.[41] Sprays of malation and diazinon controlled fowl ticks when applied to wooden feeding troughs on large, range-type commercial turkey feedlots[79] or when applied to all parts of hen houses and to floor litter.[80] A premises spray plus a fowl treatment of carbaryl controlled *A. persicus,* sprays of naled and ronnel gave less conclusive results, and trichlorfon was ineffective.[51]

VI. CONTROL OF NORTHERN FOWL MITES

A. Early Treatment Technology

The northern fowl mite, first collected on poultry in the U.S. in 1917,[81] but identified as a variety of the tropical fowl mite, was controlled by treating poultry with sulfur dip or dust, pyrethrins dust, or nicotine sulfate dip. This new mite, then called the feather mite, was recognized as a serious problem, although the taxonomic status was yet unclear,[82] and was controlled by dipping poultry in sodium fluoride. A reveiw of the uncertain taxonomic status, life history, and control of *O. sylviarum* was presented by Cameron,[83] who recommended treating roosts or chickens with nicotine sulfate to control the mite. Dipping fowl in an emulsion of Volck® oil eliminated infestations of the northern fowl mite.[14,15]

Nicotine sulfate painted on perches and roosts controlled northern fowl mites on roosting fowl by fumigant action,[84,85] but a single application of nicotine sulfate as a roost paint was not always completely effective.[16] Treating poultry topically with nicotine sulfate spray or sulfur dusts or dips was more effective against the northern fowl mite than nicotine sulfate roost paints.[86] Naphthalene or paradichlorobenzene ointments applied to poultry controlled northern fowl mites.[87]

The 1939 edition of Bulletin No. 801[17] discussed the frequent occurrence of the northern fowl mite in the U.S. and listed thorough dipping or dusting with sulfur or painting of roosts with nicotine sulfate as control measures. The 1942 *Yearbook of Agriculture*[21] listed the northern fowl mite as "an occassional but serious pest of chickens" and recommended dipping or dusting of fowl in sulfur and painting nicotine sulfate on roosts.

B. Organochlorine Treatments

DDT dust controlled northern fowl mites but was not as effective as a nicotine sulfate treatment.[88] Nicotine sulfate applied to roosters by the "drop method" controlled northern fowl mites, but dusts of sodium fluoride, Lethane A-70®, DDT, sabadella, and BHC gave short-term control.[89] Spraying of the vents of chickens with BHC failed to control northern fowl mites, but sprays or dusts of Lethane A-70® were effective.[34]

Neotran® dusts or sprays afforded inconsistent control, sulfur dust was effective, and dusts of methoxychlor, DDT, and lindane were ineffective.[90] Sulfenone sprays, dusts, or dips also controlled northern fowl mites, but thorough treatment was necessary.[91]

C. Organophosphorus and Carbamate Treatments

The first organophosphorus insecticide that controlled the northern fowl mite was malathion[39,43,92,93] applied as a dust to poultry, to litter, or nest boxes. Reed et al.[94] cautioned that although malathion was highly effective against lice, it was much less effective against the northern fowl mite. The 1956 *Yearbook of Agriculture*[45] recommended treating fowl with sulfur dust or dip, painting roosts with nicotine sulfate, or treating litter with malathion dust to control northern fowl mites. Furman and Coates[95] stated that malathion "exhibited many of the characteristics of the perfect insecticide'' the poultry industry was seeking to control the northern fowl mite. Malathion sprayed onto community-type wire mesh cages controlled the northern fowl mite.[47] Dusts of ronnel and carbophenothion were highly effective, but sulfenone was less effective against the northern fowl mite.[49]

Of nine newly introduced chemicals, sprays of coumaphos, naled, ronnel, and carbaryl controlled northern fowl mites.[51] Coumaphos and malathion sprays applied to poultry were the most consistent toxicants of a number of older and newer insecticides tested against northern fowl mites, and carbaryl was slightly less effective.[55] Ronnel, trichlorfon, and coumaphos dusts applied directly to poultry controlled the northern fowl mite.[96] Ronnel sprays applied to turkeys or malathion sprays or dusts applied to turkey houses controlled northern fowl mite.[54] Malathion dust used to treat only infested hens (''spot'' treatment), as determined by numbers of northern fowl mites on eggs, controlled the infestation at costs much less than those incurred in treating all caged hens.[97] Malathion placed in self-treatment dust-bath boxes in cages or on range controlled northern fowl mites.[98]

Beginning in 1960, malathion failed to control northern fowl mites in New York, but roost treatments, dusts, and mist sprays of ronnel, carbaryl, and coumaphos were effective treatments.[99] Resistance to malathion by the northern fowl mite was documented in California in 1961 and cross-resistance to other organophosphorus insecticides, but not carbaryl, was also detected.[100]

Northern fowl mites were controlled in human dwellings with topical application of a sorptive dust, Dri Die® 67, to birds' nests, structures, and furnishings.[101] Coumaphos, carbaryl, and malathion dusts or coumaphos spray applied to poultry or coumaphos and carbaryl dusts applied to litter were effective.[59] Dichlorvos spray applied to roosting areas controlled northern fowl mites on range turkeys.[102]

Sprays of carbaryl and stirofos applied to caged poultry gave economical, effective control of northern fowl mites.[103] Stirofos dusts or sprays or sprays of a combination of stirofos and dichlorvos were more effective than carbaryl spray, the standard treatment for control of northern fowl mites on caged layers.[104] Chlorpyrifos was highly effective against the northern fowl mite when applied as a spray directly to poultry.[62] Matthysse et al.,[105] in a complete study on the relationships of northern fowl mites to hosts, recommended insecticidal treatments to control mites because costs of control were less than the losses in egg production as a result of mite infestation.

D. Other Treatment Technologies

In a national survey of poultry raisers, DeVaney[106] reported that carbaryl was the most used insecticide; others used were stirofos, malathion, and sulfur, and many users felt that the northern fowl mite was becoming resistant to carbaryl, malathion, and stirofos.

Chlordimeform and stirofos sprays controlled northern fowl mites on caged layers, and a high-pressure spray application was more effective than low-pressure application.[107,108]

Permethrin and fenvalerate sprays controlled northern fowl mites that were resistant to malathion.[109] Both materials were as effective as carbaryl for control of northern fowl mites.[110,111]

DeVaney and Beerwinkle[112] reduced populations of the northern fowl mite on hens (but not roosters) by clipping feathers in the vent area to 2 to 3 mm in length.

Carbaryl and stirofos sprayed onto caged laying hens were more effective then coumaphos or malathion against northern fowl mites, and mites appeared to be resistant to malathion.[113] Amitraz and carbaryl sprays were initially as effective as a permethrin spray but did not possess the residual activity of permethrin for control of the northern fowl mite.[114] Permethrin sprays were more effective than coumaphos or carbaryl treatments, while malathion failed to substantially reduce populations of northern fowl mites on poultry.[115]

Although carbaryl and stirofos wettable powders used undiluted as dusts controlled mites on laying hens, the excessive treatment with wettable powders was uneconomical and little more effective than dust formulations.[116] Dusts or sprays of permethrin were more effective then those of stirofos and carbaryl for control of northern fowl mites.[117]

One problem associated with infestations of northern fowl mites on poultry is the fact that often the mites leave their hosts in large numbers and cause discomfort and irritation to egg handlers. Also, these mites are spread from premises to premises as they cling to cages, egg flats, trucks, and other objects. Fumigation of inanimate objects with methyl bromide was safe to use and controlled mites, sulfur dioxide had an irritating odor, and phosphine gas was too slow in its killing action.[118,119]

Complete submersion of hens in stirofos, carbaryl, and malathion controlled northern fowl mites, but hens dipped in a combination of stirofos and dichlorvos were poisoned. This method protected flocks for 4 to 6 weeks and reduced the quantity of insecticide, likelihood of resistance, and labor and equipment needs.[120] Treatments of permethrin, stirofos, and egg oil gave variable results, and carbaryl sprays were generally unsatisfactory for the control of the northern fowl mite, an indication of possible resistance to carbaryl in California.[121]

Polyvinyl plastic strips impregnated with permethrin and attached to legs of hens or to floors or tops of cages containing laying hens provided long-term control of northern fowl mites.[122-124] Permethrin in acetone permeated through vinyl tubing and afforded less than complete control of northern fowl mites on caged hens.[125]

Most issues of *Insecticide and Acaricide Tests* since 1976 have contained one or more reports on the use of insecticides for the control of northern fowl mites on poultry. In these reports, carbaryl, stirofos, bendiocarb, fenvalerate, and permethrin sprays or dusts were generally effective. A summary of progress in research on the control of the northern fowl mite on laying hens highlighted control on inanimate objects, dipping of hens, use of systemic insecticides in feed, and breeding of mite-tolerant hens as potential new control technologies.[126]

VII. SYSTEMIC INSECTICIDES

In an extensive study to determine if poultry parasites could be controlled systemically, a variety of chemicals and proprietary products were administered orally by capsule or in feed or water to chickens, and none, including sulfur, adequately controlled lice, mites, and ticks of poultry.[127] In preliminary tests, lice were eliminated on hens which fed on sulfur, and sulfur dusted into poultry houses controlled sticktight fleas, fowl ticks, and chicken mites.[128] In more extensive trials, when sulfur was given to chickens by capsule to prevent external contamination, lice were not controlled, but sulfur dusts were effective as external treatments.[129] Although externally applied sulfur dusts or sprays were very effective, oral sulfur in capsules or in the feed did not control lice.[130]

In the late 1950s, modern systemic insecticides were tested to determine their activity against arthropod pests of poultry. Single oral doses of ronnel given to hens via a catheter controlled shaft louse infestations, but hens refused to eat ronnel in feed so that therapeutic levels were not obtained.[131] Single oral treatments of carbaryl, ronnel, coumaphos, dimethoate, and crufomate failed to control lice.[56] Carbaryl, which did not exhibit systemic activity in other animals, in the feed of hens was systemically active against the northern fowl mice.[132] The systemic activity of carbaryl was confirmed by a bioassay in which a rat mite, *Haemogamassus liponysoides hesperus* Radovsky, was killed when fed on blood of hens given carbaryl orally.[133]

Sulfaquinoxalene added to the feed of poultry to control coccidiosis also controlled northern fowl mites.[134,135] Sulfonamides as feed additives eliminated northern fowl mites in 14 of 15 treated flocks.[136] Coumaphos in feed for 10 weeks did not control infestations of the chicken body louse.[137] Single or multiple oral doses or feed additives of coumaphos, crufomate, famphur, phosmet, and ronnel were not systemically active.[138] Nine anticoccidials were ineffective as feed additives.[139] In *Insecticide and Acaricide Tests,* oral treatments of diflubenzuron, bacitracin, zinc bacitracin, Closantel, and Larvadex® and oral, subcutaneous, or intramuscular treatments of ivermectin were not effective systemically.

VIII. CONTROL OF THE TURKEY CHIGGERS

Neoschongastia americana (Hirst), the turkey chigger, which attacks turkeys that range on heavy clay soils in the southern and western U.S., has been successfully controlled by the application of acaricides to the soil. Chlorpyrifos, stirofos, phosmet, diazinon, and ethion provided the necessary 4 weeks of control so that feeding lesions could heal before turkeys were processed.[140-144] Chlorpyrifos was labeled for use as a turkey chigger control treatment.[145]

IX. CONTROL OF BITING FLIES

Special mention should be made of the control of the *Simulium* vectors of a *Leucocytozoon* disease of turkeys. In several counties of South Carolina, of several species of *Simulium* and *Cnephia pecuarum* (Riley) feeding on turkeys, only *S. slossonae* (Dyer and Knab) was shown to be a vector of *L. smithi*.[146] When streams were treated with a DDT-oil solution applied by aircraft to kill black fly larvae, there was excellent control of black fly larvae and pupae and feeding of adult flies was reduced.[147] However, the additional *Leucocytozoon* infections suggested that other blood-sucking Diptera could be vectors. Temephos controlled black fly larvae and was most efficient when streams were treated with temephos granules applied by helicopter.[148] Temephos granular treatment on a large scale[149] afforded effective and economical prevention of *Leucocytozoon* disease in a large-scale turkey breeder operation.

X. OVERVIEW AND CURRENT TECHNOLOGY

There has been an evolution in the importance of arthropod pests of poultry that has paralleled the evolution in poultry production practices. Pests, such as the chicken mite, *Knemidokoptes* mites, lice, sticktight fleas, fowl ticks, and bed bugs, which were subjects of control measures before the advent of modern poultry production practices, are no longer important problems to the poultry industry. These species were controlled by a variety of technologies that applied insecticides to poultry or their environment. Seldom are these arthropods encountered today, except in small "backyard" flocks of poultry.

The caged layer, brooder, and breeder production systems in use today have created an environment that is favorable for the production of massive infestations of the northern fowl mite. These mites are controlled by the application of insecticides directly to poultry. Malathion was used extensively until mites developed resistance to it and has been replaced by carbaryl and a number of other insecticides, especially stirofos. It appears that, for the forseeable future, topical applications of acaricides to poultry will be the only practical technology available for the control of northern fowl mites. Experimentally, some materials were systemically active against northern fowl mites when consumed in the feed of poultry, but none has been developed into a control technology.

The turkey chigger can easily be controlled by applying acaricides to the soil upon which turkeys graze. However, much of the commercial production of turkeys has been moved to areas with sandy soils which are unsuitable for the production of chiggers. There is little need to pursue further development of control technologies for this species.

The control of the black fly vectors of *Leucocytozoon* disease of turkeys is obtained by treating streams with appropriate larvicides.

REFERENCES

1. **Loomis, E. C.,** External parasites, in *Diseases of Poultry,* Hofstad, M. S., Colnek, B. W., Helmboldt, C. F., Reid, W. M., and Yoder, H. W., Eds., Iowa State University Press, Ames, 1984, 586.
2. **Axtell, R. C.,** Arthropod pests of poultry, in *Livestock Entomology,* Williams R. E., Hall, R. D., Broce, A. B., and Scholl, P. J., Eds., John Wiley & Sons, New York, 1985, 269.
3. **Osborn, H.,** Insects affecting domestic animals: an account of the species of importance in North America with mention of related forms occurring on other animals, *U.S. Dep. Agric. Bull.,* 5, 1896.
4. **Banks, N.,** Mites and lice on poultry, *U.S. Dep. Agric. Bur. Entomol. Circ.,* 92, 1907.
5. **Herrick, G. W.,** Some external parasites of poultry with special reference to Mallophaga, with directions for their control, *Cornell Agric. Exp. Stn. Bull.,* 359, 1915.
6. **Lamson, G. H. and Manter, J. A.,** Some lice and mites of the hen, *Storrs Agric. Exp. Stn. Bull.,* 86, 171, 1916.
7. **Moore, W.,** Fumigation of animals to destroy their external parasites, *J. Econ. Entomol.,* 9, 71, 1916.
8. **Bishopp, F. C. and Wood, H. P.,** Mites and lice on poultry, *U.S. Dep. Agric. Farmers' Bull.,* 801, 1917.
9. **Abbott, W. S.,** Naphthalene vs. chicken lice, *J. Econ. Entomol.,* 12, 397, 1919.
10. **Wood, H. P.,** The depluming mite of chickens: its complete eradication from a flock by one treatment, *J. Econ. Entomol.,* 12, 402, 1919.
11. **Abbott, W. S.,** Results of experiments with miscellaneous substances against chicken lice and the dog flea, *U.S. Dep. Agric. Bull.,* 888, 1920.
12. **Wells, R. W., Bishopp, F. C., and Laake, E. W.,** Derris as a promising insecticide, *J. Econ. Entomol.,* 15, 90, 1922.
13. **Davidson, W. M.,** Results of experiments with miscellaneous substances against the chicken mite, *U.S. Dep. Agric. Bull.,* 1228, 1924.
14. **Bruce, W. G.,** The use of Volck against external parasites of domestic animals, *J. Kans. Entomol. Soc.,* 1, 74, 1928.
15. **Caler, H. L.,** Volck special emulsion number 2 as a control for external parasites of animals, *J. Kans. Entomol. Soc.,* 4, 77, 1931.
16. **Bishopp, F. C. and Wagner, R. D.,** Nicotine in the control of ecto-parasites of poultry, *J. Econ. Entomol.,* 24, 56, 1931.
17. **Bishopp, F. C. and Wood, H. P.,** Mites and lice on poultry, *U.S. Dep. Agric. Farmers' Bull.,* No. 801, 1939.
18. **Parish, H. E.,** Effects of phenothiazine on chicken lice, *J. Econ. Entomol.,* 33, 700, 1940.
19. **Hamilton, C. M.,** A "delousing leg band" for chickens, *Vet. Med.,* 37, 178, 1942.
20. **Bishopp, F. C.,** Poultry lice and their control, *U.S. Dep. Agric. Yearb. Agric.,* 1048, 1942.
21. **Bishopp, F. C.,** Poultry mites, *U.S. Dep. Agric. Yearb. Agric.,* 1055, 1942.
22. **Parish, H. E.,** Sodium fluosilicate to control poultry lice, *J. Econ. Entomol.,* 36, 353, 1943.
23. **Telford, H. S.,** Chicken louse control, *Soap Sanit. Chem.,* 20, 113, 1944.
24. **Telford, H. S.,** New insecticides for chicken louse control, *J. Econ. Entomol.,* 38, 573, 1945.
25. **Warren, D. S.,** The value of DDT for the control of the common chicken louse, *Poultry Sci.,* 25, 473, 1945.
26. **Telford, H. S.,** DDT as a chicken lice control, *J. Econ. Entomol.,* 38, 700, 1945.
27. **Alicata, J. E., Holdaway, F. G., Quisenberry, J. H., and Jensen, D. C.,** Observations on the comparative efficacy of certain old and new insecticides in the control of lice and mites of chickens, *Poultry Sci.,* 25, 376, 1946.
28. **Quigley, G. D. and Cory, E. N.,** The utility of DDT for the control of poultry ectoparasites, *Poultry Sci.,* 25, 419, 1946.
29. **Telford, H. S.,** Benzene hexachloride to control certain insects affecting domestic animals, *J. Econ. Entomol.,* 40, 918, 1947.
30. **Roberts, I. H. and Peterson, H. O.,** Hexachlorocyclohexane — a fumigant for the control of chicken lice, *Poultry Sci.,* 26, 588, 1947.
31. **Hixson, E. and Muma, M. H.,** Toxicity of certain insecticides to the chicken mite, *J. Econ. Entomol.,* 40, 596, 1947.
32. **Alicata, J. E., Kartman, L., Nishida, T., and Palafox, A. L.,** Efficacy of certain sprays in control of lice and mites of chickens, *J. Econ. Entomol.,* 40, 922, 1947.
33. **Creighton, J. T., Hetrick, L. A., Hunt, P. J., and Duncan, D. U.,** The application of chlorinated hydrocarbons to the soil and roosts effectively controls lice of poultry, *Poultry Sci.,* 26, 674, 1947.
34. **Peterson, E. H.,** Field tests of some insecticides in the control of the common red mite of poultry and of the northern fowl mite, *Poultry Sci.,* 28, 411, 1949.
35. **Edgar, S. A., Walsh, W. L., and Johnson, L. W.,** Comparative efficacy of several insecticides and methods of application in the control of lice on chickens, *Poultry Sci.,* 28, 320, 1949.

36. **Smith, C. L.,** Field tests of insecticides against ectoparasites of poultry, *J. Econ. Entomol.,* 45, 748, 1952.
37. **Moore, S., III,** Control and eradication of chicken lice with lindane. *Poultry Sci.,* 31, 444, 1952.
38. **Fairchild, H. E. and Dahm, P. A.,** Lice control on chickens with chlorinated hydrocarbon insecticides, *J. Econ. Entomol.,* 48, 141, 1955.
39. **Moore, S., III and Schwardt, H. H.,** The control of external parasites of chickens in New York State, *Poultry Sci.,* 33, 1230, 1954.
40. **Smith, C. L. and Richards, R.,** Evaluations of some new insecticides against lice on livestock and poultry, *J. Econ. Entomol.,* 48, 566, 1955.
41. **Furman, D. P. and Weinmann, C. J.,** Toxicity of malathion to poultry and their ectoparasites, *J. Econ. Entomol.,* 49, 447, 1956.
42. **Harding, W. C., Jr. and Quigley, G. D.,** Litter treatment with malathion to control the chicken body louse, *J. Econ. Entomol.,* 49, 806, 1956.
43. **Hoffman, R. A.,** Control of the northern fowl mite and two species of lice on poultry, *J. Econ. Entomol.,* 49, 347, 1956.
44. **Raun, E. S.,** Chicken louse and mite control with malathion formulations, *J. Econ. Entomol.,* 49, 628, 1956.
45. **Roberts, I. H. and Smith, C. L.,** Mites on poultry, *U.S. Dep. Agric. Yearb. Agric.,* 493, 1956.
46. **Rodriguez, J. L., Jr., and Riehl, L. A.,** Control of the chicken body louse on hens by self-treatment with malathion dust, *J. Econ. Entomol.,* 50, 64, 1957.
47. **Rodriguez, J. L., Jr. and Riehl, L. A.,** Malathion for control of chicken mites on hens in wire cages, *J. Econ. Entomol.,* 51, 158, 1958.
48. **Rodriguez, J. L., Jr. and Riehl, L. A.,** Comparisons of diazinon, dicapthon, chlorobenzilate and kelthane for control of the chicken mite in hen houses, *J. Econ. Entomol.,* 51, 911, 1958.
49. **Linkfield, R. L. and Reid, W. M.,** Newer acaricides and insecticides in the control of ectoparasites of poultry, *J. Econ. Entomol.,* 51, 188, 1958.
50. **Gless, E. E. and Raun, E. S.,** Insecticidal control of the chicken body louse on range turkeys, *J. Econ. Entomol.,* 51, 229, 1958.
51. **Kraemer, P.,** Relative efficacy of several materials for control of poultry ectoparasites, *J. Econ. Entomol.,* 52, 1195, 1959.
52. **Rodriguez, J. L., Jr. and Riehl, L. A.,** The malathion dust-bath for control of five species of lice on chickens, *J. Econ. Entomol.,* 53, 328, 1960.
53. **Rodriguez, J. L., Jr. and Riehl, L. A.,** Malathion dust for chicken mite control, *J. Econ. Entomol.,* 53, 328, 1960.
54. **Bigley, W. S., Roth, A. R., and Eddy, G. W.,** Laboratory and field tests against mites and lice attacking poultry, *J. Econ. Entomol.,* 53, 12, 1960.
55. **Hoffman, R. A.,** The control of poultry lice and mites with several organic insecticides, *J. Econ. Entomol.,* 53, 160, 1960.
56. **Hoffman, R. A.,** Experiments on the control of poultry lice, *J. Econ. Entomol.,* 54, 1114, 1961.
57. **Hoffman, R. A. and Drummond, R. O.,** Control of lice on livestock and parasites on poultry with General Chemical 4072, *J. Econ. Entomol.,* 54, 1052, 1961.
58. **Knapp, F. W.,** Co-Ral as a litter and nest dust to control the chicken body louse, *J. Econ. Entomol.,* 55, 571, 1962.
59. **Simco, J. S. and Lancaster, J. L., Jr.,** Control of common external parasites on commerical layers and hatchery flocks, *Univ. Arkansas Agric. Exp. Stn. Bull.,* 703, 1965.
60. **Kunz, S. E. and Hogan, B. F.,** Dichlorvos-impregnated resin strands for control of chicken lice on laying hens, *J. Econ. Entomol.,* 63, 263, 1970.
61. **Hoffman, R. A. and Hogan, B. F.,** Control of chicken body, shaft, and wing lice on laying hens by self-treatment with insecticide dusts and granules, *J. Econ. Entomol.,* 60, 1703, 1967.
62. **Simco, J. S. and Lancaster, J. L., Jr.,** Controlling external parasites on laying hens with Dursban, *Arkansas Farm Res.,* 22, 9, 1973.
63. **Hoffman, R. A. and Gingrich, R. E.,** Dust containing *Bacillus thuringiensis* for control of chicken body, shaft, and wing lice, *J. Econ. Entomol.,* 61, 85, 1968.
64. **Meinecke, C. F.,** Potential biological control of poultry lice, *Poultry Sci.,* 47, 2017, 1968.
65. **Sell, J. L., Rose, R. J., Johnson, R. L., and Mork, I. J.,** Evaluation of a biological insecticide for control of poultry mites, *Poultry Sci.,* 49, 557, 1970.
66. **Bishopp, F. C.,** Fleas as pests to man and animals, with suggestions for their control, *U.S. Dep. Agric. Farmers' Bull.,* 683, 1915.
67. **Bishopp, F. C.,** Fleas, *U.S. Dep. Agric. Bull.,* 248, 1915.
68. **Bishopp, F. C.,** Fleas and their control, *U.S. Dep. Agric. Farmers' Bull.,* 897, 1917.
69. **Bishopp, F. C.,** Fleas and their control, *U.S. Dep. Agric. Farmers' Bull.,* 897, 1921.
70. **Eads, R. B.,** Control of the sticktight flea on chickens, *J. Econ. Entomol.,* 39, 659, 1946.

71. **Rodriguez, J. L. and Riehl, L. A.,** Sticktight flea control on chickens with malathion dust self-treatment, *J. Econ. Entomol.,* 54, 1212, 1961.

72. **Marlatt, C. L.,** The bedbug, *U.S. Dep. Agric. Farmers' Bull.,* 754, 1916.

73. **Back, E. A. and Bishopp, F. C.,** Bedbugs as pests of poultry, *U.S. Dep. Agric. Yearb. Agric.,* 1068, 1942.

74. **Kulash, W. M. and Maxwell, J. M.,** DDT and bedbugs in chicken houses, *J. Econ. Entomol.,* 38, 606, 1945.

75. **Bishopp, F. C.,** The fowl tick and how premises may be freed from it, *U.S. Dep. Agric. Farmers' Bull.,* 1070, 1919.

76. **Bishopp, F. C.,** The fowl tick and how premises may be freed from it, *U.S. Dep. Agric. Farmers' Bull.,* 1070, 1941.

77. **Bishopp, F. C.,** The fowl tick, *U.S. Dep. Agric. Yearb. Agric.,* 1062, 1942.

78. **Edgar, S. A., Little, C. D., and Herndon, J. F.,** Control of the fowl tick, *Argas persicus* (Oken), on an Alabama poultry farm, *J. Am. Vet. Med. Assoc.,* 123, 446, 1953.

79. **Rodriguez, J. L., Jr. and Riehl, L. A.,** Four pesticides tested against the fowl tick infesting turkeys in feed lots, *J. Econ. Entomol.,* 49, 713, 1956.

80. **Rodriguez, J. L., Jr., and Riehl, L. A.,** Malathion spray for fowl tick control, *J. Econ. Entomol.,* 50, 41, 1957.

81. **Wood, H. P.,** Tropical fowl mite in the United States, *U.S. Dep. Agric. Circ.,* 79, 1920.

82. **Cleveland, C. R.,** A new parasite threatens the poultry industry, *Poultry Sci.,* 2, 129, 1923.

83. **Cameron, D.,** The northern fowl mite (*Liponyssus sylviarum* C. & F., 1877) investigations at McDonald College, Que., with a summary of previous work, *Can. J. Res.,* 16, 230, 1938.

84. **Cutright, C. R.,** A valuable aid to the control of the feather mite, *Liponyssus sylviarum, J. Econ. Entomol.,* 22, 422, 1929.

85. **Payne, L. F.,** A new method for controlling feather mites, *J. Econ. Entomol.,* 22, 819, 1929.

86. **Maw, W. A.,** The northern fowl mite, *Liponyssus sylviarum,* of poultry, *Sci. Agric.,* 11, 710, 1931.

87. **Maw, W. A., Whitehead, W. E., and Bemont, L. H.,** The northern fowl mite and its control, *Sci. Agric.,* 16, 79, 1935.

88. **Povar, M. L.,** Value of DDT for the control of the northern feather mite *(Liponyssus sylviarum), Cornell Vet.,* 36, 91, 1946.

89. **Ritcher, P. O. and Insko, W. M., Jr.,** Control of the northern fowl mite, *J. Econ. Entomol.,* 41, 123, 1948.

90. **Furman, D. P.,** Control of the northern fowl mite, *J. Econ. Entomol.,* 45, 926, 1952.

91. **Furman, D. P.,** Comparative evaluation of control procedures against the northern fowl mite, *J. Econ. Entomol.,* 46, 822, 1953.

92. **Vincent, L. E., Lindgren, D. L., and Krone, H. E.,** Toxicity of malathion to the northern fowl mite, *J. Econ. Entomol.,* 47, 943, 1954.

93. **Harding, W. C., Jr.,** Malathion to control the northern fowl mite, *J. Econ. Entomol.,* 48, 605, 1955.

94. **Reid, W. M., Linkfield, R. L., and Lewis, G.,** Limitations of malathion in northern fowl mite and louse control, *Poultry Sci.,* 35, 1397, 1956.

95. **Furman, D. P. and Coates, W. S.,** Northern fowl mite control with malathion, *Poultry Sci.,* 36, 252, 1957.

96. **Knapp, F. W. and Krause, G. F.,** Control of the northern fowl mite, *Ornithonyssus sylviarum* (C. & F.), with ronnel, Bayer L 13/59 and Bayer 21/199, *J. Econ. Entomol.,* 53, 4, 1960.

97. **Rodriguez, J. L., Jr. and Riehl, L. A.,** Spot treatments with malathion dust for control of the northern fowl mite on hens in individual wire cages, *J. Econ. Entomol.,* 52, 13, 1959.

98. **Rodriguez, J. L., Jr. and Riehl, L. A.,** Control of northern fowl mite in community wire cages with malathion in special dust-bath-boxes, *J. Econ. Entomol.,* 53, 701, 1960.

99. **Foulk, J. D. and Matthysse, J. G.,** Experiments on control of the northern fowl mite, *J. Econ. Entomol.,* 56, 321, 1963.

100. **Rodriquez, J. L. and Riehl, L. A.,** Northern fowl mites tolerant to malathion, *J. Econ. Entomol.,* 56, 509, 1963.

101. **Tarshis, I. B.,** A sorptive dust for control of the northern fowl mite, *Ornithonyssus sylviarum,* infesting dwellings, *J. Econ. Entomol.,* 57, 110, 1964.

102. **Lancaster, J. L., Jr. and Simco, J. S.,** Northern fowl mite control on mature turkeys on range, *J. Econ. Entomol.,* 61, 1471, 1968.

103. **Furman, D. P. and Lee, D.,** Experimental control of the northern fowl mite, *J. Econ. Entomol.,* 62, 1246, 1969.

104. **Nelson, C. B., Bramhall, E. L., Miller, W. V., and Simkover, H. G.,** Control of the northern fowl mite on laying hens with Shell SD-8447, *J. Econ. Entomol.,* 62, 47, 1969.

105. **Matthysse, J. G., Jones, C. J., and Purnasiri, A.,** Development of northern fowl mite populations on chickens, effects on the host and immunology, *Search Agric.,* 4, 1, 1974.

106. **DeVaney, J. A.,** A survey of poultry ectoparasite problems and their research in the United States, *Poultry Sci.,* 57, 1217, 1978.

107. **Hall, R. D., Townsend, L. H., Jr., and Turner, E. C., Jr.,** The use of chlordimeform against northern fowl mites on caged laying hens, *Vet. Parasitol.,* 1, 185, 1975.

108. **Christensen, C. M., Knapp, F. W., and Tuttle, J. W.,** The efficacy of chlordimeform for the control of the northern fowl mite, *Ornithonyssus sylvarium* (Canestrini and Fanzago) (Acarina, Dermanyssidae), *Poultry Sci.,* 56, 79, 1977.

109. **Hall, R. D., Townsend, L. H., Jr., and Turner, E. C., Jr.,** Laboratory and field tests to compare the effectiveness of organophosphorus, carbamate, and synthetic pyrethroid acaricides against northern fowl mites, *J. Econ. Entomol.,* 71, 315, 1978.

110. **Loomis, E. C., Bramhall, E. L., and Dunning, L. L.,** Comparative effectiveness of fenvalerate and carbaryl sprays against the northern fowl mite, *J. Econ. Entomol.,* 72, 856, 1979.

111. **Williams, R. E. and Berry, J. G.,** Control of northern fowl mite with permethrin and fenvalerate, two synthetic pyrethroid compounds, *Poultry Sci.,* 59, 1211, 1980.

112. **DeVaney, J. A. and Beerwinkle, K. R.,** A nonchemical method of controlling the northern fowl mite, *Ornithonyssus sylviarum* (Canestrini and Fanzago), on caged white leghorn hens, *Poultry Sci.,* 59, 1226, 1980.

113. **Hall, R. D., Vandepopuliere, J. M., English, L. M., Jaynes, W., Lyons, J. J., Doisy, K. E., and Foehse, M. C.,** Comparative evaluation of four registered acaricides for field control of northern fowl mites on caged laying hens, *Poultry Sci.,* 59, 2424, 1980.

114. **Collison, C. H., Danka, R. G., and Kennell, D. R.,** An evaluation of permethrin, carbaryl, and amitraz for the control of northern fowl mites on caged chickens, *Poultry Sci.,* 60, 1812, 1981.

115. **Braun, H. E., Surgeoner, G. A., Stanek, J., and Ralley, W. E.,** Efficacy and dissipation of permethrin for the control of the northern fowl mite in hens, *Can. Vet. J.,* 22, 291, 1981.

116. **Hall, R. D., Foehse, M. C., and Vandepopuliere, J. M.,** Application phenomena and efficacy of concentrated acaricide dusts for northern fowl mite control on caged laying hens, *Poultry Sci.,* 60, 1187, 1981.

117. **Arthur, F. H. and Axtell, R. C.,** Comparisons of permethrin formulations and application methods for northern fowl mite control on caged laying hens, *Poultry Sci.,* 61, 879, 1982.

118. **Beerwinkle, K. R. and DeVaney, J. A.,** Control of the northern fowl mite on inanimate objects by fumigation: laboratory studies, *Poultry Sci.,* 62, 38, 1982.

119. **DeVaney, J. A. and Beerwinkle, K. R.,** Control of the northern fowl mite on inanimate objects by fumigation: field studies, *Poultry Sci.,* 62, 43, 1982.

120. **DeVaney, J. A., Beerwinkle, K. R., and Ivie, G. W.,** Residual activity of selected pesticides on laying hens treated for northern fowl mite control by dipping, *Poultry Sci.,* 61, 1630, 1982.

121. **McKeen, W. D., Loomis, E. C., and Dunning, L. L.,** Effectiveness of Ectiban, egg oil, Rabon, or Sevin for control of northern fowl mites on laying hens, *Poultry Sci.,* 62, 2343, 1983.

122. **Hall, R. D., Vandepopuliere, J. M., Fischer, F. J., Lyons, J. J., and Doisy, K. E.,** Comparative efficacy of plastic strips impregnated with permethrin and permethrin dust for northern fowl mite control on caged laying hens, *Poultry Sci.,* 62, 612, 1983.

123. **Jones, E. M. and Kissam, J. B.,** The effectiveness of polyvinyl chloride plastic bands impregnated with permethrin as a control for the northern fowl mite, *Ornithonyssus sylviarum* (Canestrini and Fanzago), infesting laying chickens, *Poultry Sci.,* 62, 1113, 1983.

124. **Hall, R. D., Vandepopuliere, J. M., Jaynes, W., and Fischer, F. J.,** Prophylactic efficiency and longevity of polyvinyl chloride strips containing permethrin for control of northern fowl mites (Acari: Macronyssidae) on caged chickens, *J. Econ. Entomol.,* 77, 1224, 1984.

125. **Hall, R. D., Vandepopuliere, J. M., Fischer, F. J., Lyons, J. J., and Van Horn, J. D.,** A new in-cage treatment system for control of northern fowl mites on laying hens, *Poultry Sci.,* 63, 628, 1984.

126. **DeVaney, J. A.,** Progress on control of northern fowl mites on caged laying hens, *Vet. Parasitol.,* 18, 289, 1985.

127. **Parman, D. C., Abbott, W. S., Culver, J. J., and Davidson, W. M.,** Ineffectiveness of internal medication of poultry for the control of external parasites, *U.S. Dep. Agric. Tech. Bull.,* 60, 1928.

128. **Emmel, M. W.,** Sulfur in the control of external parasites of chickens, *J. Am. Vet. Med. Assoc.,* 91, 201, 1937.

129. **Emmel, M. W.,** Field experiments in the use of sulfur to control lice, fleas and mites of chickens, *Univ. Fla. Agric. Exp. Stn. Bull.,* 374, 1942.

130. **Creighton, J. T., Dekle, G. W., and Russel, J.,** The use of sulfur and sulfur compounds in the control of poultry lice, *J. Econ. Entomol.,* 36, 413, 1943.

131. **Raffensperger, E. M.,** The effects of Dow ET-57 on chicken shaft louse infestations, *J. Econ. Entomol.,* 51, 558, 1958.

132. **Kraemer, P. and Furman, D. P.,** Systemic activity of Sevin in control of *Ornithonyssus sylviarum* (C. & F.), *J. Econ. Entomol.,* 52, 170, 1959.

133. **Furman, D. P. and Pieper, G. R.,** Systemic acaricidal effects of Sevin in poultry, *J. Econ. Entomol.,* 55, 355, 1962.

134. **Furman, D. P. and Stratton, V. S.,** Control of northern fowl mites, *Ornithonyssus sylviarum,* with sulfaquinoxaline, *J. Econ. Entomol.,* 56, 904, 1963.

135. **Furman, D. P. and Stratton, V. S.,** Systemic activity of sulfaquinoxaline in control of northern fowl mites, *Ornithonyssus sylviarum, Poultry Sci.,* 43, 1263, 1964.

136. **Goldhaft, T. M.,** The use of a combined sulfonamide feed additive for the control of a fowl feather mite *(Ornithonyssus sylviarum), Refu. Vet.,* 26, 167, 1969.

137. **Quigley, G. D. and Harding, W. C., Jr.,** Use of Co-Ral as a systemic insecticide for layers, *Poultry Sci.,* 42, 1247, 1963.

138. **DeVaney, J. A. and Ivie, G. W.,** Systemic activity of coumaphos, famphur, crufomate, ronnel and phosmet given orally to hens for control of the northern fowl mite, *Ornithonyssus sylviarum* (Canestrini and Fanzago), *Poultry Sci.,* 59, 1208, 1980.

139. **DeVaney, J. A.,** Activity of selected anticoccidials as feed additives for control of the northern fowl mite, *Ornithonyssus sylviarum* (Canestrini and Fanzago), *Poultry Sci.,* 60, 2033, 1981.

140. **Lancaster, J. L., Jr. and Simco, J. S.,** Turkey chigger control, *Arkansas Farm Res.,* 19, 5, 1970.

141. **Price, M. A. and Kunz, S. E.,** Insecticidal screening for chemicals to control the chigger *Neoschongastia americana* on turkeys, *J. Econ. Entomol.,* 63, 373, 1970.

142. **Price, M. A., Kunz, S. E., and Matter, J. J.,** Use of Dursban® to control *Neoschongastia americana,* a turkey chigger, in experimental pens, *J. Econ. Entomol.,* 63, 377, 1970.

143. **Kunz, S. E., Price, M. A., and Everett, R.,** Evaluation of insecticides to control the chigger *Neoschongastia americana* on turkeys, *J. Econ. Entomol.,* 64, 900, 1971.

144. **Kunz, S. E., Price, M. A., and Everett, R. E.,** Large-scale testing of chlorpyrifos for control of *Neoschongastia americana* on turkeys, *J. Econ. Entomol.,* 65, 1207, 1972.

145. **Smith, P. E. and McGregor, W. S.,** Effective turkey chigger control, *Pract. Nutr.,* 9, 16, 1975.

146. **Jones, C. M. and Richey, D. J.,** Biology of the black flies in Jasper County, South Carolina, and some relationships to a *Leucocytozoon* disease of turkeys, *J. Econ. Entomol.,* 49, 121, 1956.

147. **Anthony, D. W. and Richey, D. J.,** Influence of black fly control on the incidence of *Leucocytozoon* disease in South Carolina turkeys, *J. Econ. Entomol.,* 51, 845, 1958.

148. **Kissam, J. B., Noblet, R., and Moore, H. S., IV,** *Simulium*: field evaluation of Abate larvacide for control in an area endemic for *Leucocytozoon smithi* of turkeys, *J. Econ. Entomol.,* 66, 426, 1973.

149. **Kissam, J. B., Noblet, R., and Garris, G. I.,** Large-scale aerial treatment of an endemic area with Abate® granular larvicide to control black flies (Diptera: Simuliidae) and suppress *Leucocytozoon smithi* of turkeys, *J. Med. Entomol.,* 12, 359, 1975.

Chapter 16

CONTROL OF FLIES AND OTHER ARTHROPOD PESTS THAT BREED IN POULTRY MANURE*

I. INTRODUCTION

A dramatic change has taken place in the commercial production of poultry in the past 40 years. The concentration of large numbers of fowl, especially laying hens in cages in a confined area, has created a situation that is ideal for the production of nuisance or filth flies. Manure that accumulates on the floor of poultry houses is an ideal habitat for the breeding of pest flies, primarily the house fly♦, *Musca domestica* Linnaeus, and the little house fly♦, *Fannia canicularis* (Linnaeus). Other species include the coastal fly, *F. femoralis* (Stein); the black garbage fly, *Ophyra leucostoma* (Wiedemann), *O. aenescens* (Wiedemann); the stable fly♦, *Stomoxys calcitrans* (Linnaeus); and the black soldier fly♦, *Hermetia illucens* (Linnaeus). Several species of blow flies may be found in poultry manure, but usually they have developed on broken eggs or the flesh of dead animals. Also, poultry manure may be infested with larvae and adults of the lesser mealworm♦, *Alphitobius diaperinus* (Panzer).

The primary technology used to eliminate fly breeding in manure is the frequent removal of the manure. If manure cannot be removed sufficiently or in a timely manner, it is necessary to institute other control measures. The rapid drying of manure will provide a poor environment for fly larvae and also a habitat that can be readily populated by predators and parasites of fly eggs and larvae. Predacious and parasitic mites, beetles, wasps, and other arthropods may provide a natural, biological control of pest flies. The use of these organisms, including the augmentation of naturally occurring species with the release of introduced parasites and/or predators, is addressed in Chapter 21. The final technology available to control arthropod pests in poultry manure is the use of insecticides. Insecticides may be applied to the surface of the manure to control fly larvae, or larvae may be controlled by placing insecticides and other chemicals in the feed or water of poultry so that their manure is toxic to or affects the development of fly larvae. Finally, insecticides may be used as space sprays, mists, fogs, or aerosols as residual sprays applied to structures or with baits to attract and control adult flies. The integration of cultural, biological, and chemical control technologies into a fly management system should be a necessary part of any efficient poultry production program. An excellent discussion of the various aspects of fly control in poultry manure is presented in a chapter in *Livestock Entomology*.[1]

Because the technologies that have been or are used to control adults of the house fly and other filth-breeding flies are essentially the same for all types of animal housing structures, including poultry houses, they are discussed in detail in Chapter 18. This chapter will concentrate only on technologies used to control fly larvae in poultry manure, specifically the direct treatment of manure and the treatment of manure by oral treatment of poultry.

II. CONTROL OF FLY LARVAE BY TREATING MANURE

Early poultry production practices, in which small flocks were maintained on the ground with free access to nests and roosts, did not allow for the production of flies, for the manure was scattered and did not accumulate. Also, poultry continually sought out and fed on fly

---

* Common names of insects and acarines, as listed in *Common Names of Insects and Related Organisms* (published by the Entomological Society of America), are marked with a ♦ the first time they are cited preceding the scientific name.

larvae — an excellent control technique. Thus, early literature on the control of larvae of the house fly and other flith-breeding species focused on horse (or cow) manure as a breeding site. This subject is also addressed in Chapter 18.

A. Organochlorine Treatments

DDT sprayed onto the surface of turkey manure that accumulated under wire turkey sunporches controlled house fly larvae as well as phenothiazine and better then thiourea and borax which are used to control house fly larvae in cattle and horse manure.[2] DDT sprayed onto manure beneath batteries containing laying hens was highly effective against larvae of the house fly and other species of flies and beetles;[3] a dust formulation was ineffective and a spray of an emulsion was four times more effective than a spray of a suspension.

B. Organophosphorus Treatments

The appearance of resistance in house fly adults and larvae to DDT and other chlorinated hydrocarbon insecticides in the early 1950s necessitated the substitution of other materials, especially organophosphorus insecticides, to control house fly larvae. A spray or a granular formulation of malathion applied to manure rapidly killed adult house flies and was also highly effective against larvae of the house fly and black soldier fly.[4,5] Malathion sprayed onto the surface of turkey manure that accumulated beneath porches or under wire racks controlled house fly larvae.[6] Diazinon or trichlorfon sprays were more effective than sprays of malathion, dicapthon, and chlorthion for control of fly larvae in manure under caged layers.[7] Each of eight organophosphorus insecticides sprayed onto poultry manure controlled house fly larvae for 2 days to 2 weeks. The most effective material, diazinon, was more effective as a dust than as a spray, presumably because the dust helped dry the manure, making it less favorable for fly breeding.[8] Diazinon, mevinphos, and ronnel were more effective than trichlorfon or azinphosmethyl when sprayed onto poultry manure.[9] Ronnel was also more effective than malathion.[10] Sprays of emulsifiable concentrates of diazinon, trichlorfon, ronnel, carbophenothion, and malathion in deodorized kerosene controlled house fly larvae and did not liquify the manure as often happened with aqueous sprays.[11] Fenthion applied as a spray, dust, or granular formulation was the most effective of eight larvicides tested.[12] Calcium arsenate suspension was also effective.

Although certain soil fumigants applied as sprays or granules to poultry manure controlled fly larvae, lack of residual toxicity made them less than satisfactory practical treatments.[13] Diazinon wettable powder mixed with agricultural gypsum and applied as a dust weekly to manure gave excellent control of larvae of the little house fly and the false stable fly♦, *Muscina stabulans* (Fallen), but not the house fly because of resistance to diazinon.[14] Dimethoate sprays were more effective than sprays of coumaphos, diazinon, and six other organophosphorus insecticides for the control of larvae of the little house fly.[15] Of 16 newer materials sprayed onto manure, only stirofos was as effective as the standard treatment of dimethoate, and none was effective for 1 week.[16] Chlorfenvinphos and propoxur were also as effective as dimethoate as larvicides.[17]

In tests with a field strain of house fly larvae that was 120 times (at LC_{90}) less susceptible to diazinon than susceptible larvae, only dimethoate, stirofos, formothion, and Bay-62863 were effective larvicides for 1 week.[18]

Low-volume aqueous sprays (5 to 8 mℓ/m^2 of manure) of insecticides were more effective and less expensive to apply than high-volume, conventional sprays (100 mℓ/m^2) for the control of house fly larvae.[19] Three applications of a slow release, plastic formulation of dichlorvos to the surface of poultry manure controlled both larval and adult house flies for about 7 weeks.[20]

C. Other Treatment Materials

Methoprene, an insect growth regulator, was ineffective when applied topically to poultry manure.[21] Diflubenzuron, a compound that inhibits chitin synthesis in insects, decreased the emergence of house flies and was less detrimental to the natural parasitoids than dimethoate.[22] Thiourea sprayed onto poultry manure was effective both as a larvicide and as a chemosterilant for adults.[23] Erythrosin B, a xanthene dye, sprayed onto poultry manure reduced populations of house fly larvae and did not affect populations of the black soldier fly.[24] Larvadex®, a triazine compound, was effective as a spray applied topically to poultry manure.[25-27]

D. Integrated Control Technology

Through the years, there continued to be research on use of technologies other than chemicals for the control of fly larvae in poultry manure. The covering of stockpiled poultry manure with black polyethylene tarpaulins not only controlled fly larvae but also retained major fertilizer elements of the manure.[28] The composting of poultry manure in windrows decreased oviposition by flies and populations of larvae.[29]

Other studies investigated the integration of the use of chemicals with other technologies for the control of fly larvae in poultry manure. Axtell[30] determined that 12 insecticides applied to poultry manure controlled house fly larvae but also eliminated populations of a predaceous mite, *Macrocheles muscaedomestica* (Scopoli). Because such treatments controlled fly larvae only for a short period of time and populations of larvae increased much more rapidly than the mite populations, he advocated a selective program of controlling adult flies rather than larvae in order to allow for biological control of larvae. Larvicides applied to manure at concentrations below the LC_{50} for *M. muscaedomestica* combined with trichlorfon or Bomyl® baits to control adult flies was an effective integrated control technique.[31] Weekly larviciding of manure under caged layers with insecticides gave satisfactory fly control, but was more expensive and time-consuming than less frequent adulticiding with residual sprays or baits and the utilization of natural parasites and predators to control manure-breeding flies.[32]

Frequency of removal of poultry manure had an effect on populations of fly larvae and their arthropod predators.[33] Excellent control of flies, especially the little house fly, was obtained by early-season removal of manure plus the use of residual sprays and baits to control adults.[34] *Bacillus thuringiensis* (BT) sprayed onto manure controlled fly larvae, but not predaceous mites, and house flies were controlled by a combination of naled or ronnel baits and the mites, with or without the BT treatment.[35]

Applying dimethoate to manure as a larvicide and using a chemosterilant bait for adults were more effective than the insecticide treatment alone for control of house flies.[36] A residual spray of diflubenzuron applied to house fly resting surfaces plus release of parasitoids and minimum use of dimethoate as a larvicide provided greater control of house flies than did the use of insecticides alone.[37]

Control of larvae of the black soldier fly, a natural competitor with house fly larvae in moist manure,[38] allowed for an increase of house flies, which had been unable to live as larvae in the manure made liquid by the action of the black soldier fly larvae.[39] Treatment of manure with Larvadex® prevented development of black soldier fly and house fly larvae, and the addition of water to untreated manure encouraged development of large numbers of black soldier fly larvae, which provided almost complete control of larvae of the house fly and the little house fly.[40]

In climate-controlled, caged-layer poultry houses in the northern U.S., biological control agents did not prevent the buildup of house fly populations, and larviciding was necessary to reduce fly populations not controlled by adulticiding.[41] In warmer climates, there is a need for habitat stability and supervised fly control (manure removal plus baits for adult flies) in order to maximize the benefits of naturally occurring parasites and predators.[42]

An excellent summary of the benefits gained by properly integrating cultural, biological, and chemical methods to control house flies and filth flies in poultry manure was presented by Axtell.[43] He emphasized keeping poultry manure dry, the timing and extent of manure removal, developing stable populations of predators and parasites, and the careful use of insecticides with the emphasis on adulticides.

III. TREATING POULTRY ORALLY TO CONTROL FLY LARVAE IN MANURE

A. First Effective Treatments

The first report of the effectiveness of a material given orally to caged layers to control house fly larvae in poultry manure was that of Burns et al.,[44] who found that Polybor 3®, in feed, controlled house fly larvae, but boron residues were present in eggs and tissues of treated hens.

The feeding of preparations of spores and crystalline inclusion bodies of BT to chickens reduced the emergence of house flies.[45,46] Different commercially prepared, spore-powder formulations of BT provided variable control of house fly larvae when fed to caged layers, and certain dosages were toxic to the hens.[47] Commercial formulations of spores of BT fed to Japanese quail were effective against house fly larvae, and increased moisture in manure enhanced the effectiveness of the treatment.[48] The treating of larval medium with BT and selection of survivors resulted in house fly larvae 8- to 14-fold less susceptible to BT than unselected larvae.[49] Preparations of sodium and calcium salts of β-exotoxin of BT fed to hens and pullets were toxic to the fowl and did not control house fly larvae in manure. House fly larvae developed 30-fold resistance to BT after 6 months of selection in treated manure.[50]

B. Organophosphorus Treatments

Single oral treatments of malathion, trichlorfon, and ronnel controlled house fly larvae in chick manure for 1 to 6 days posttreatment.[51] Coumaphos, diazinon, trichlorfon, and ronnel controlled fly larvae in manure when fed continuously to chickens, but malathion and phenothiazine were ineffective.[52] Trichlorfon, when added to the water of chicks, controlled fly larvae in their manure, but conversion of trichlorfon to dichlorvos under alkaline conditions decreased larvicidal activity.[53] Although fenthion, ronnel, and several experimental insecticides controlled house fly larvae when fed to broilers, several also caused a decrease in feed consumption.[54]

Coumaphos in the diet of hens controlled larvae of the house fly[55,56] and the little house fly, but the dosage needed in the feeding tests was 70 times the dosage needed when coumaphos was mixed directly with manure.[57] Coumaphos in the diet of laying hens generally afforded moderate to poor control of larvae of the little house fly, the false stable fly, and the house fly, but good to excellent control of larvae of *F. femoralis* and black garbage fly.[58]

Of 44 insecticides administered to chicks in daily diet, several were highly toxic to larvae of the house fly, *Chrysomya megacephala* (Fabricius), *Parasarcophaga argyrostoma* (Robineau-Desvoidy), and the chicken dung fly*, *F. pusio* (Wiedeman), and some were also toxic to the chicks.[59] Propyl thiopyrophosphate in the diet of hens controlled larvae of the house fly and *C. megacephala*.[60] Stirofos in the feed of laying hens controlled larvae of three species listed above, but not *F. pusio*, and also caused a reduction in egg production and affected egg flavor.[61] Chlorpyrifos in the feed of laying hens afforded excellent control of larvae of three species listed above and of *Boettcherisca peregrina* (Robineau-Desvoidy), but only moderate control of larvae of *P. argyrostoma* and did not affect hens or their eggs.[62] Shell® SD-8211 and SD-8280 controlled larvae of all five species of flies listed above.[63]

The feeding of an encapsulated formulation of stirofos decreased metabolism of the insecticide by poultry and provided excellent control of both susceptible and organophosphorus-resistant house fly larvae.[64]

C. Other Treatment Materials

An insect growth regulator, methoprene, almost eliminated emergence of house flies when added to feed of hens,[21] and an encapsulated formulation was ten times more effective then unencapsulated, technical methoprene.[65] Although methoprene in feed reduced emergence of flies from manure of some 18,000 pullets held in large cage-rearing houses, numbers of flies caught on sticky paper or numbers of fly defecation spots on cards were not reduced, presumably the result of immigrating flies.[66] When encapsulated methoprene as a feed additive failed to control house fly larvae, comparative bioassays indicated that the larvae were resistant to methoprene.[67] Diflubenzuron, when added to the feed of laying hens, controlled fly larvae in manure, but residues of the chemical were found in eggs.[68] The feeding of an encapsulated formulation of permethrin to hens controlled house fly larvae.[69]

Feed additives of three experimental triazine insect growth regulators, CGA-19255, CGA-34296, and Larvadex®, prevented emergence of house flies and little house flies, but not the latrine fly♦, *F. scalaris* (Fabricius).[25,26,70-72] A feed additive of Larvadex® prevented larval development and adult emergence of house flies, *F. femoralis,* and the false stable fly.[73] The treatment also controlled larvae of the black soldier fly but did not affect populations of predatory mites and beetles.[74] A feed additive of another insect growth regulator, Bay Vi-7533, prevented emergence of house flies,[75] but high levels in the diet reduced egg production and, at all levels tested, residues of Bay Vi-7533 were detected in the eggs of treated hens.[76,77] *Insecticide and Acaricide Tests* from 1975 to 1985 contain a number of reports on the effectiveness of stirofos, diflubenzuron, three triazine compounds, methoprene, and Bay Vi-7533 as feed-through or water treatments for the control of larvae of several species of flies in poultry manure.

Miller and Miller[78] reviewed progress on research on feed-through treatments for the control of fly larvae in poultry manure and listed ten chemicals that were effective larvicides. The only feed additive to become commercially available for control of fly larvae in poultry manure is Larvadex®.

IV. OVERVIEW AND CURRENT TECHNOLOGY

With the advent of large, complex breeder and caged-layer poultry production systems, the need to control flies in poultry manure has become a critical problem to poultry raisers. The millions of flies that can be produced from manure at large poultry production sites can become a serious nuisance to nearby residential areas. Persons living in these areas can apply public and legal pressure to the poultry producers to eliminate fly breeding or discontinue operations.

The treatment of poultry manure topically with chlorinated hycrocarbon insecticides provided control of house fly larvae for only a short period of time because of the resistance that developed in the flies and larvae. A number of organophosphorus insecticides are effective as topical treatments. However, broad-spectrum insecticides applied to manure to control fly larvae also control parasites, predators, and competitors of the larvae, which, if not affected by the treatment, can provide some control of fly larvae in manure.

A number of insecticides and insect growth regulators were effective against fly larvae when added to the feed or water supply of poultry. Larvadex® is currently registered for that use in the U.S.

The most critical aspect of the control of fly larvae in poultry manure is the proper management of manure. Control of fly breeding in poultry houses can be obtained by integration of chemical, biological, and cultural methods.

REFERENCES

1. **Axtell, R. C.**, Arthropod pests of poultry, in *Livestock Entomology*, Williams, R. E., Hall, R. D., Broce, A. B., and Scholl, P. J., Eds., John Wiley & Sons, New York, 1985, 269.

2. **Wolfenbarger, D. O. and Hoffmann, E.**, Uses of DDT on the poultry farm, *Poultry Sci.*, 23, 545, 1944.

3. **Tanada, Y., Holdaway, F. G., and Quisenberry, J. H.**, DDT to control flies breeding in poultry manure, *J. Econ. Entomol.*, 43, 30, 1950.

4. **Mayeux, H. S.**, Malathion for house fly control, *Fla. Entomol.*, 37, 97, 1954a.

5. **Mayeux, H. S.**, Granular insecticidal baits against flies, *Fla. Entomol.*, 37, 171, 1954b.

6. **Dicke, R. J., Lugthart, G. J., and Jones, R. H.**, Control of maggots in turkey dung with malathion, *J. Econ. Entomol.*, 48, 342, 1955.

7. **Hoffman, R. A. and Monroe, R. E.**, Control of house fly larvae in poultry droppings, *J. Econ. Entomol.*, 49, 704, 1956.

8. **Wilson, H. G. and Gahan, J. B.**, Control of house fly larvae in poultry houses, *J. Econ. Entomol.*, 50, 613, 1957.

9. **Hoffman, R. A. and Monroe, R. E.**, Further tests on the control of fly larvae in poultry and cattle manure, *J. Econ. Entomol.*, 50, 515, 1957.

10. **Knapp, F. W., Terhaar, C. J., and Roan, C. C.**, Dow ET-57 as a fly larvicide, *J. Econ. Entomol.*, 51, 361, 1958.

11. **Wilson, H. G. and LaBrecque, G. C.**, Test with organophosphorus compounds as house fly larvicides in poultry houses, *Fla. Entomol.*, 41, 5, 1958.

12. **Wilson, H. G. and LaBrecque, G. C.**, Tests with larvicides for the control of house flies in poultry houses, *Fla. Entomol.*, 43, 19, 1960.

13. **Smith, W. W.**, Field tests of some soil fumigants as house fly larvicides, *J. Econ. Entomol.*, 55, 1001, 1962.

14. **Bell, D. D., Bowen, W. R., Deal, A. S., and Loomis, E. C.**, Diazinon dust for fly control in poultry manure, *Calif. Agric.*, 19, 8, 1965.

15. **Eversole, J. W., Lilly, J. H., and Shaw, F. R.**, Comparative effectiveness and persistence of certain insecticides in poultry droppings against larvae of the little house fly, *J. Econ. Entomol.*, 58, 704, 1965.

16. **Brady, U. E., Jr. and LaBrecque, G. C.**, Larvicides for the control of house flies in poultry houses, *J. Econ. Entomol.*, 59, 1521, 1966.

17. **Morgan, P. B., LaBrecque, G. C., and Wilson, H. G.**, Tests with larvicides for the control of house flies, *Musca domestica* (Diptera: Muscidae), in poultry houses, *Fla. Entomol.*, 49, 91, 1966.

18. **Bailey, D. L., Meifert, D. W., and Bishop, P. M.**, Control of house flies in poultry houses with larvicides, *Fla. Entomol.*, 51, 107, 1968.

19. **Bailey, D. L., LaBrecque, G. C., and Whitfield, T. L.**, Insecticides applied as low-volume and conventional sprays to control larvae of the house fly in poultry houses, *J. Econ. Entomol.*, 63, 891, 1970.

20. **Bailey, D. L., LaBrecque, G. C., and Whitfield, T. L.**, House fly control in a poultry house with insecticides in slow-release plastic formulations, *J. Econ. Entomol.*, 64, 138, 1971.

21. **Morgan, P. B., LaBrecque, G. C., Weidhaas, D. E., and Benton, A.**, The effect of methoprene, an insect growth regulator, on *Musca domestica* (Diptera: Muscidae), *Can. Entomol.*, 107, 413, 1975.

22. **Ables, J. R., West, R. P., and Shepard, M.**, Response of the house fly and its parasitoids to Dimilin (TH-6040), *J. Econ. Entomol.*, 68, 622, 1975.

23. **Hall, R. D., Vandepopuliere, J. M., and Lyons, J. J.**, Laboratory response of susceptible house flies to thiourea as a larvicide and chemosterilant, *J. Econ. Entomol.*, 72, 204, 1979.

24. **Pimprikar, G. D., Fondren, J. E., Jr., and Heitz, J. R.**, Small- and large-scale field tests of erythrosin B for house fly control in caged layer chicken houses, *Environ. Entomol.*, 9, 53, 1980.

25. **Williams, R. E. and Berry, J. G.**, Evaluation of CGA 72662 as a topical spray and feed additive for controlling house flies breeding in chicken manure, *Poultry Sci.*, 59, 2207, 1980.

26. **Hall, R. D. and Foehse, M. C.**, Laboratory and field tests of CGA-72662 for control of the house fly and face fly in poultry, bovine, or swine manure, *J. Econ. Entomol.*, 73, 564, 1980.

27. **Mulla, M. S. and Axelrod, H.**, Evaluation of Larvadex, a new IGR for the control of pestiferous flies on poultry ranches, *J. Econ. Entomol.*, 76, 520, 1983.

28. **Eastwood, R. E., Kada, J. M., and Schoenburg, R. B.**, Plastic tarpaulins for controlling flies in stockpiled poultry manure fertilizer, *J. Econ. Entomol.*, 59, 1507, 1966.

29. **Eastwood, R. E., Kada, J. M., Schoenburg, R. B., and Brydon, H. W.**, Investigations on fly control by composting poultry manures, *J. Econ. Entomol.*, 60, 88, 1967.

30. **Axtell, R. C.**, Integrated house fly control: populations of fly larvae and predaceous mites, *Macrocheles muscaedomesticae,* in poultry manure after larvicide treatment, *J. Econ. Entomol.*, 61, 245, 1968.

31. **Rodriguez, J. G., Singh, P., and Taylor, B.**, Manure mites and their role in fly control, *J. Med. Entomol.*, 7, 335, 1970.

32. **Axtell, R. C.,** Fly control in caged-poultry houses: comparison of larviciding and integrated control programs, *J. Econ. Entomol., 63,* 1734, 1970.
33. **Peck, J. H. and Anderson, J. R.,** Influence of poultry-manure-removal schedules on various Diptera larvae and selected arthropod predators, *J. Econ. Entomol., 63,* 82, 1970.
34. **Axtell, R. C.,** Integrated fly-control program for caged-poultry houses, *J. Econ. Entomol., 63,* 400, 1970.
35. **Wicht, M. C., Jr. and Rodriguez, J. G.,** Integrated control of muscid flies in poultry houses using predator mites, selected pesticides and microbial agents, *J. Med. Entomol., 7,* 687, 1970.
36. **Meifert, D. W. and LaBrecque, G. C.,** Integrated control for the suppression of a population of house flies, *Musca domestica* L., *J. Med. Entomol., 8,* 43, 1971.
37. **Shepard, M. and Kissam, J. B.,** Integrated control of house flies on poultry farms: treatment of house fly resting surfaces with diflubenzuron plus releases of the parasitoid, *Muscidifurax raptor, J. Ga. Entomol. Soc., 16,* 222, 1981.
38. **Furman, D. P., Young, R. D., and Catts, E. P.,** *Hermetia illucens* (Linnaeus) as a factor in the natural control of *Musca domestica* Linnaeus, *J. Econ. Entomol., 52,* 917, 1959.
39. **Axtell, R. C. and Edwards, T. D.,** *Hermetia illucens* control in poultry manure by larviciding, *J. Econ. Entomol., 63,* 1786, 1970.
40. **Sheppard, C.,** House fly and lesser fly control utilizing the black soldier fly in manure management systems for caged laying hens, *Environ. Entomol., 12,* 1439, 1983.
41. **Matthysse, J. G. and McClain, D.,** House fly control in climate-controlled caged-hen layer houses, *J. Econ. Entomol., 66,* 927, 1973.
42. **Legner, E. F. and Dietrick, E. I.,** Effectiveness of supervised control practices in lowering population densities of synanthropic flies on poultry ranches, *Entomophaga, 19,* 467, 1974.
43. **Axtell, R. C.,** Fly management in poultry production: cultural, biological, and chemical, *Poultry Sci., 65,* 657, 1986.
44. **Burns, E. C., Tower, B. A., Bonner, F. L., and Austin, H. C.,** Feeding Polybor 3 for fly control under caged layers, *J. Econ. Entomol., 52,* 446, 1959.
45. **Briggs, J. D.,** Reduction of adult house-fly emergence by the effects of *Bacillus* spp. on the development of immature forms, *J. Insect Pathol., 2,* 418, 1960.
46. **Harvey, T. L. and Brethour, J. R.,** Feed additives for control of house fly larvae in livestock feces, *J. Econ. Entomol., 53,* 774, 1960.
47. **Burns, E. C., Wilson, B. H., and Tower, B. A.,** Effect of feeding *Bacillus thuringiensis* to caged layers for fly control, *J. Econ. Entomol., 54,* 913, 1961.
48. **Borgatti, A. L. and Guyer, G. E.,** The effectiveness of commercial formulations of *Bacillus thuringiensis* Berliner on house-fly larvae, *J. Insect Pathol., 5,* 377, 1963.
49. **Harvey, T. L. and Howell, D. E.,** Resistance of the house fly to *Bacillus thuringiensis* Berliner, *J. Invert. Pathol., 7,* 92, 1965.
50. **Barker, R. J. and Anderson, W. F.,** Evaluation of β-exotoxin of *Bacillus thuringiensis* Berliner for control of flies in chicken manure, *J. Med. Entomol., 12,* 103, 1975.
51. **Sherman, M. and Ross, E.,** Toxicity of house fly larvae to insecticides administered as single oral dosages to chicks, *J. Econ. Entomol., 52,* 719, 1959.
52. **Sherman, M. and Ross, E.,** Toxicity to house fly larvae of droppings from chickens fed insecticide-treated rations, *J. Econ. Entomol., 53,* 429, 1960.
53. **Sherman, M. and Ross, E.,** Toxicity to house fly larvae of droppings from chicks given Dipterex-treated water, *J. Econ. Entomol., 53,* 1066, 1960.
54. **Dorough, H. W. and Arthur, B. W.,** Toxicity of several organophosphates administered in the diet of broilers to house fly larvae in the feces, *J. Econ. Entomol., 54,* 1117, 1961.
55. **Quigley, G. D. and Harding, W. C., Jr.,** Use of Co-Ral as a systemic insecticide for layers, *Poultry Sci., 42,* 1247, 1963.
56. **Simco, J. S. and Lancaster, J. L., Jr.,** Field test to determine the effectiveness of coumaphos as a feed additive to control house fly larvae under caged layers, *J. Econ. Entomol., 59,* 671, 1966.
57. **Eversole, J. W., Lilly, J. H., and Shaw, F. R.,** Toxicity of droppings from coumaphos-fed hens to little house fly larvae, *J. Econ. Entomol., 58,* 709, 1965.
58. **Loomis, E. C., Deal, A. S., and Bowen, W. R.,** The relative effectiveness of coumaphos as a poultry feed additive to control synanthropic fly larvae in manure, *J. Econ. Entomol., 61,* 904, 1968.
59. **Sherman, M., Komatsu, G. H., and Ikeda, J.,** Larvicidal activity to flies of manure from chicks administered insecticide-treated feed, *J. Econ. Entomol., 60,* 1395, 1967.
60. **Sherman, M., Chang, M. T. Y., and Herrick, R. B.,** Fly control, chronic toxicity, and residues from feeding propyl thiopyrophosphate to laying hens, *J. Econ. Entomol., 62,* 1494, 1969.
61. **Sherman, M. and Herrick, R. B.,** Fly control, chronic toxicity, and residues from feeding Rabon to laying hens, *J. Econ. Entomol., 64,* 1159, 1971.
62. **Sherman, M. and Herrick, R. B.,** Fly control and chronic toxicity from feeding Dursban® (0,0-diethyl 0-3, 5, 6-trichloro-2-pyridyl phosphorothioate) to laying hens, *Poultry Sci., 52,* 741, 1973.

63. **Sherman, M. and Herrick, R. B.**, Fly control and chronic toxicity from feeding two chlorinated organophosphorus insecticides to laying hens, *J. Econ. Entomol.*, 66, 139, 1973.

64. **Wasti, S. S., Mkwaila, B. D., and Shaw, F. R.**, Residues of encapsulated Rabon in poultry manure and its larvicidal activity to house flies, *J. Econ. Entomol.*, 64, 225, 1971.

65. **Breeden, G. C., Turner, E. C., Jr., and Beane, W. L.**, Methoprene as a feed additive for control of the house fly breeding in chicken manure, *J. Econ. Entomol.*, 68, 451, 1975.

66. **Adams, A. W., Jackson, M. E., and Pitts, C. W.**, A feed additive to control flies in poultry manure, *Poultry Sci.*, 55, 2001, 1976.

67. **Breeden, G. C., Turner, E. C., Jr., Beane, W. L., Miller, R. W., and Pickens, L. C.**, The effect of methoprene as a feed additive on house fly emergence in poultry houses, *Poultry Sci.*, 60, 556, 1981.

68. **Miller, R. W., Corley, C., and Hill, K. R.**, Feeding TH 6040 to chickens: effect on larval house flies in manure and determination of residues in eggs, *J. Econ. Entomol.*, 68, 181, 1975.

69. **Townsend, L. H., Jr. and Turner, E. C., Jr.**, Encapsulated Ectiban® permethrin as a feed additive for control of house flies breeding in chicken manure, *J. Ga. Entomol. Soc.*, 15, 460, 1980.

70. **Miller, R. W., Corley, C., and Pickens, L. G.**, CGA-19255: a promising new insect growth regulator tested as a poultry feed additive for control of flies, *Southwest. Entomol.*, 2, 197, 1977.

71. **Christensen, C. M., Knapp, F. W., and Tuttle, J. W.**, The efficacy of two azidotriazine compounds as poultry feed-through fly larvicides, *Poultry Sci.*, 58, 1167, 1979.

72. **Miller, R. W. and Corley, C.**, Feed-through efficacy of CGA-19255 and CGA-72662 against manure-breeding flies and other arthropods and residues in feces, eggs, and tissues of laying hens, *Southwest. Entomol.*, 5, 144, 1980.

73. **Mulla, M. S. and Axelrod, H.**, Evaluation of the IGR Larvadex as a feed-through treatment for the control of pestiferous flies on poultry ranches, *J. Econ. Entomol.*, 76, 515, 1983.

74. **Axtell, R. C. and Edwards, T. D.**, Efficacy and nontarget effects of Larvadex® as a feed additive for controlling house flies in caged-layer poultry manure, *Poultry Sci.*, 62, 2371, 1983.

75. **Miller, R. W.**, Bay Vi 7533 tested in cattle and poultry as a feed-through compound against flies, *Southwest. Entomol.*, 7, 130, 1982.

76. **Beck, A. F., Vaughan, J. A., and Turner, E. C., Jr.**, Bay VI-7533 insect growth regulator: effect on house fly adult emergence and caged-layer egg production when administered in layer feed, *J. Ga. Entomol. Soc.*, 18, 159, 1983.

77. **Miller, R. W., Wong, Y., and Thomas, O. P.**, Feeding BAY Vi 7533 to hens, *Poultry Sci.*, 63, 1748, 1984.

78. **Miller, R. W. and Miller, J. A.**, Feed-through chemicals for insect control in animals, in *Agricultural Chemicals of the Future*, Hilton, J. L., Ed., Rowman and Allanheld, Totowa, N. J., 1984, 355.

Chapter 17

AREA CONTROL OF TICKS AND CHIGGERS*

I. INTRODUCTION

The control of tick and chigger pests of livestock has generally been accomplished by the application of acaricides directly onto the host animals (see Chapter 11). Because all species of ticks and chiggers spend much or a portion of their life cycle off of the host, there has been some interest and research activity to develop technologies for the area control of these acarines. Chapter 15 discusses control of the fowl tick✦, *Argas persicus* (Oken), by applying acaricides to poultry structures or by constructing poultry houses so as to eliminate hiding places of the off-the-host stages. Chapter 15 discusses control of the turkey chigger✦, *Neoschongastia americana* (Hirst), by applying acaricides to the pens and soil where turkeys are held.

This chapter will focus on the use of acaricides and other control measures to control ticks and chiggers in pastures and recreational areas. These area control technologies have been directed primarily against those species that are of more importance to man because of tick-borne disease, such as Rocky Mountain spotted fever, Lyme disease, or babesiosis or because ticks are nuisance problems.

II. CONTROL OF TICKS

Control of the Rocky Mountain wood tick✦, *Dermacentor andersoni* Stiles, a vector of Rocky Mountain spotted fever, was accomplished by dipping livestock in acaricides. Other control technologies included destroying the rodent hosts of immature stages of the tick, removing livestock from pastures, burning pastures, and clearing and developing forest land.[1]

Eradication of the cattle tick✦, *Boophilus annulatus* (Say), from the U.S. was accomplished by the dipping of cattle in arsenic and the removing of cattle from infested pastures for a period of time sufficient to allow for the death of the larvae of this one-host species.[2] No mention is made of the treatment of pastures with acaricides, presumably because of the large areas involved.

A. Acaricides

1. Organochlorine Treatments

After World War II, Smith and Gouck[3] published their pioneering research on application of acaricides to the environment to control the American dog tick✦, *Dermacentor variabilis* (Say); the blacklegged tick✦, *Ixodes scapularis* Say; and the lone star tick✦, *Amblyomma americanum* (Linnaeus). Sprays of nicotine sulfate, a mixture of nicotine sulfate and sodium fluoride, dinitroorthocyclohexylphenyl, and pyrethrins gave an immediate reduction in tick abundance but had limited residual activity. DDT sprays or dusts not only gave excellent initial kill of ticks but also had considerable residual effectiveness.[4,5]

In their classic study on the American dog tick, Smith et al.[6] listed control measures as treating dogs and cattle with acaricides, treating vegetation (ticks tended to occur in abundance along sides of roads and paths and the treating of these limited areas would kill a

---

* Common names of insects and acarines, as listed in *Common Names of Insects and Related Organisms* (published by the Entomological Society of America), are marked with a ✦ the first time they are cited preceding the scientific name.

high proportion of host-seeking ticks), eradication of meadow mice, and burning grass in the tick habitat. Large-scale application of DDT controlled the American dog tick, the lone star tick, and blacklegged tick for several months.[7] DDT plus pyrethrins applied by a ground-operated thermal aerosol fog generator controlled questing American dog tick adults; benzene hexachloride (BHC) and nicotine were also effective.[8] Aerial application of DDT or ground application of DDT or BHC sprays or dusts to vegetation along roadsides or trails controlled host-seeking American dog ticks.[9] DDT applied to vegetation to control adult American dog ticks had sufficient residual activity to kill larvae that hatched from eggs laid in the treated area.[10] In small plot tests, dieldrin was as effective as DDT; toxaphene and chlordane were slightly less effective and parathion was effective but had a very short residual activity.[11] Sprays of chlordane and toxaphene were as effective as DDT for the control of the lone star tick;[12] BHC was less effective and nicotine and isobornyl thiocyanoacetate were ineffective. Dusts of BHC, toxaphene, chlordane, and parathion were as effective as DDT. Large-scale testing with DDT indicated that large treated areas became reinfested much more slowly than small experimental plots. If roadside vegetation was treated with DDT early in the year, a second treatment may be necessary to provide season-long control of the American dog tick.[13]

Dusts of dieldrin were more effective against the lone star tick than those of aldrin, lindane, DDT, and chlordane.[14] A granular formulation of dieldrin provided long-term control of lone star ticks, and heptachlor and chlordane were less effective.[15] Sprays of dieldrin and heptachlor became effective against Rocky Mountain wood ticks by 3 weeks posttreatment although initial rate of kill was low.[16] The spraying of roadside vegetation with combinations of DDT or lindane with the herbicides, 2,4-D and 2,4,5-T, not only killed American dog ticks, but also the woodside vegetation on which the ticks ascended to await hosts; DDT afforded longer residual control than lindane.[17]

2. Organophosphorus Treatments

High-volume applications (77 ℓ/ha) of chlorpyrifos, diazinon, fenthion, and fenitrothion were as effective as DDT, and aerial ultra-low-volume (ULV) (0.2 to 2.2 kg/ha) applications of fenthion were less effective then ground ULV applications of fenthion or propoxur.[18]

The carbamate, carbaryl, controlled the tropical bont tick, *Amblyomma variegatum* (Fabricius), in the U.S. Virgin Islands.[19] Carbaryl was applied with turbine blowers and sprayers carried on jeeps, and areas inaccessible to ground vehicles were treated with carbaryl applied by aircraft. The area treatment plus dipping or spray dipping of cattle and other livestock in coumaphos eradicated *A. variegatum* in a campaign of only 8 months.

ULV (0.2-4.7 ℓ/ha) applications of chlorpyrifos, fenthion, naled, propoxur, fenitrothion, and stirofos were as effective against the lone star tick as high-volume applications of the same acaricides and offered the advantages of small volume and simpler application equipment.[20] Diazinon or chlorpyrifos applied as granules were slightly less effective than ULV applications of these acaricides for the control of lone star ticks.[21] In limited field tests, sprays of the pyrethroids, NRDC-161 and permethrin, were as effective as sprays of the standard treatment of chlorpyrifos for control of lone star ticks; diazinon sprays were also highly effective, while carbaryl was less effective and a slow release granular formulation of chlorpyrifos was ineffective.[22]

Both naled and chlorpyrifos were highly toxic to larvae of the American dog tick,[23] and, in field tests, naled sprays reduced populations of questing ticks.[24] It was necessary to apply naled three to four times to vegetation to control the American dog tick during its activity period.[25]

High-volume sprays of permethrin, propoxur, diazinon, and naled as well as granules of diazinon were generally as effective against overwintered free-living nymphs and adults as sprays of chlorpyrifos or stirofos, which were labeled for use for the area control of lone star ticks.[26] Chlorpyrifos or stirofos applied with a tractor-mounted air blast sprayer at a volume of 47 ℓ/ha provided satisfactory area control of lone star ticks.[27]

Treatment of vegetation with one to three applications of high-volume sprays of chlorpyrifos, diazinon, or stirofos or granules of diazinon in the late summer controlled lone star tick larvae.[28] Aerial application of diazinon granules was as effective as ground application of similar rates of treatment.[29] An ULV (0.34 to 1.2 ℓ/ha) mist application was as effective as a low-volume (47 ℓ/ha) application of chlorpyrifos for control of lone star ticks.[30] Applications of chlorpyrifos, diazinon, or stirofos were more effective in May than in March, indicating an age-related increase in acaricide susceptibility of lone star ticks.[31] Sprays of propetamphos, but not diazinon or bendiocarb, were as effective as the chlorpyrifos standard.[32]

A unique, baited pesticide treatment station was described by Sonenshine and Haines[33] in which the small mammal hosts of the American dog tick were attracted into baited containers and, while there, were treated with carbaryl dust or diazinon oil. This technique controlled the ticks and could be used in areas of high human population density where other methods of tick control would be unacceptable.

Ticks on baled hay, hides, or in quarantine facilities were controlled by fumigation with methyl bromide; dichlorvos vapors were only partially effective and immersion in salt solution was ineffective.[34-36]

B. Nonchemical and Integrated Technologies

Control of lone star ticks in recreation areas was reviewed by Hair and Howell,[37] who suggested that an integrated program of vegetative alteration and acaricide treatment could suppress populations of lone star ticks in recreation areas. The mechanical clearing of undergrowth plus the use of stirofos spray was the most effective of a variety of treatments, including acaricide spray alone, clearing plus application of the herbicide, 2,4,5-T, the herbicide only, or clearing only.[38] Cleared areas became rapidly reinfested when the secondary growth of new vegetation attracted tick-infested deer into the area. In a 4-year study, the clearing of vegetation mechanically or by herbicide application, with or without the application of stirofos, reduced all stages of the lone star tick.[39] The mechanical clearing of trails plus the application of chlorpyrifos as a spray or granules along cleared trails provided satisfactory control of lone star ticks in recreation areas.[40]

Wilkinson,[41] in an analysis of methods that could be used to prevent paralysis of cattle by *D. andersoni*, listed vegetation modification, reduction of ticks on rodents, and acaricide treatments in order to reduce the total number of ticks in the environment. The treatment of certain shrubs with a spray of a mixture of 2,4-D and picloram or with pellets of picloram did not reduce numbers of Rocky Mountain wood ticks.[42] In a review of the ecological aspects of managing ixodid ticks, Wilkinson[43] discussed most of the techniques listed above to control ticks in the environment and suggested future research needs and prospects for practical tick control.

Removal of understory vegetation, partial removal of overstory, and frequent mowing to maintain grass at less than 15 cm controlled all stages, especially larvae, of the lone star tick.[44] Habitat modification, which involved the clearing of land and establishment of new pasture, significantly reduced numbers of lone star ticks on the pasture and on cattle and was more effective and profitable than the use of fences to exclude cattle from favorable tick habitats or standard spraying of cattle for tick control.[45]

Controlled burning is used to alter the habitat by incinerating the standing vegetation, surface leaf litter, and duff layer, which is the lower, compact, decaying forest litter. Such burning did not kill lone star ticks in pastures because many of the ticks in the duff layer were not exposed to the high temperatures of the fire in the burning leaf litter.[46] In contrast, numbers of lone star ticks infesting turkeys that grazed on recently burned plots were significantly fewer than numbers on turkey poults that grazed on unburned plots.[47] Fewer adult blacklegged ticks were collected from tick drags on pine-palmetto flatwood areas for 3 years after burning.[48] Populations of the Gulf Coast tick♦, *Amblyomma maculatum* Koch, were reduced for two seasons following burning of large (12,000-ha) areas, but not small (1-ha) areas.[49] A prescribed burn in the spring in Canada killed ca. 97% of engorged female winter tick♦, *D. albipictus* (Packard), and also reduced the number of larvae recovered.[50]

The mechanical flaming of vegetation, flaming plus the exclusion of bovine hosts, and the use of herbicides to control woody plants were evaluated as methods to reduce populations of lone star ticks.[51] Treatment with herbicide was more effective against the ticks, less costly then flaming, and allowed for additional forage areas and, thus, was the treatment of choice.

In 1984, a pilot test was initiated at selected sites in Tennessee Valley Authority Land Between The Lakes to evaluate integrated technology to manage lone star ticks in recreation areas. That test involves the use of management of the hosts (especially deer) of the adult ticks, alteration of the habitat by management of vegetation, and the use of acaricides applied to the environment.[52]

III. CONTROL OF CHIGGERS

Chiggers, more of a pest of man than of livestock, are generally controlled by the application of acaricides to the soil. In 1921, *U.S. Dep. Agric. Bulletin* No. 986[53] reviewed the early literature on chiggers, described a number of personal protective measures to prevent chiggers from reaching the skin of humans, and listed several area control measures, such as the destruction of breeding places by mowing, grazing of sheep or cattle to eat the grass, brush removal, and applying sulfur dust to limited ground areas. Chigger control consisted of applying sulfur to heavily infested areas, cleaning up leaves and litter, and applying sulfur to the skin and clothing of persons.[54]

During the 1940s, there was considerable interest in the testing of acaricides applied to the ground for the control of chiggers. In tests with *Acariscus masoni* (Ewing), dusts of DDT, sulfur and dinitro-*o*-cresol were more effective than those of cryolite, sodium fluoride, phenazine, and diphenylamine, and dusts of DDT and sulfur were also effective against *Eutrombicula alfreddugesi* (Oudemans).[55] Dusts or sprays of hydroxypentamethylflaven, sulfur, benzene hexachloride (BHC), and sprays of chlordane and toxaphene were all highly effective.[56] Of about 75 materials tested as dusts or sprays, the most effective were BHC, Valone®, and pentachlorophenol, while DDT and sulfur were less effective than a number of the compounds tested.[57] Both BHC and cyclohexanone afforded excellent chigger control, and, because BHC was effective by fumigant action, control was obtained when BHC was inpregnated onto coarse materials which penetrated the ground cover.[58]

Ground treatments with dusts of DDT or sprays of DDT, diphenylamine, or diphenylene oxide in diesel oil were no more effective than sprays of the diesel oil alone to control chiggers.[59] Both dieldrin and aldrin sprays provided practical, efficient control of chiggers.[60] In the U.S., in small plot tests, the more effective treatments were toxaphene, dieldrin, lindane, and BHC, and tepp, diazinon, malathion, and parathion were less effective.[61]

In tests with alternative, biodegradable acaricides, ULV (1.5 to 16.7 ℓ/ha) application of propoxur provided control of chiggers equal to that provided by high-volume (473 ℓ/ha) application.[62] Chlorpyrifos, applied as an ULV spray or as a granular formulation, was as effective as the standard propoxur ULV spray.[63] The granules gave excellent penetration of foliage and could be applied with less complex equipment than the sprays. Permethrin and NRDC-161, as ULV sprays or granular formulation (NRDC-161 only), were not as effective as the standard propoxur ULV spray.[64]

Burning of forest litter reduced populations of chiggers for only 2 days, and thereafter populations increased steadily.[65]

IV. OVERVIEW AND CURRENT TECHNOLOGY

Historically, there has been limited use of technologies for area control of ticks. Pasture vacation was an area control strategy that was employed as one aspect of the national campaign that eradicated cattle ticks from the U.S. Because of the large number of alternative hosts (such as native and exotic deer and other game) found on many ranches today, the use of pasture vacation alone is being questioned as an appropriate technique.

In the 1940s and 1950s, chlorinated hydrocarbon acaricides were evaluated as area treatments for the control of ticks of importance to humans. From the 1960s to the 1980s, a limited number of organophosphorus acaricides were also tested. Both chlorpyrifos and stirofos became commercially available for area control of ticks. In addition, other methods (such as burning of pastures and clearing of vegetation) have been used alone or integrated with acaricides for the area control of ticks. Treatment technology has advanced through research to the point that low-volume or ultra-low-volume applications of acaricides to control ticks or chiggers are as effective as high-volume sprays and are more easily applied.

Integrated tick control or management strategies, including vegetative management, area application of acaricides, and livestock management have the potential to significantly reduce the numbers of ticks on cattle. These methods are expensive and normally are not cost-effective for the livestock producer. In general, the use of area control methods for ticks or chiggers is limited to areas that are used by humans and where ticks or chiggers are a nuisance or the disease-carrying aspects of ticks pose a potential human problem.

REFERENCES

1. **Burgdorfer, W.,** Tick-borne diseases in the United States: Rocky Mountain spotted fever and Colorado tick fever, *Acta Trop., 34,* 103, 1977.
2. **Graybill, H. W.,** Methods of exterminating the Texas-fever tick, *U.S. Dep. Agri. Farmers' Bull.,* 498, 1912.
3. **Smith, C. N. and Gouck, H. K.,** Sprays for the control of ticks about houses or camps, *J. Econ. Entomol.,* 37, 85, 1944.
4. **Smith, C. N. and Gouck, H. K.,** Effectiveness of DDT in the control of ticks on vegetation, *J. Econ. Entomol.,* 37, 128, 1944.
5. **Smith, C. N. and Gouck, H. K.,** DDT to control ticks on vegetation, *J. Econ. Entomol.,* 38, 553, 1945.
6. **Smith, C. N., Cole, M. M., and Gouck, H. K.,** Biology and control of the American dog tick, *U.S. Dep. Agric. Tech. Bull.,* 905, 1946.
7. **Gouck, H. K. and Smith, C. N.,** DDT to control wood ticks, *J. Econ. Entomol.,* 40, 303, 1947.
8. **Glasgow, R. D. and Collins, D. L.,** Control of the American dog tick, a vector of Rocky Mountain spotted fever: preliminary tests, *J. Econ. Entomol.,* 39, 235, 1946.
9. **Glasgow, R. D. and Collins, D. L.,** Ecological, economic and mechanical considerations relating to the control of ticks and Rocky Mountain spotted fever on Long Island, *J. Econ. Entomol.,* 41, 427, 1948.
10. **Collins, D. L. and Nardy, R. V.,** Effects of DDT spray residues on larvae of the tick *Dermacentor variabilis* Say, *J. Econ. Entomol.,* 43, 861, 1950.
11. **Gouck, H. K. and Fluno, J. A.,** Field tests on control of American dog tick in Massachusetts, *J. Econ. Entomol.,* 43, 698, 1950.
12. **McDuffie, W. C., Eddy, G. W., Jr., Clark, J. C., and Husman, C. N.,** Field studies with insecticides to control the lone star tick in Texas, *J. Econ. Entomol.,* 43, 520, 1950.
13. **Collins, D. L. and Nardy, R. V.,** The development and application of spray procedures for controlling the tick *Dermacentor variabilis* Say, *N.Y. State Mus. Circ.,* 26, 1951.
14. **Therrien, A. A., Hunter, G. W., III, Moon, A. P., and Adams, A. L.,** Tests of potential acaricides against the lone star tick, *J. Econ. Entomol.,* 47, 76, 1954.
15. **Lancaster, J. L., Jr.,** Preliminary studies of granular insecticides against the lone star tick, *J. Kans. Entomol. Soc.,* 30, 41, 1957.

16. **Curtis, L. C.**, Control of the Rocky Mountain wood tick, *Dermacentor andersoni* Stiles (Acarina:Ixodidae), with ground sprays of dieldrin and heptachlor, *Proc. Entomol. Soc. Br. Col.*, 56, 13, 1959.

17. **McKiel, J. A., Dever, D. A., Proctor, J. R., and Garvie, M. B.**, Herbicide-insecticide formulations for control of the American dog tick, *J. Econ. Entomol.*, 60, 1570, 1967.

18. **Mount, G. A., Hirst, J. M., McWilliams, J. G., Lofgren, C. S., and White, S. A.**, Insecticides for control of the lone star tick tested in the laboratory and as high- and ultra-low-volume sprays in wooded areas, *J. Econ. Entomol.*, 61, 1005, 1968.

19. **Hourrigan, J. L., Strickland, R. K., Kelsey, O. L., Knisely, B. E., Crago, C. C., Whittaker, S., and Gilhooly, D. J.**, Eradication efforts against tropical bont tick, *Amblyoma variegatum*, in the Virgin Islands, *J. Am. Vet. Med. Assoc.*, 154, 540, 1969.

20. **Grothaus, R. H., Mount, G. A., Hirst, J. M., and Keenan, W. T.**, ULV and HV lone star tick control, *Pest Control*, 43, 18, 1975.

21. **Mount, G. A., Grothaus, R. H., Reed, J. T., and Baldwin, K. F.**, *Amblyomma americanum:* area control with granules or concentrated sprays of diazinon, propoxur, and chlorpyrifos, *J. Econ. Entomol.*, 69, 257, 1976.

22. **Roberts, R. H., Zimmerman, J. H., and Mount, G. A.**, Evaluation of potential acaricides as residues for the area control of the lone star tick, *J. Econ. Entomol.*, 73, 506, 1980.

23. **White, D. J. and Benach, J. L.**, Control of *Dermacentor variabilis*. 1. Larval and adult susceptibility to selected insecticides, *J. N.Y. Entomol. Soc.*, 139, 16, 1981.

24. **White, D. J., Benach, J. L., Smith, L. A., and Ouyang, S. P.**, Control of *Dermacentor variabilis*. III. An analytical study of the effect of low volume spray frequency on insecticide-stressed and nonstressed populations, *J. N.Y. Entomol. Soc.*, 139, 23, 1981.

25. **White, D. J., Benach, J. L., Smith, L. A., and Ouyang, S. P.**, Analysis of a chemical control study for *Dermacentor variabilis*, in *Rickettsiae and Rickettsial Diseases*, Burgdorfer, W. and Anacker, R. L., Eds., Academic Press, New York, 1981, 603.

26. **Mount, G. A.**, *Amblyoma americanum:* area control of overwintered nymphs and adults in Oklahoma with acaricides, *J. Econ. Entomol.*, 74, 24, 1981.

27. **Mount, G. A.**, *Amblyomma americanum:* control in Oklahoma parks with air-blast sprayer applications of acaricides, *J. Econ. Entomol.*, 74, 27, 1981.

28. **Mount, G. A.**, Area control of larvae of the lone star tick (Acari: Ixodidae) with acaricides, *J. Econ. Entomol.*, 76, 113, 1983.

29. **Mount, G. A.**, Aerial application of diazinon granules for area control of the lone star tick (Acari: Ixodidae), *J. Econ. Entomol.*, 77, 1211, 1984.

30. **Mount, G. A. and Whitney, R. W.**, Ultralow-volume mists of chlorpyrifos from a tractor-mounted blower for area control of the lone star tick (Acari: Ixodidae), *J. Econ. Entomol.*, 77, 1219, 1984.

31. **Mount, G. A.**, Effect of age, application date, and life stage on the susceptibility of free-living lone star ticks (Acari: Ixodidae) to acaricides, *J. Econ. Entomol.*, 77, 1214, 1984.

32. **Roberts, R. H., Breeden, G. C., Zimmerman, J. H., and Kline, D. L.**, Small plot evaluation of potential residual acaricides against the lone star tick, *J. Agric. Entomol.*, 1, 64, 1984.

33. **Sonenshine, D. E. and Haines, G.**, A convenient method for controlling populations of the American dog tick, *Dermacentor variabilis* (Acari: Ixodidae), in the natural environment, *J. Med. Entomol.*, 22, 577, 1985.

34. **Barnett, S. F. and Parsons, B. T.**, The control of ticks on fodder and bedding using methyl bromide, *Vet. Rec.*, 75, 1213, 1963.

35. **Roth, H.**, Fumigants for quarantine control of the adult brown dog tick: laboratory studies, *J. Econ. Entomol.*, 66, 1283, 1973.

36. **Gladney, W. J.**, Preliminary tests with methyl bromide and dichlorvos as fumigants for *Boophilus* spp. ticks at quaratine stations, ARS-S-102, U.S. Department of Agriculture, Washington, D. C., 1976.

37. **Hair, J. A. and Howell, D. E.**, Lone star ticks their biology and control in Ozark recreation areas, *Okla. State Agric. Exp. Stn. Bull.*, B-679, 1970.

38. **Clymer, B. C., Howell, D. E., and Hair, J. A.**, Environmental alteration in recreational areas by mechanical and chemical treatment as a means of lone star tick control, *J. Econ. Entomol.*, 63, 504, 1970.

39. **Hoch, A. L., Barker, R. W., and Hair, J. A.**, Further observations on the control of lone star ticks (Acarina: Ixodidae) through integrated control procedures, *J. Med. Entomol.*, 8, 731, 1971.

40. **Cooney, J. C. and Pickard, E.**, Comparative tick control field tests — Land between the Lakes, *Down Earth*, 28, 9, 1972.

41. **Wilkinson, P. R.**, Pest-management concepts and control of tick paralysis in British Columbia, *J. Entomol. Soc. Br. Col.*, 65, 3, 1968.

42. **Wilkinson, P. R.** Effect of herbicidal killing of shrubs on abundance of adult *Dermacentor andersoni* (Acarina: Ixodidae) in British Columbia, *J. Med. Entomol.*, 13, 713, 1977.

43. **Wilkinson, P. R.**, Ecological aspects of pest management of ixodid ticks, in *Recent Advances in Acarology*, Vol. 2, Rodriguez, J. G., Ed., Academic Press, New York, 1979, 25.

44. **Mount, G. A.,** Control of the lone star tick in Oklahoma parks though vegetative management, *J. Econ. Entomol.,* 74, 173, 1981.
45. **Meyer, J. A., Lancaster, J. L., Jr., and Simco, J. S.,** Comparison of habitat modification, animal control, and standard spraying for control of the lone star tick, *J. Econ. Entomol.,* 75, 524, 1982.
46. **Hoch, A. L., Semtner, P. J., Barker, R. W., and Hair, J. A.,** Preliminary observations on controlled burning for lone star tick (Acari: Ixodidae) control in woodlots, *J. Med. Entomol.,* 9, 446, 1972.
47. **Jacobson, H. A. and Hurst, G. A.,** Prevalence of parasitism by *Amblyomma americanum* on wild turkey poults as influenced by prescribed burning, *J. Wildlife Dis.,* 15, 43, 1979.
48. **Rogers, A. J.,** The abundance of *Ixodes scapularis* Say as affected by burning, *Fla. Entomol.,* 38, 17, 1955.
49. **Oldham, T. W., Scifres, C. J., and Drawe, D. L.,** Gulf Coast tick response to prescribed burning on the coastal prairie, Brush Management: Range Improvement Research 1980—81, Progress Report 3993, Texas A & M University, College Station, 1982, 153.
50. **Drew, M. L., Samuel, W. M., Lukiwski, G. M., and Willman, J. N.,** An evaluation of burning for control of winter ticks, *Dermacentor albipictus,* in Central Alberta, *J. Wildlife Dis.,* 21, 313, 1985.
51. **Barnard, D. R.,** Density perturbation in populations of *Amblyomma americanum* (Acari: Ixodidae) in beef cattle forage areas in response to two regimens of vegetation management, *J. Econ. Entomol.,* 79, 122, 1986.
52. **Anon.,** USDA-TVA team tackles ticks, *Impact,* 7, 2, 1984.
53. **Ewing, H. E.,** Studies on the biology and control of chiggers, *U.S. Dep. Agric. Bull.,* 986, 1921.
54. **Ewing, H. E.,** Recent developments in regard to the control of chiggers, *J. Wash. Acad. Sci.,* 17, 182, 1927.
55. **Smith, C. N. and Gouck, H. K.,** DDT, sulfur, and other insecticides for the control of chiggers, *J. Econ. Entomol.,* 37, 131, 1944.
56. **Smith, C. N. and Gouck, H. K.,** The control of chiggers in woodland plots, *J. Econ. Entomol.,* 40, 790, 1947.
57. **Linduska, J. P., Morton, F. A., and McDuffie, W. C.,** Tests of materials for the control of chiggers on the ground, *J. Econ. Entomol.,* 41, 43, 1948.
58. **Linduska, J. P. and Morton, F. A.,** Benzene hexachloride for area control of trombiculid mites, *Am. J. Trop. Med.,* 27, 771, 1947.
59. **Bushland, R. C.,** Insecticides applied to forest litter to control New Guinea chiggers, *J. Econ. Entomol.,* 39, 344, 1946.
60. **Traub, R., Newson, H. D., Walton, B. C., and Audy, J. R.,** Efficacy of dieldrin and aldrin in area control of the chigger vectors of scrub typhus, *J. Econ. Entomol.,* 47, 429, 1954.
61. **Keller, J. C. and Gouck, H. K.,** Small-plot tests for the control of chiggers, *J. Econ. Entomol.,* 50, 141, 1957.
62. **Mount, G. A., Grothaus, R. H., Baldwin, K. F., and Haskins, J. R.,** ULV sprays of propoxur for control of *Trombicula alfreddugesi, J. Econ. Entomol.,* 68, 761, 1975.
63. **Mount, G. A., Grothaus, R. H., Reed, J. T., and Baldwin, K. F.,** Area control of chigger mites with granules and concentrated sprays of chlorpyrifos, *J. Econ. Entomol.,* 71, 27, 1978.
64. **Roberts, R. H. and Zimmerman, J. H.,** Chigger mites: efficacy of control with two pyrethroids, *J. Econ. Entomol.,* 73, 811, 1980.
65. **Reed, J. T., Passingham, L. H., and Grothaus, R. H.,** The effect of forest litter burning on populations of the chigger *Eutrombicula alfreddugesi* (Acarina: Trombiculidae), *J. Med. Entomol.,* 14, 134, 1977.

Chapter 18

CONTROL OF FLIES IN LIVESTOCK MANURE AND AROUND STRUCTURES*

I. INTRODUCTION

Most chapters of this book focus on the technology of applying insecticides, acaricides, and other chemicals directly to livestock to control arthropod pests that spend some, most, or all of their lives on livestock. However, there are a number of arthropods, especially the filth-breeding flies, that spend little or none of their lives on livestock, yet are also considered important pests. These arthropods breed in manure, filth, and wastes that accumulate around livestock structures. The control of these species depends upon measures that decrease or eliminate larval breeding or are effective against the adult stage of the species. Chapter 16 addresses the control of flies and other arthropods that breed in poultry manure. Sections of Chapters 2 and 6 address the control of larvae of the horn fly*, *Haematobia irritans* (Linnaeus), and of the face fly*, *Musca autumnalis* De Geer, which develop in fresh, intact cattle manure.

In this chapter, we shall review the technology used to control larvae and adults of filth- and waste-breeding flies found in livestock manure and in or around structures that house livestock. The most important pest species found in this environment are the house fly*, *Musca domestica* Linnaeus, and the stable fly*, *Stomoxys calcitrans* (Linnaeus). Species of flies in other genera, such as *Muscina, Ophyra, Fannia, Hermetia*, which may become problems, also breed in that habitat. Because of the importance and ubiquitous nature of the house fly, it has been the object of a number of books on its biology and control and, thus, the literature and knowledge base are enormous. We shall not try to review all this information but will focus on the house fly and its association with livestock. Thus, control technologies reviewed will be both selected and limited to the veterinary aspects of the species. In contrast, the literature on control of the stable fly and other pest flies found around livestock structures is much more limited and will be reviewed in depth. Some aspects of the biological control of these species are addressed in Chapter 21.

The most important and effective technology to eliminate breeding of flies in manure and other wastes associated with confined livestock is the constant removal of manure from the premises and spreading of the removed manure on fields for use as fertilizer. Dry manure is not attractive to ovipositing flies and is not a suitable medium for larval growth. If manure cannot be removed, then other measures must be used in order to control fly larvae.

The first part of this chapter will be devoted to a review of control measures applied to manure topically. Because of its uniqueness, the treatment of manure to control fly larvae by the addition of chemicals to the diet or water of cattle and other livestock will be discussed next. Finally, there is a section on the treatment of adults in structures.

II. TREATMENT OF MANURE TOPICALLY

A. Early Treatment Technology

Historically, the most important larval medium for the breeding of house flies and stable flies was horse manure when mixed with straw, hay, feed, and other materials. Early studies

---

* Common names of insects and acarines, as listed in *Common Names of Insects and Related Organisms* (published by the Entomological Society of America), are marked with a * the first time they are cited preceding the scientific name.

in the U.S. on the control of the house fly focused on the control of larvae in horse manure. *U.S. Dep. Agric. Farmers' Bulletin* No. 459 in 1911[1] stated that the first measure to control house flies was the prompt gathering and spreading of horse manure. Treatment of manure piles to control fly larvae with chloride of lime was expensive, but effective, and treatment with kerosene was cheap, but ineffective on a large scale. Also, holding manure in a fly-tight closet provided some control of flies.

There was a considerable increase in the amount of information on the control of house flies between 1911 and 1920. Following observations[2] that house fly larvae migrated from moist manure to dryer manure in order to pupate, a maggot trap was designed[3,4] so that larvae leaving moist manure placed on a wooden platform above a concrete basin fell into the water-filled basin and drowned. Manure had to be kept moistened and the basin had to be kept free of debris that fell from the platform.

The use of chemicals to treat horse manure, which was defined as horse urine and feces mixed with feed, hay, straw, and other debris, to kill fly larvae was reviewed in 1914 in *U.S. Dep. Agric. Bulletin* No. 118.[5] This bulletin reported that borax (sodium borate) or calcined colemanite (crude calcium borate) killed larvae and did not affect fertilizing properties of the manure, but that applying greater than 15 tons of treated manure per acre may affect plant growth. *U.S. Dep. Agric. Bulletin* No. 245 in 1915[6] reported that powdered hellebore (*Veratrum album* and *V. viride*), an alkaloid, was as effective as borax. A mixture of calcium cyanamid, acid phosphate, and kainit controlled larvae and increased the fertilizing value of the manure.[7]

In 1915, *U.S. Dep. Agric. Farmers' Bulletin* No. 679,[8] which superseded Bulletin No. 459, contained a large section on preventive and control measures for fly larvae. It included rules for construction and care of stables, use of fly-tight manure pits or bins, removal of horse manure two times per week in rural areas and daily in suburban areas, treating manure with powdered hellebore or borax, and a detailed description of the maggot trap. In 1917, *U.S. Dep. Agric. Farmers' Bulletin* No. 851[9] superseded Bulletin No. 679, listed all the previous control technologies, and added that the treating of manure with a mixture of calcium cyanamid and acid phosphate plus compact heaping of manure made the manure heap unfavorable for larval development. In 1924, *U.S. Dep. Agric. Farmers' Bulletin* No. 1408[10] superseded Bulletin No. 851 and a 1926 revision of Bulletin No. 1408[11] contained no changes in control technology.

In the 1930s and early 1940s there was little published on new technologies to control flies in manure and around livestock structures. During this period the numbers of horses rapidly decreased due to the widespread use of the automobile. Beef cattle feedlots and confined dairy cattle, two present major sources of bovine manure, had not become very widespread. Sodium fluosilicate was as effective as borax for controlling fly larvae and had no detrimental effect on the growth of certain plants, as was the case with borax-treated manure.[12] The forming of manure piles into ricks with perpendicular sides and covering the ricks with tar roofing paper or creosote-oil impregnated burlap for 4 to 5 days controlled house fly larvae.[13]

B. Organochlorine Treatments

Preliminary tests showed that DDT was extremely effective as a larvicide when sprayed onto cow manure.[14] In large-scale tests, treatment of manure piles with DDT was only partially effective and not of much practical value.[15] Muma and Hixon[16] reviewed this "DDT era" and found that sanitation, although dismissed by some entomologists as unimportant because DDT and other chlorinated hydrocarbon insecticides were so effective against flies, affected the length of residual effectiveness of these treatments.

After finding that house flies became resistant faster and had higher levels of resistance to DDT when both larvae and adults were treated, Bruce and Decker[17] recommended that adulticides should not contaminate manure and larvicides should not be related to the adulticiding chemical. Larvae of a strain of house flies resistant as adults to DDT were also resistant to DDT.[18] House fly larvae were controlled by treating manure and other breeding sites with aldrin, heptachlor, and chlordane. However, the treatments did not reduce the numbers of adults, and treatment of larvae resulted in much faster development of resistance in adults than the treatment of adults.[19]

C. Organophosphorus Treatments

There had been little research on the control of fly larvae in manure since the advent of DDT and other effective insecticides to control adults and the recognition that treatment of larvae would rapidly increase resistance in adults. A number of commonly available insecticides and fumigants[20-22] were toxic (many were not) to house fly larvae, but no treatments were used in large-scale field tests. Diazinon applied to manure controlled house fly larvae.[23] The effectiveness of a diazinon treatment of cattle manure was related to the amount of penetration by the insecticide of the crust that forms on the surface of the manure.[24] In a review of the chemicals applied directly to manure or as feed additives, Miller[25] noted that in 1970, diazinon, dichlorvos, dimethoate, phenothiazine, ronnel, and stirofos were registered by the U.S. Department of Agriculture (USDA) for direct application to cattle manure as larvicides.

D. Other Manure Treatments

In the middle 1970s, several juvenile hormone analogues and a compound that inhibits chitin synthesis in insects, diflubenzuron, showed considerable promise as manure treatments to control stable flies and house flies.[26,27] The crust that formed on the surface of manure in feedlots inhibited penetration by a surface treatment of Stauffer® R-20458 to the site of larval activity and, thus, effectiveness was diminished.[28] Diflubenzuron, R-20458, methoprene, and *Bacillus thuringiensis* (BT) were as effective as stirofos, dichlorvos, and other insecticides applied topically to feedlot manure in inhibiting emergence of stable flies. However, the effects of these insect growth regulator (IGR) treatments were decreased because they did not affect the later instar larvae and the pupae.[29] The problem of crusting of manure was overcome by mechanical disking or hoeing of the manure before application of treatment. Larvadex®, a triazine insect growth regulator, when applied to the surface of poultry, bovine, or swine manure, prevented the emergence of several species of pest flies.[30]

A study by Meyer and Peterson[31] showed that sanitation, which included cleaning drainage ditches, covering or vertical stacking of silage, elimination of spilled feed, and removal of manure, greatly reduced fly breeding around feedlots and dairies.

III. TREATMENT OF MANURE BY ORAL TREATMENT OF CATTLE

A. Early Treatments

Eddy et al.[32] determined that benzene hexachloride (BHC), lindane, chlordane, and toxaphene did not control house fly larvae in the manure of treated cattle, but manure from cattle fed dieldrin and aldrin was toxic to house fly, horn fly, and stable fly larvae. Daily feeding of Polybor 3® was ineffective, but *Bacillus thuringiensis* prevented development of house fly larvae in manure of treated cattle.[33,34]

B. Organophosphorus Treatments

Daily oral treatments of coumaphos, ronnel, and Bayer® 22408 controlled face fly and house fly larvae in manure.[35] Of 25 insecticides fed to cattle, coumaphos and Bayer® 22408 were the most effective against house fly larvae.[36] Low levels of coumaphos in the feed of cattle were highly effective against house fly larvae.[37] Chlorfenvinphos, stirofos, bromophos,

Bayer® 37341, and Bayer® 37342 controlled house fly larvae and famphur was only partially effective.[38,39] Polyvinyl chloride resin formulations of dichlorvos controlled face fly larvae and house fly larvae.[40] Coumaphos and stirofos controlled house fly larvae when added to the diet of dairy cows.[41,42]

In his review, Miller[25] noted that phenothiazine, ronnel, and coumaphos were registered as feed additives for beef cattle and only coumaphos was registered for beef and lactating dairy cattle. BT was partially effective as a feed additive to control house fly larvae, and the dosage needed for control was 100 times that of stirofos.[43] The encapsulation of stirofos prevented the loss of activity while passing through the digestive tract of cattle, allowed a greater amount to be deposited in the manure, and was markedly more effective than nonencapsulated stirofos.[44] Long-term feeding of stirofos controlled house fly larvae and did not adversely effect the health or reproductive performance of dairy cows.[45] A feed additive of stirofos was superior to coumaphos and ronnel for the control of house fly larvae, and no treatment caused a decrease in natural biodegradation of manure pats.[46] In a practical field trial, stirofos feed additive controlled horn fly populations, but not house fly and stable fly populations because of the large numbers of larvae found in untreated wet straw bedding.[47] In other practical trials, stirofos in the feed of dairy cattle reduced numbers of house fly larvae in manure by 87%, but numbers of adults by only 27%.[48]

C. Other Treatment Materials

Methoprene, an insect growth regulator prevents emergence of flies from pupae, as a feed additive, reduced the number of house flies and face flies that emerged from treated manure.[49] The dosage needed to control house flies was several times greater than those needed to control face flies and horn flies.[50,51] In contrast, the same oral dosage of diflubenzuron, an inhibitor of chitin synthesis in insects, that controlled face fly larvae also controlled house fly larvae.[52] House fly development was inhibited in manure of cattle given diflubenzuron in mineral blocks[53] or added to feed.[54] A triazine insect growth regulator, Larvadex®, when fed to cattle, gave only partial and variable control of house fly larvae at dosages that were effective against flies in swine and poultry manure.[30]

Ivermectin, a chemically modified form of a fermentation product of the fungus, *Streptomyces avermitilis,* when given to cattle orally or subcutaneously at very low dosages, controlled horn fly and face fly larvae and was partially active against stable fly and house fly larvae.[55]

In a comprehensive study of fly control in feedlots and dairies, Stevenson[56] recommended the use of oral larvicides for the most economical, efficient, and effective fly control program.

The recent developments on feed-through chemicals were reviewed by Miller and Miller,[57] who noted that coumaphos, methoprene, phenothiazine, ronnel, and stirofos were registered for control of manure-breeding flies. Such treatments are especially effective against horn flies and face flies that breed in undiluted manure and thus are subjected to greater doses of treatments than house flies or stable flies that breed in diluted manure and other wastes. They discussed the development and use of a intrarumenal sustained-release bolus to provide long-term release of chemicals into the manure (see Chapter 2).

IV. CONTROL OF FLIES IN STRUCTURES

A. Early Treatment Technology

From 1910 to 1922, limited research was conducted on the effectiveness of attractants and poisons for use in fly traps to control adult house flies. *U.S. Dep. Agric. Farmers' Bulletin* No. 459 in 1911[1] contained two sentences on the control of adult house flies with traps. Vinegar was an excellent bait and a good poison when mixed with formalin; other attractants were beer, milk, and alcohol.[58] The original issue of *U.S. Dep. Agric. Farmers'*

Bulletin No. 734 in 1915[59] described conical hoop traps, tent traps, garbage-can traps, manure-box traps, and window traps and listed a number of baits for house flies and other species.

In 1915, *U.S. Dep. Agric. Farmers' Bulletin* No. 679,[8] which superseded Bulletin No. 459, stated that sticky papers, poisons (formalin and milk in a shallow dish), burning fresh pyrethrins powder, and fly traps provided only temporary fly control unless there was control of larvae at breeding sites. In 1917, *U.S. Dep. Agric. Farmers' Bulletin* No. 851[9] superseded Bulletin No. 679 and contained a description of a fly trap, selection of proper baits for the trap, and information on fly papers and fly poisons which often contained arsenic. In 1924, *U.S. Dep. Agric. Farmers' Bulletin* No. 1408 superseded Bulletin No. 851[10] and contained no changes in control technology. The 1926 revision of Bulletin No. 1408[11] added a brief section on the use of sprays of an extract of pyrethrins in kerosene to control flies in buildings. A revision of Bulletin No. 734[60] in 1928 eliminated recommendations on tent traps and garbage-can traps and warned that fly traps afford only partial relief, even though they caught many flies. Electrified traps and electric screens in windows of buildings showed promise as control measures for flies.[61]

B. Organochlorine Treatments

The availability of DDT and other organochlorine insecticides after World War II shifted emphasis from control of flies with traps and poisons to the use of toxicants as residual sprays to control adults. DDT applied as an residual spray to surfaces of barns controlled stable flies[62] and house flies.[63,64] DDT needed to be applied only to a cloth or to specific limited areas (the "spot" treatment) where flies congregated to be effective.[65-67] DDT sprayed in dairies controlled house flies and stable flies.[15] Both DDT and TDE applied to limited portions of dairy barns controlled both house flies and stable flies.[68] There was considerable optimism and enthusiasm that spraying both cattle and barns with DDT or BHC would eliminate flies as pests of cattle.[69] Sprays of DDT, TDE, methoxychlor, toxaphene, and chlordane were all equally effective against house flies and stable flies, but weather conditions and sanitation affected the residual effectiveness of the treatments.[16]

The discovery of residues of DDT in milk of dairy cattle sprayed with DDT[70] or held in DDT-sprayed rooms,[71] plus the fact that house flies had become resistant to DDT[72,73] led to the use of other insecticides as residual sprays. Methoxychlor, lindane, chlordane, and dieldrin controlled DDT-resistant house flies.[74] Methoxychlor, toxaphene, and lindane had longer residual activity than pyrethrins plus piperonyl butoxide.[75] Residual sprays or spot treatments of most organochlorine insecticides were effective, but thermal aerosol application of toxaphene to cows and barns gave unsatisfactory results.[76] "Space" sprays of DDT, chlordane, and synergized pyrethrins applied with an aerosol generator to barns and stanchioned dairy cattle controlled house flies and a variety of other "barn" flies, but not stable flies.[77] Treating of screen wire strips with insecticides and hanging them in barns for fly resting sites controlled house flies; dieldrin was the most effective insecticide.[78] Lindane applied continuously as a vapor from electrically heated vaporizers gave better house fly control than a residual spray.[79,80] By 1952, resistance in house flies to lindane, methoxychlor, chlordane, and dieldrin made them ineffective as residual sprays.[39] Because of resistance, only limited control was obtained with residual sprays or spot applications of DDT, lindane, and methoxychlor, strip treatments of screen wire, mosquito cloth, crinoline or twine with dieldrin, lindane, or DDT, and vapors of lindane.[82] The appearance of house flies resistant to most organochlorine insecticides reemphasized the need for sanitation, proper treatment and handling of manure, and use of baits and other control techniques.

C. Organophosphorus and Carbamate Treatments

1. Residual Sprays

First reports on residual sprays of organophosphorus and carbamate insecticides appeared in 1953. Diazinon residual sprays controlled resistant and nonresistant house flies, but pyrolan and pyramat did not have sufficient residual activity.[23,83] Residual sprays of diazinon, coumaphos, chlorthion, trichlorfon, and malathion controlled flies for 2 days to 2 weeks, and addition of sugar to the spray appeared to prolong the residual activity.[84] A spray of DDT plus Dilan® afforded longer residual activity against resistant house flies than sprays of propyl thiopyrophosphate or malathion.[85]

Sanitation was absolutely necessary to prevent buildup of fly populations and reduce use of insecticides.[86] Fogging of stanchioned cattle in barns with a spray of synergized pyrethrins in kerosene 75 to 100 times a summer controlled a variety of flies in the barns and on cattle.[87]

Residual sprays of dicapthion, chlorthion, methoxychlor, malathion, and lindane controlled house flies and stable flies for several weeks.[88] Residual sprays of isochlorthion, chlorthion, diazinon, penthion, and pirazinon killed house flies, but only diazinon also controlled stable flies.[89] Residual sprays of both diazinon and pirazinon controlled house flies for 40 to 50 days or longer.[90] Diazinon was more effective than ronnel, dicapthion, chlorthion, or malathion as a residual spray.[91] Residual sprays of diazinon, chlorthion, dicapthion, and coumaphos applied with a garden hose sprayer were as effective as sprays applied with a high-pressure hydraulic sprayer, and spot treatments were as effective as whole barn treatments.[92] Residual sprays of diazinon, malathion, and methoxychlor controlled house flies, and a varnish bait containing trichlorfon killed flies for 3 weeks.[93] Residual sprays of malathion, diazinon, dicapthion, chlorthion, pirazinon, and trichlorfon controlled house flies.[94] Residual sprays of malathion, chlorthion, dicapthion, diazinon, and trichlorfon with sugar added provided 7 to 11 weeks control of house flies, but coumaphos spray was not satisfactory.[95]

Knipling and McDuffie[96] reviewed the literature on the control of flies in dairy barns and listed sanitation as an absolute necessity for adequate control of house flies and stable flies. They recommended residual sprays of methoxychlor, lindane, malathion, chlorthion, and diazinon for use inside dairy barns, and DDT, chlordane, BHC, and dieldrin for use outside buildings. Of 30 organophosphorus insecticides evaluated in the laboratory, the most effective residual treatments in field trials against house flies were diazinon, ronnel, and dicapthion.[97] Sprays of diazinon and trichlorfon with sugar added had longer residual effectiveness against resistant house flies than sprays without sugar; other effective treatments were ronnel and a mixture of EPN and DDT.[98]

Resistance of house flies in the U.S. to diazinon was first observed in 1956.[99] Certain diazinon-resistant strains were also resistant to a variety of other organophosphorus and organochlorine insecticides,[100] and, although malathion and dimethoate failed to control resistant flies, they controlled nonresistant flies. A residual spray of fenthion controlled resistant house flies.[101] Dimethoate sprayed onto barns and loafing pens controlled house flies and stable flies as well as horn flies on cattle using these structures.[102] Pyrethrins plus piperonyl butoxide applied to cattle and barns with a compressed air fogger controlled house flies and horn flies but not stable flies or horse flies. The fogging was two to four times more expensive than residual spraying of barns or dusting of cattle with methoxychlor.[103] Chlorfenvinphos residual spray controlled stable flies for >30 days.[104]

The development of house fly resistance to diazinon, ronnel, and malathion was generally related to the history of treatment and breeding potential within barns.[105] A residual spray of an "antiresistant DDT", which was DDT plus WARF antiresistant, provided two to three times longer control than sprays of DDT alone of house flies that were 250 times as resistant to DDT as susceptible flies.[106]

House fly control was improved over that obtained in previous years by applying residual sprays of ronnel or dimethoate shortly before flies were noticeable in the spring.[107] Residual sprays of fenthion, chlorfenvinphos, and dimethoate all afforded satisfactory control of house flies.[108] Residual sprays of chlorfenvinphos were effective at low dosages and sprays of

Hooker® HRS-1422 also provided satisfactory control of house flies.[109] Residual sprays of stirofos, Stauffer® N-2404, and Hooker® HRS-1422 gave satisfactory control of house flies.[110]

Of a number of insecticides tested as residual sprays in dairy barns, dimethoate was more effective than any other insecticide tested.[111] Residual sprays of diazinon, ronnel, and dimethoate gave variable control of resistant flies, and stirofos showed promise as a new insecticide.[112] Of nine insecticides field tested as residual sprays, dimethoate was the most effective treatment, and Spencer S-6900 and Mobam® were also effective for 1 week or more.[113] Residual sprays of Mobam® and stirofos and selective treatments of resting areas with Mobam® controlled house flies.[114]

Early-season residual sprays of stirofos, stirofos plus dichlorvos, and iodofenphos controlled house flies, but failed later in the season because of resistance that developed during the season; resmethrin, a pyrethroid, gave excellent knockdown but little residual activity.[115]

Stable flies were controlled with residual sprays of stirofos, Mobam®, and propoxur, but mist blower-applied space sprays of dichlorvos or naled gave only partial control for 1 day.[116] Residual sprays of dimethoate, iodofenphos, resmethrin, crotoxyphos, and Mobam® failed to control house flies for 2 weeks, but space sprays of naled and resmethrin were effective.[117]

In an excellent overview of the problems of flies, odors, and dusts as a result of animal confinement operations, Loomis[118] discussed sanitation (or lack of it), proper use of insecticides, and the need for an integrated control program.

Most issues of *Insecticide and Acaricide Tests* since 1978 have contained one or more reports on tests with chemicals to control flies. Of particular interest were reports on the effectiveness of residual sprays of permethrin, cypermethrin, and fenvalerate and a fog treatment of permethrin for the control of house flies in barns.

2. Baits and Traps

During the early 1950s there was renewed interest in the use of baits containing an attractant and a toxicant for the control of house flies. A bait that contained tepp was highly toxic to flies and people as well.[119] A garden sprinkling can was used to apply a mixture of corn syrup, tepp, and lindane to floors and other horizontal surfaces every 2 to 3 days.[120] The treatment controlled house flies and also horn flies on cows that remained in the treated area for at least 1 hr. Baits of brewers' malt and blackstrap molasses with sodium arsenate placed in pans controlled DDT-resistant house flies and were easier and safer to use than baits of tepp with or without lindane sprinkled onto floors.[121] Malathion as a dry granular bait scattered on the floor or as a liquid bait in honey applied to burlap or in narrow bands on hard surfaces controlled house flies in dairy barns.[122,123] Liquid baits containing sugar or molasses and diazinon, trichlorfon, and malathion gave excellent fly control.[124,125] Dry sugar baits containing diazinon, malathion, and trichlorfon controlled resistant flies.[126]

Wet and dry baits of diazinon and trichlorfon and dry baits of chlorthion controlled house flies, but not *Fannia* spp. or stable flies.[88] Insoluble granular baits containing malathion and chlorthion were effective and did not have the disadvantages of liquid baits, which dried rapidly or soaked into porous surfaces, or dry sugar baits, which dissolved on contact with moisture and were less effective in high humidity.[127] Bait stations, which consisted of wooden tongue depressors stapled to paper coasters or pieces of screen coated with a slurry of sugar, other ingredients, and trichlorfon or malathion, controlled house flies, if enough were used and sanitation was at least fair.[128] Dichlorvos as a liquid or dry bait was very effective when treatments were repeated at 2- to 5-day intervals.[129] Dry and wet baits of diazinon and trichlorfon[91] and malathion, dicapthion, chlorthion, and pirazinon used twice a week controlled house flies.[94] Dry baits containing malathion and dichlorvos placed in large plywood trays failed to control the little house fly♦, *F. canicularis* (Linnaeus).[130] Sugar baits containing dimetilan controlled organophosphorus-resistant house flies.[131]

A chicken watering device was used as a semiautomatic dispenser to dispense liquid fly baits for as long as 6 weeks without retreatment.[132] This dispenser was improved[133] by the addition of a sponge that prevented accumulation of dead flies on the liquid.

A dry bait containing Bomyl® afforded excellent control of house flies, and a combination of dichlorvos liquid bait plus cords impregnated with parathion and diazinon was also effective.[115] Dry sugar baits of dimethoate, fenthion, formothion, naled, ronnel, and trichlorfon were all about equally effective, even though the house flies were resistant to trichlorfon.[134]

The addition of a house fly sex pheromone, muscalure, increased the attractiveness and effectiveness of fly paper strips, panels painted with adhesives, sugar baits, and electric grid traps from 2.8- to 12.4-fold.[135] Muscalure increased attractiveness of sugar-based dichlorvos and trichlorfon bait in relation to the amount of pheromone added.[136] Another attractant, freeze-dried fermented whole egg solids, increased effectiveness of dichlorvos sugar bait threefold.[137] A slow-release formulation of four or five chemicals attracted more house flies than did a commercial sugar bait toxicant with muscalure.[138]

3. Treated Cords and Plastic Strands

Cotton cords impregnated with parathion or diazinon and hung inside structures gave excellent control of house flies.[139,140] A commercially available fly cord, impregnated with parathion and diazinon, controlled house flies and little house flies,[130] and a severe house fly problem was controlled with the use of double the recommended amount of fly cord.[141]

Ronnel-treated cords were as effective as parathion- or diazinon-treated cords for control of house flies.[142] Diazinon-parathion-treated cords gave season-long control of little house flies, but needed supplemental treatments with malathion sugar baits to control house flies.[143] Cords treated with ronnel, diazinon, or fenthion satisfactorily controlled house flies.[144] Organophosphorus-resistant flies were controlled with fly ribbons and cords treated with dimetilan[131] and with dimetilan-treated fly bands or ronnel-treated cords.[101]

Dichlorvos-impregnated resin strands hung from the rafters of buildings reduced populations of house flies at two of three locations treated.[109] In tests the next year, dichlorvos-impregnated resin strands failed to control house flies[110] because the formulation had a faster vaporization rate than the earlier-tested formulation. Dichlorvos-impregnated resin strips reduced fly populations, but cords treated with parathion and diazinon combined with liquid baits containing trichlorfon gave excellent control of house flies.[115]

D. Other Treatments

1. Chemosterilants

A bait containing tepa reduced a house fly population at an isolated refuse dump,[145] and a bait containing metepa applied to poultry manure caused a decrease in hatching rate of house fly eggs and some reduction in house fly numbers.[146] A liquid sugar bait containing apholate, available in dispensers, lowered numbers of ovipositing females and hatchability of eggs but did not affect numbers of house flies.[110] In an enclosed, screened hog farrowing-weaning barn, a sugar syrup bait containing metepa greatly reduced a house fly population in 7 weeks.[147]

2. Pyrethroid Insecticides

CO_2 was used to expell micronized resmethrin dust as a space treatment for cattle in a closed barn to control house flies, stable flies, and little house flies; the treatment was effective for less than 24 hr.[148] Details of an improved dust gun and treatment system were presented by Morgan and Retzer.[149] The application of the dust was automated so that an ULV treatment could be applied on command or by programmed timer.[150]

An automatic piped aerosol system that dispensed synergized pyrethrins throughout a poultry breeding facility provided excellent control of house flies.[151]

Pyrethrins and the pyrethroids, tetramethrin, and NIA-17370, applied as residual sprays controlled house flies in closed barns.[152] The pyrethroids were less irritating to humans than the pyrethrins. Permethrin applied as a residual spray or aerosol mist fog reduced house fly populations to below nuisance levels for $3^1/_2$ to 5 weeks or longer.[153]

3. Traps

A renewed interest in traps led to the testing of cage or electrocutor traps to control house flies and stable flies attracted to blacklight fluorescent lamps.[154,155] Increasing the number of traps increased the number of house flies captured, but a large increase in trap numbers would be needed to catch any remaining flies.[156] Muscalure improved catches of flies in traps; color of traps did not affect attractiveness; location of the trap and other factors did affect the numbers of flies trapped.[157]

Stable flies, although generally pests of livestock, have also been a serious problem to humans on beaches in northwest Florida (see Chapter 3). A description of an integrated pest management (IPM) program to control stable flies, called "dog flies", was presented by Hogsette et al.[158] Of interest is the research that led to the development of a trap to sample stable fly populations and could be used to control stable flies. Alsynite® fiberglass panels coated with sticky material attracted and trapped many stable flies,[159] and coating these traps with permethrin reduced populations of stable flies by 84 to 90% in 7 to 8 days if used at the rate of one trap for five animals.[160] Narrow fiberglass strips coated with permethrin (called an attractant-toxicant device) suspended from the ceiling reduced house fly populations below nuisance level (ca. 75% control).[161] The addition of muscalure to the attractant-toxicant device, which was then named the pheromone-toxicant device, caused an early decline in house fly numbers but did not provide effective control, apparently because the many flies attracted from surrounding resting sites were not all killed by the toxicant.[162]

V. OVERVIEW AND CURRENT TECHNOLOGY

The vast quantities of horse manure found in the U.S. and Canada until the advent of the automobile were a constant source of house flies and stable flies. The major technology used to prevent the breeding of flies in manure was the prompt collection and dispersal of manure, making it unsuitable for fly larvae. Other control technologies, such as treatment of manure with chemicals and use of fly traps, were used when proper sanitation was not possible.

More modern sources of manure are feedlots and confined dairy and swine production systems. Sanitation remains as the first priority for fly control, for without sanitation to reduce or eliminate fly breeding, the effectiveness of other control measures can be greatly reduced. A number of insecticides and other materials can be added to manure to kill fly larvae.

The use of oral treatments to control fly larvae in manure of cattle has only recently become a widespread technology. Insecticides and insect growth regulators are effective by this method of treatment which may become more widespread with the advent of a variety of new, highly effective treatment materials. These treatments are only effective against flies breeding in manure from the treated cattle and do not affect immigrating flies.

House flies and other flies around structures may be controlled with a variety of insecticides applied as residual sprays to structures, on treated cords or plastic strands, or as attractive baits. Each of these technologies can be used to advantage for the control of flies around structures. Control of flies around structures and in manure can be accomplished with the integration of cultural, biological, and chemical technologies.

REFERENCES

1. **Howard, L. O.,** House flies, *U.S. Dep. Agric. Farmers' Bull.,* 459, 1911.
2. **Hutchison, R. H.,** The migratory habit of housefly larvae as indicating a favorable remedial measure. An account of progress, *U.S. Dep. Agric. Bull.,* 14, 1914.
3. **Levy, E. C. and Tuck, W. T.,** The maggot trap — a new weapon in our warfare against the typhoid fly, *Am. J. Public Health,* 3, 657, 1913.
4. **Hutchison, R. H.,** A maggot trap in practical use; an experiment in house-fly control, *U.S. Dep. Agric. Bull.,* 200, 1915.
5. **Cook, F. C., Hutchison, R. H., and Scales, F. M.,** Experiments in the destruction of fly larvae in horse manure, *U.S. Dep. Agric. Bull.,* 118, 1914.
6. **Cook, F. C., Hutchison, R. H., and Scales, F. M.,** Further experiments in the destruction of fly larvae in horse manure, *U.S. Dep. Agric. Bull.,* 245, 1915.
7. **Cook, F. C. and Hutchison, R. H.,** Experiments during 1915 in the destruction of fly larvae in horse manure, *U.S. Dep. Agric. Bull.,* 408, 1916.
8. **Howard, L. O. and Hutchison, R. H.,** House flies, *U.S. Dep. Agric. Farmers' Bull.,* 679, 1915.
9. **Howard, L. O.,** The house fly, *U.S. Dep. Agric. Farmers' Bull.,* 851, 1917.
10. **Howard, L. O. and Bishopp, F. C.,** The house fly and how to suppress it, *U.S. Dep. Agric. Farmers' Bull.,* 1408, 1924.
11. **Howard, L. O. and Bishopp, F. C.,** The house fly and how to suppress it, *U.S. Dep. Agric. Farmers' Bull.,* 1408, 1926.
12. **Marcovitch, S. and Anthony, M. V.,** A preliminary report on the effectiveness of sodium fluosilicate as compared with borax in controlling the house fly (*Musca domestica* Linne), *J. Econ. Entomol.,* 24, 490, 1931.
13. **Fay, R. W.,** A control for the larvae of houseflies in manure piles, *J. Econ. Entomol.,* 32, 851, 1939.
14. **Simmons, S. W. and Wright, M.,** The use of DDT in the treatment of manure for fly control, *J. Econ. Entomol.,* 37, 135, 1944.
15. **Bruce, W. G. and Blakeslee, E. B.,** DDT to control insect pests affecting livestock, *J. Econ. Entomol.,* 39, 367, 1946.
16. **Muma, M. H. and Hixson, E.,** Effects of weather, sanitation and chlorinated chemical residues on house and stable fly populations on Nebraska farms, *J. Econ. Entomol.,* 42, 231, 1949.
17. **Bruce, W. N. and Decker, G. C.,** House fly tolerance for insecticides, *Soap Sanit. Chem.,* 26, 122, 1950.
18. **Pimentel, D. and Dewey, J. E.,** Laboratory tests with house flies and house fly larvae resistant to DDT, *J. Econ. Entomol.,* 43, 105, 1950.
19. **Hadjinicolagu, J. and Hansens, E. J.,** Chlorinated hydrocarbon insecticides to control house fly larvae, *J. Econ. Entomol.,* 46, 34, 1953.
20. **Standifer, L. N.,** Larvicides for control of the house fly, *J. Econ. Entomol.,* 48, 731, 1955.
21. **Sampson, W. W.,** Insecticides used to control house fly larvae, *J. Econ. Entomol.,* 49, 74, 1956.
22. **Smith, W. W.,** Laboratory tests of some soil fumigants as house fly larvicides, *J. Econ. Entomol.,* 55, 265, 1962.
23. **Wingo, C. W.,** House fly control with diazinon, *J. Econ. Entomol.,* 47, 632, 1954.
24. **Hoffman, R. A. and Monroe, R. E.,** Further tests on the control of fly larvae in poultry and cattle manure, *J. Econ. Entomol.,* 50, 515, 1957.
25. **Miller, R. W.,** Larvicides for fly control — a review, *Bull. Entomol. Soc. Am.,* 16, 154, 1970.
26. **Wright, J. E., Campbell, J. B., and Hester, P.,** Hormones for control of livestock arthropods: evaluation of two juvenile hormone analogues applied to breeding materials in small plot tests in Nebraska and Florida for control of the stable fly, *Environ. Entomol.,* 2, 69, 1973.
27. **Wright, J. E.,** Insect growth regulators: laboratory and field evaluations of Thompson-Hayward TH-6040 against the house fly and the stable fly, *J. Econ. Entomol.,* 67, 746, 1974.
28. **Wright, J. E., Campbell, J. B., and Oehler, D. D.,** Insect growth regulators: large plot field tests against the stable fly in cattle feedlots, *J. Econ. Entomol.,* 67, 459, 1974.
29. **Campbell, J. B. and Wright, J. E.,** Field evaluations of insect growth regulators, insecticides, and a bacterial agent for stable fly control in feedlot breeding areas, *J. Econ. Entomol.,* 69, 566, 1976.
30. **Hall, R. D. and Foehse, M. C.,** Laboratory and field tests of CGA-72662 for control of the house fly and face fly in poultry, bovine, or swine manure, *J. Econ. Entomol.,* 73, 564, 1980.
31. **Meyer, J. A. and Petersen, J. J.,** Characterization and seasonal distribution of breeding sites of stable flies and house flies (Diptera: Muscidae) on eastern Nebraska feedlots and dairies, *J. Econ. Entomol.,* 76, 103, 1983.
32. **Eddy, G. W., McGregor, W. S., Hopkins, D. E., and Dreiss, J. M.,** Effects on some insects of the blood and manure of cattle fed certain chlorinated hydrocarbon insecticides, *J. Econ. Entomol.,* 47, 35, 1954.

33. **Harvey, T. L. and Brethour, J. R.,** Feed additives for control of house fly larvae in livestock feces, *J. Econ. Entomol.,* 53, 774, 1960.

34. **Dunn, P. H.,** Control of house flies in bovine feces by a feed additive containing *Bacillus thuringiensis* var. *thuringiensis* Berliner, *J. Insect Pathol.,* 2, 13, 1960.

35. **Anthony, D. W., Hooven, N. W., and Bodenstein, O.,** Toxicity to face fly and house fly larvae of feces from insecticide-fed cattle, *J. Econ. Entomol.,* 54, 406, 1961.

36. **Eddy, G. W. and Roth, A. R.,** Toxicity to fly larvae of the feces of insecticide-fed cattle, *J. Econ. Entomol.,* 54, 408, 1961.

37. **Skaptason, J. S. and Pitts, C. W.,** Fly control in feces from cattle fed Co-Ral, *J. Econ. Entomol.,* 55, 404, 1962.

38. **Drummond, R. O.,** Toxicity to house flies and horn flies of manure from insecticide-fed cattle, *J. Econ. Entomol.,* 56, 344, 1963.

39. **Drummond, R. O., Whetstone, T. M., and Ernst, S. E.,** Control of larvae of the house fly and the horn fly in manure of insecticide-fed cattle, *J. Econ. Entomol.,* 60, 1306, 1967.

40. **Pitts, C. W. and Hopkins, T. L.,** Toxicological studies on dichlorvos feed-additive formulations to control house flies and face flies in cattle feces, *J. Econ. Entomol.,* 57, 881, 1964.

41. **Miller, R. W., Gordon, C. H., Morgan, N. O., Bowman, M. C., and Beroza, M.,** Coumaphos as a feed additive for the control of house fly larvae in cow manure, *J. Econ. Entomol.,* 63, 853, 1970.

42. **Miller, R. W., Gordon, C. H., Bowman, M. C., Beroza, M., and Morgan, N. O.,** Gardona as a feed additive for control of fly larvae in cow manure, *J. Econ. Entomol.,* 63, 1420, 1970.

43. **Miller, R. W., Pickens, L. G., and Gordon, C. H.,** Effect of *Bacillus thuringiensis* in cattle manure on house fly larvae, *J. Econ. Entomol.,* 64, 902, 1971.

44. **Miller, R. W. and Gordon, C. H.,** Encapsulated Rabon for larval house fly control in cow manure, *J. Econ. Entomol.,* 65, 455, 1972.

45. **Miller, R. W. and Gordon, C. H.,** Effect of feeding Rabon to dairy cows over extended periods, *J. Econ. Entomol.,* 66, 135, 1973.

46. **Miller, R. W. and Pickens, L. G.,** Feeding of coumaphos, ronnel, and Rabon to dairy cows: larvicidal activity against house flies and effect on insect fauna and biodegradation of fecal pats, *J. Econ. Entomol.,* 66, 1077, 1973.

47. **Miller, R. W. and Pickens, L. G.,** Feed additives for control of flies on dairy farms (Diptera: Muscidae), *J. Med. Entomol.,* 12, 141, 1975.

48. **Hurd, M. A., Olton, G. S., and Ware, G. W.,** Impact of stirofos oral larvicide on the seasonal abundance of house flies in dairy cow manure in central Arizona, *J. Econ. Entomol.,* 72, 184, 1979.

49. **Miller, R. W. and Uebel, E. C.,** Juvenile hormone mimics as feed additives for control of the face fly and house fly, *J. Econ. Entomol.,* 67, 69, 1974.

50. **Harris, R. L., Frazar, E. D., and Younger, R. L.,** Horn flies, stable flies, and house flies: development in feces of bovines treated orally with juvenile hormone analogues, *J. Econ. Entomol.,* 66, 1099, 1973.

51. **Miller, R. W. and Pickens, L. G.,** Evaluation of methoprene formulations for fly control, *J. Econ. Entomol.,* 68, 810, 1975.

52. **Miller, R. W.,** TH 6040 as a feed additive for control of the face fly and house fly, *J. Econ. Entomol.,* 67, 697, 1974.

53. **Wright, J. E.,** Insect growth regulators: development of house flies in feces of bovines fed TH 6040 in mineral blocks and reduction in field populations by surface treatments with TH 6040 or a mixture of stirofos and dichlorvos at larval breeding areas, *J. Econ. Entomol.,* 68, 322, 1975.

54. **Barker, R. W. and Newton, G. L.,** Dimilin: evaluation as a livestock dietary feed additive for control of *Musca domestica* larvae in cattle waste, *J. Ga. Entomol. Soc.,* 11, 71, 1976.

55. **Miller, J. A., Kunz, S. E., Oehler, D. D., and Miller, R. W.,** Larvicidal activity of Merck MK-933, an avermectin, against the horn fly, stable fly, face fly, and house fly, *J. Econ. Entomol.,* 74, 608, 1981.

56. **Stevenson, D. E.,** Fly control in feedlot, dairy, and poultry operations, *Bull. Soc. Vector Ecol.,* 8, 25, 1983.

57. **Miller, R. W. and Miller, J. A.,** Feed-through chemicals for insect control in animals, in *Agricultural Chemicals of the Future, BARC Symposium 8,* Hilton, J. L., Ed., Rowman & Allanheld, Totowa, N.J., 1985, 27.

58. **Morrill, A. W.,** Experiments with house-fly baits and poisons, *J. Econ. Entomol.,* 7, 268, 1914.

59. **Bishopp, F. C.,** Flytraps and their operation, *U.S. Dep. Agric. Farmers' Bull.,* 734, 1915.

60. **Bishopp, F. C.,** Flytraps and their operation, *U.S. Dep. Agric. Farmers' Bull.,* 734, 1928.

61. **Wells, R. W.,** Some observations on electrified screens and traps, *J. Econ. Entomol.,* 24, 1242, 1931.

62. **Blakeslee, E. B.,** DDT as a barn spray in stablefly control, *J. Econ. Entomol.,* 37, 134, 1944.

63. **Lindquist, A. W., Madden, A. H., Wilson, H. G., and Jones, H. A.,** The effectiveness of DDT as a residual spray against houseflies, *J. Econ. Entomol.,* 37, 132, 1944.

64. **Van Leeuwen, E. R.,** Residual effect of DDT against houseflies, *J. Econ. Entomol.,* 37, 134, 1944.

65. **Lindquist, A. W., Madden, A. H., Wilson, H. G., and Knipling, E. F.,** DDT as a residual-type treatment for control of houseflies, *J. Econ. Entomol.,* 38, 257, 1945.

66. **Brett, C. H. and Fenton, F. A.,** DDT as a residual insecticide for fly control in barns, *J. Econ. Entomol.,* 39, 397, 1946.

67. **Sweetman, H. L.,** DDT as a spot treatment for flies, *J. Econ. Entomol.,* 39, 380, 1946.

68. **Sweetman, H. L.,** Comparative effectiveness of DDT and DDD for control of flies, *J. Econ. Entomol.,* 40, 565, 1947.

69. **Cory, E. N. and Langford, G. S.,** Fly control in dairy barns and on livestock by cooperative spray services, *J. Econ. Entomol.,* 40, 425, 1947.

70. **Carter, R. H., Wells, R. W., Radeleff, R. D., Smith, C. L., Hubanks, P. E., and Mann, H. D.,** The chlorinated hydrocarbon content of milk from cattle sprayed for control of horn flies, *J. Econ. Entomol.,* 42, 116, 1949.

71. **Claborn, H. V., Beckman, H. F., and Wells, R. W.,** Excretion of DDT and TDE in milk from cows treated with these insecticides, *J. Econ. Entomol.,* 43, 850, 1950.

72. **Hansens, E. J., Schmitt, J. B., and Barber, G. W.,** Resistance of house flies to residual applications of DDT in New Jersey, *J. Econ. Entomol.,* 41, 802, 1948.

73. **King, W. V. and Gahan, J. B.,** Failure of DDT to control house flies, *J. Econ. Entomol.,* 42, 405, 1949.

74. **Hansens, E. J.,** House fly control in dairy barns, *J. Econ. Entomol.,* 43, 852, 1950.

75. **Laake, E. W., Howell, D. E., Dahm, P. A., Stone, P. C., and Cuff, R. L.,** Relative effectiveness of various insecticides for control of house flies in dairy barns and horn flies on cattle, *J. Econ. Entomol.,* 43, 858, 1950.

76. **Pimentel, D., Schwardt, H. H., and Norton, L. B.,** House fly control in dairy barns, *J. Econ. Entomol.,* 43, 510, 1950.

77. **Morrison, H. E., Lauderdale, R. W., Crowell, H. H., and Mote, D. C.,** Space spraying for fly control in dairy barns, *J. Econ. Entomol.,* 43, 846, 1950.

78. **Pimentel, D., Schwardt, H. H., and Norton, L. B.,** New methods of house fly control in dairy barns, *Soap Sanit. Chem.,* 27, 102, 1951.

79. **Sweetman, H. L., Wells, L. F., Jr., Toczydlowski, A. H., and Moore, S., III,** Mange and fly control with lindane in a piggery, *J. Econ. Entomol.,* 44, 112, 1951.

80. **Moore, S., III, Toczydlowski, A. H., and Sweetman, H. L.,** Fly control experiments in Massachusetts in 1950, *J. Econ. Entomol.,* 44, 731, 1951.

81. **Hansens, E. J.,** Failure of residual insecticides to control house flies, *J. Econ. Entomol.,* 46, 246, 1953.

82. **Goodwin, W. J. and Schwardt, H. H.,** House fly control in New York state dairy barns, *J. Econ. Entomol.,* 46, 299, 1953.

83. **Hansens, E. J. and Bartley, C. E.,** Three new insecticides for housefly control in barns, *J. Econ. Entomol.,* 46, 372, 1953.

84. **Hoffman, R. A. and Cohen, N. W.,** House fly control with residual sprays of organic phosphorus insecticides, *J. Econ. Entomol.,* 47, 701, 1954.

85. **Kilpatrick, J. W. and Schoof, H. F.,** House fly control in dairies near Savannah, Georgia, with residual applications of CS-708, NPD, and malathion, *J. Econ. Entomol.,* 47, 999, 1954.

86. **Hoffman, R. A.,** Observations on fly control by sanitation, *J. Econ. Entomol.,* 47, 194, 1954.

87. **Fisher, E. H.,** A dairy-barn fogging method for fly control, *J. Econ. Entomol.,* 48, 330, 1955.

88. **Hansens, E. J., Granett, P., and O'Connor, C. T.,** Fly control in dairy barns in 1954, *J. Econ. Entomol.,* 48, 306, 1955.

89. **Dahm, P. A. and Raun, E. S.,** Fly control on farms with several organic thiophosphate insecticides, *J. Econ. Entomol.,* 48, 317, 1955.

90. **Hansens, E. J. and Scott, R.,** Diazinon and pirazinon in fly control, *J. Econ. Entomol.,* 48, 337, 1955.

91. **Hansens, E. J.,** Control of house flies in dairy barns with special reference to diazinon, *J. Econ. Entomol.,* 49, 27, 1956.

92. **Goodwin, W. J. and Gressette, F. R., Jr.,** Residual house fly control in dairy and beef barns in South Carolina, *J. Econ. Entomol.,* 49, 622, 1956.

93. **DeFoliart, G. R.,** Fly control in Wyoming barns, *J. Econ. Entomol.,* 49, 341, 1956.

94. **Johnson, W. T., Langford, G. S., and Lall, B. S.,** Tests with organic phosphorus insecticides for fly control, *J. Econ. Entomol.,* 49, 77, 1956.

95. **Kilpatrick, J. W. and Schoof, H. F.,** House fly control in dairy barns with residual treatments of phosphorus compounds, *J. Econ. Entomol.,* 50, 36, 1957.

96. **Knipling, E. F. and McDuffie, W. C.,** Controlling flies on dairy cattle and in dairy barns, *Bull. WHO,* 16, 865, 1957.

97. **Gahan, J. B., Wilson, H. G., Keller, J. C., and Smith, C. N.,** Organic phosphorus insecticides as residual sprays for the control of house flies, *J. Econ. Entomol.,* 50, 789, 1957.

98. **Schoof, H. F. and Kilpatrick, J. W.,** Organic phosphorus compounds for the control of resistant house flies in dairy barns, *J. Econ. Entomol.,* 51, 20, 1958.

99. **Hansens, E. J.,** House fly resistance to diazinon, *J. Econ. Entomol.,* 51, 497, 1958.

100. **Hansens, E. J.,** Field studies of house fly resistance to organophosphorus insecticides, *J. Econ. Entomol.,* 53, 313, 1960.

101. **Weinburgh, H. B., Kilpatrick, J. W., and Schoof, H. F.,** Field studies on the control of resistant house flies, *J. Econ. Entomol.,* 54, 114, 1961.

102. **Cheng, T. H., Frear, D. E. H., and Enos, H. F., Jr.,** Fly control in dairy barns sprayed with dimethoate and the determination of dimethoate residues in milk, *J. Econ. Entomol.,* 54, 740, 1961.

103. **DeFoliart, G. R. and Eschle, J. L.,** Barn fogging as a fly control method, *J. Econ. Entomol.,* 54, 862, 1961.

104. **Roberts, R. H., Wrich, M. J., Hoffman, R. A., and Jones, C. M.,** Control of horn flies and stable flies with three General Chemical compounds, *J. Econ. Entomol.,* 54, 1047, 1961.

105. **Hansens, E. J. and Morris, A. P.,** Field studies of house fly resistance to diazinon, ronnel, and other insecticides, *J. Econ. Entomol.,* 55, 702, 1962.

106. **Bell, D. and Daehnert, R. H.,** Control of house flies on poultry ranches with antiresistant/DDT, *J. Econ. Entomol.,* 55, 817, 1962.

107. **DeFoliart, G. R.,** Preventive spraying schedules for dairy farm fly control, *J. Econ. Entomol.,* 56, 649, 1963.

108. **Kilpatrick, J. W. and Schoof, H. F.,** Adult house fly control with residual treatments of six organophosphorus compounds, *J. Econ. Entomol.,* 56, 79, 1963.

109. **Mathis, W. and Schoof, H. F.,** Field tests of dichlorvos, General Chemical 4072, Hooker Compound 1422, and synergized DDT against *Musca domestica, J. Econ. Entomol.,* 57, 256, 1964.

110. **Mathis, W. and Schoof, H. F.,** Studies on housefly control, *J. Econ. Entomol.,* 58, 291, 1965.

111. **Brady, U. E., Jr., Meifert, D. W., and LaBrecque, G. C.,** Residual sprays for the control of house flies in field tests, *J. Econ. Entomol.,* 59, 1522, 1966.

112. **Hansens, E. J., Benezet, H. J., and Evans, E. S., Jr.,** House fly control and insecticide resistance with continued use of diazinon, ronnel, and dimethoate, *J. Econ. Entomol.,* 60, 1057, 1967.

113. **Bailey, D. L., LaBrecque, G. C., and Bishop, P. M.,** Residual sprays for the control of house flies, *Musca domestica,* in dairy barns, *Fla. Entomol.,* 50, 161, 1967.

114. **Mathis, W. and Schoof, H. F.,** Chemical control of house flies in dairy barns and chicken ranches, *J. Econ. Entomol.,* 61, 1071, 1968.

115. **Hansens, E. J. and Anderson, W. F.,** House fly control and insecticidal resistance in New Jersey, *J. Econ. Entomol.,* 63, 1924, 1970.

116. **Campbell, J. B. and Hermanussen, J. F.,** Efficacy of insecticides and methods of insecticidal application for control of stable flies in Nebraska, *J. Econ. Entomol.,* 64, 1188, 1971.

117. **Mathis, W., Flynn, A. D., and Schoof, H. F.,** House fly resistance in the Savannah, Georgia, area and its influence on chemical-control measures, *J. Econ. Entomol.,* 65, 748, 1972.

118. **Loomis, E. C.,** Agricultural sanitation of livestock manures for control of flies, odors, and dusts, *J. Milk Food Technol.,* 36, 57, 1973.

119. **Farrar, M. D. and Brannon, C. C.,** Fly control on dairy farms, *J. Econ. Entomol.,* 46, 172, 1953.

120. **Thompson, R. K., Whipp, A. A., Davis, D. L., and Batte, E. G.,** Fly control with a new bait application method, *J. Econ. Entomol.,* 46, 404, 1953.

121. **Gahan, J. B., Anders, R. S., Highland, H., and Wilson, H. G.,** Baits for the control of resistant flies, *J. Econ. Entomol.,* 46, 965, 1953.

122. **Mayeux, H. S.,** Granular insecticidal baits against flies, *Fla. Entomol.,* 37, 171, 1954.

123. **Mayeux, H. S.,** Malathion for house fly control, *Fla. Entomol.,* 37, 97, 1954.

124. **Langford, G. S., Johnston, W. T., and Harding, W. C.,** Bait studies for fly control, *J. Econ. Entomol.,* 47, 438, 1954.

125. **Gahan, J. B., Wilson, H. G., and McDuffie, W. C.,** Organic phosphorus compounds as toxicants in house fly baits, *J. Econ. Entomol.,* 47, 335, 1954.

126. **Gahan, J. B., Wilson, H. G., and McDuffie, W. C.,** Dry sugar baits for the control of houseflies, *J. Agric. Food Chem.,* 2, 425, 1954.

127. **Keller, J. C. and Wilson, H. G.,** Granular baits for the control of house flies, *J. Econ. Entomol.,* 48, 642, 1955.

128. **Keller, J. C., Wilson, H. G., and Smith, C. N.,** Bait stations for the control of house flies, *J. Econ. Entomol.,* 49, 751, 1956.

129. **Kilpatrick, J. W. and Schoof, H. F.,** DDVP as a toxicant in poison baits for house fly control, *J. Econ. Entomol.,* 48, 623, 1955.

130. **Ogden, L. J. and Kilpatrick, J. W.,** Control of *Fannia canicularis* (L.) in Utah dairy barns, *J. Econ. Entomol.,* 51, 611, 1958.

131. **Smith, C. N., LaBrecque, G. C., Wilson, H. G., Hoffman, R. A., Jones, C. M., and Warren, J. W.,** Dimetilan baits, fly ribbons and cords for the control of house flies, *J. Econ. Entomol.,* 53, 898, 1960.

132. **Kilpatrick, J. W. and Schoof, H. F.**, A semiautomatic liquid fly bait dispenser, *J. Econ. Entomol.*, 52, 775, 1959.

133. **Kilpatrick, J. W., Maddock, D. R., and Miles, J. W.**, Modification of a semiautomatic liquid-poison bait dispenser for house fly control, *J. Econ. Entomol.*, 55, 951, 1962.

134. **Bailey, D. L., LaBrecque, G. C., and Whitfield, T. L.**, Insecticides in dry sugar baits for control of house flies in Florida dairy barns, *J. Econ. Entomol.*, 63, 2000, 1970.

135. **Carlson, D. A. and Beroza, M.**, Field evaluations of (Z)-9-tricosene, a sex attractant pheromone of the house fly, *Environ. Entomol.*, 2, 555, 1973.

136. **Morgan, P. G., Gilbert, I. H., and Fye, R. L.**, Evaluation of (Z)-9-tricosene for attractancy for *Musca domestica* in the field, *Fla. Entomol.*, 57, 136, 1974.

137. **Willson, H. R. and Mulla, M. S.**, Attractants for synanthropic flies. II. Response patterns of house flies to attractive baits on poultry ranches, *Environ. Entomol.*, 2, 815, 1973.

138. **Mulla, M. S., Hwang, Y. S., and Axelrod, H.**, Attractants for synanthropic flies: chemical attractants for domestic flies, *J. Econ. Entomol.*, 70, 644, 1977.

139. **Kilpatrick, J. W.**, The control of rural fly populations in South-eastern Georgia with parathion-impregnated cords, *Am. J. Trop. Med. Hyg.*, 4, 758, 1955.

140. **Schoof, H. F. and Kilpatrick, J. W.**, House fly control with parathion and diazinon impregnated cords in dairy barns and dining halls, *J. Econ. Entomol.*, 50, 24, 1957.

141. **Smith, A. C.**, Fly-cord studies in California, *Calif. Vector Views*, 5, 57, 1958.

142. **Kilpatrick, J. W. and Schoof, H. F.**, The effectiveness of ronnel as a cord impregnant for house fly control, *J. Econ. Entomol.*, 52, 779, 1959.

143. **Steve, P. C.**, Biology and control of the little house fly, *Fannia canicularis*, in Massachusetts, *J. Econ. Entomol.*, 53, 999, 1960.

144. **Burns, E. C. and Nipper, W. A.**, House fly control in pig parlors, *J. Econ. Entomol.*, 53, 539, 1960.

145. **LaBrecque, G. C., Smith, C. N., and Meifert, D. W.**, A field experiment in the control of house flies with chemosterilant baits, *J. Econ. Entomol.*, 55, 449, 1962.

146. **LaBrecque, G. C., Meifert, D. W., and Fye, R. L.**, A field study on the control of house flies with chemosterilant techniques, *J. Econ. Entomol.*, 56, 159, 1963.

147. **Pausch, R. D.**, Local house fly control with baited chemosterilants. 2. Field application in enclosed situations, *J. Econ. Entomol.*, 65, 449, 1972.

148. **Morgan, N. O., Sullivan, W. N., and Schechter, M. S.**, Micronized resmethrin dust for control of flies in dairy barns, *J. Econ. Entomol.*, 66, 1281, 1973.

149. **Morgan, N. O. and Retzer, H. J.**, Modified double nozzle micronized dust gun for delivering insecticides, *J. Econ. Entomol.*, 67, 563, 1974.

150. **Retzer, H. J. and Morgan, N. O.**, Automatic indoor insecticide duster, *Southwest. Entomol.*, 5, 47, 1980.

151. **Kissam, J. B. and Query, G. W.**, Accudose aerosol — an effective house fly (Diptera; Muscidae: *Musca domestica* L.) adulticide control system for cage type poultry houses, *Poultry Sci.*, 55, 1906, 1976.

152. **Adkins, T. R., Jr., Kissam, J. B., and Krebs, W. F., III**, Field evaluation of natural and synthetic pyrethroid water-based pressurized formulations against the house fly, *J. Econ. Entomol.*, 64, 459, 1971.

153. **Schmidtmann, E. T.**, Water base and aerosol concentrate application of permethrin for house fly control in New York dairy housing, *J. Econ. Entomol.*, 74, 404, 1981.

154. **Morgan, N. O., Pickens, L. G., and Thimijan, R. W.**, House flies and stable flies captured by two types of traps, *J. Econ. Entomol.*, 63, 672, 1970.

155. **Thimijan, R. W., Pickens, L. G., and Morgan, N. O.**, A trap for house flies, *J. Econ. Entomol.*, 63, 1030, 1970.

156. **Thimijan, R. W., Pickens, L. G., Morgan, N. O., and Miller, R. W.**, House fly capture as a function of number of traps in a dairy barn, *J. Econ. Entomol.*, 65, 876, 1972.

157. **Mitchell, E. R., Tingle, F. C., and Carlson, D. A.**, Effect of muscalure on house fly traps of different color and location in poultry houses, *J. Ga. Entomol. Soc.*, 10, 168, 1975.

158. **Hogsette, J. A., Ruff, J. P., and McGowan, M. J.**, Stable fly integrated pest management (IPM) in northwest Florida, *J. Fla. Anti-Mosq. Assoc.*, 52, 48, 1981.

159. **Williams, D. F.**, Sticky traps for sampling populations of *Stomoxys calcitrans*, *J. Econ. Entomol.*, 66, 1279, 1973.

160. **Meifert, D. W., Patterson, R. S., Whitfield, T., LaBrecque, G. C., and Weidhaas, D. E.**, Unique attractant-toxicant system to control stable fly populations, *J. Econ. Entomol.*, 71, 290, 1978.

161. **Patterson, R. S., Meifert, D. W., Buschman, L., Whitfield, T., and Fye, R. L.**, Control of the house fly, *Musca domestica* (Diptera: Muscidae), with permethrin-coated fiber glass strips, *J. Med. Entomol.*, 17, 232, 1980.

162. **Carlson, D. A. and Leibold, C. M.**, Field trials of pheromone-toxicant devices containing muscalure for house flies (Diptera: Muscidae), *J. Med. Entomol.*, 18, 73, 1981.

Chapter 19

RESISTANCE OF ARTHROPOD PESTS OF LIVESTOCK TO INSECTICIDES AND ACARICIDES*

I. INTRODUCTION

Because the primary focus of this book is a review of technologies using chemicals to control arthropod pests of livestock, we must address resistance to insecticides and acaricides. The appearance of resistant strains of arthropods not only may change the types of chemicals that can be used to control the arthropod but also can stimulate research on alternative control technologies if chemicals can no longer provide practical control of the pest.

We will limit our review to resistance of arthropod pests of livestock in the U.S. and Canada, which are remarkably free of species with resistant strains when compared with numbers of species with resistant strains in the rest of the world. This chapter will primarily present information on the appearance of resistance in strains of arthropods that are recognized pests of livestock. We will not review the vast literature on the resistance of mosquitoes and will only briefly review resistance in the house fly♦, *Musca domestica* Linnaeus.

II. RESISTANT SPECIES THROUGH 1980

A. Species with Documented Resistance

Reviews on resistance have usually cited publications that have documented the species, its location, and the testing undertaken to determine the resistance spectrum. The species, the spectrum of their resistance, and the literature citation for arthropod pests of livestock are listed in Table 1.

Brown[1] presented a detailed history of the appearance of resistance in house flies in the U.S. and Canada to DDT and other insecticides and reviewed resistance in mosquitoes, lice, fleas, bed bugs, flies, ticks, and other arthropod pests of man and livestock. Schoof[2] focused on mosquitoes but also reported resistance of house flies in the U.S. in 1955 to malathion, diazinon, and other organophosphorus insecticides. McDuffie[3] noted that there was no confirmed resistance of the stable fly♦ (*Stomoxys calcitrans* [Linnaeus]), the horn fly♦ (*Haematobia irritans* [Linnaeus]), the screwworm♦ (*Cochliomyia hominivorax* [Coquerel]), fleeceworms, cattle grubs, or the sheep ked♦ (*Melophagus ovinus* [Linnaeus]), to insecticides in the U.S., despite some field reports of less than satisfactory control. Harris et al.[4] also focused on resistance in livestock insects in the U.S. Graham and Harris[5] included resistance in livestock insects in their review of arthropods of public health and veterinary importance. Brown[6] included resistance in parasites of man and animals in his brief review of pest resistance to pesticides.

Brown and Pal[7] presented a comprehensive review, with extensive literature citations, of the resistance of house flies to almost all chlorinated hydrocarbon and organophosphorus insecticides and included resistance in several more livestock pests in North America. Resistance in ticks and insects of veterinary importance was reviewed by Drummond,[8] who did not present any new instances of resistance.

Lists of arthropods that have resistant strains were presented by the Food and Agriculture Organization of the United Nations (FAO)[9] and the World Health Organization (WHO).[10,11]

---

* Common names of insects and acarines, as listed in *Common Names of Insects and Related Organisms* (published by the Entomological Society of America), are marked with a ♦ the first time they are cited preceding the scientific name.

Table 1
RESISTANT STRAINS OF ARTHROPOD PESTS OF
LIVESTOCK IN U,S. AND CANADA THROUGH 1980

Species	Insecticide group	Ref.
Cochliomyia hominivorax (Coquerel)	Phenothiazine	14[a]
Glyptotendipes paripes Edwards	EPN/BHC	15[a]
Boophilus annulatus Say	Toxaphene	16[a]
Culicoides furens (Poey)	Lindane, heptachlor, and dieldrin	17[b]
Bovicola caprae (Gurlt) and *Bovicola limbatus* (Gervais)	Toxaphene	18[c]
Linognathus vituli (Linnaeus)	DDT	19[c]
Haematobia irritans (Linnaeus)	Ronnel	20[d]
Ornithonyssus sylviarum (Canestrini & Fanzago)	Malathion and other OPs	21[d]
Haematobia irritans (Linnaeus)	Ronnel	22[e]
Stomoxys calcitrans (Linnaeus)	DDT, dieldrin	23[e]
Haematopinus eurysternus (Nitzsch)	DDT, lindane	24[f]
Amblyomma americanum (Linnaeus)	BHC, cyclodienes	Footnote f
Dermacentor variabilis (Say)	DDT, lindane, and chlordane	25[f]
Hippelates collusor (Townsend)	Lindane, DDT, and dieldrin	26[f]
	Aldrin, dieldrin, and heplachlor	27[f]
Simulium venustum Say and *Prosimuluim fuscum* Lyme and Davies	DDT	28[g]
Fannia canicularis (Linnaeus)	DDT, dieldrin, and OPs	29[g]
Fannia femoralis Stein	DDT, dieldrin, and OPs	29[g]
Ophyra leucostoma (Wiedemann)	DDT, dieldrin	29[g]
Fannia canicularis (Linnaeus)	Malathion	30
Ornithonyssus sylviarum (Canestrini and Fanzago)	Malathion	31, 32

[a]   Cited in Reference 1.
[b]   Cited in Reference 2.
[c]   Cited in Reference 3.
[d]   Cited in Reference 4.
[e]   Cited in Reference 5.
[f]   Cited in Reference 6.
[g]   Cited in Reference 7.

An extensive listing of species with resistance reported through 1980[12] contained a number of arthropod pests of livestock. The subject of resistance was very broadly reviewed in *Pest Resistance to Pesticides,*[13] but new records of resistance in arthropod pests of livestock were not presented.

B. Reports Requiring Verification

With respect to North American fauna, the following listed cases of resistance obtained from the literature require verification:

Boophilus annulatus	and	Toxaphene (Knipling[16] in Brown[1])
Amblyomma americanum	and	BHC/cyclodienes (Reported in Brown[6])
Dermacentor variabilis	and	DDT and BHC/cyclodienes (N. Ward by Fishang[25] in Brown[6])
Haematopinus eurysternus	and	BHC/cyclodienes and organophosphates (Haufe by Nelson[24] in Brown[6])

Knipling[16] stated "the Oklahoma Experiment Station has reported the occurrence of toxaphene-resistant ticks". Because *B. annulatus* had been eradicated from Oklahoma for many years, the species in question is not *B. annulatus.* Brown[6] does not cite a specific reference for the resistance of *A. americanum* to BHC/cyclodienes but lists Oklahoma 1954 as the state and date. Possibly, the reference is to the Knipling[16] article. With reference to *D. variabilis,* Fishang[25] reported that Dr. Norman Ward of Worcester, Mass., noted that resistance in wood ticks had appeared to DDT and lindane in that area. In an informal newsletter, Nelson[24] reported that W. A. Haufe could kill only about one third of the *H. eurysternus* on "carrier" cattle with DDT. None of these reports contained quantitative data obtained by treating these pests with insecticides or acaricides. The WHO[11] stated that "Earlier records of resistance to DDT and dieldrin in *Amblyomma americanum* and *Dermacentor variabilis* are now considered of doubtful significance".

III. REPORTS OF RESISTANCE SINCE 1980

A. Horn Flies

Resistance in horn flies in the U.S. to ronnel[20] was very limited in its geographical distribution and did not become a major problem. Of much greater importance is the recent appearance of resistance of the horn fly to stirofos and to pyrethroid insecticides. When ear tags impregnated with stirofos failed to provide the expected 3 months of control of horn flies, resistance was thought in certain instances in Georgia[33] to be related to the use of stirofos in the diet of these same animals for the previous two summers. Resistance to stirofos did not become widespread because stirofos-impregnated ear tags were rapidly replaced by pyrethroid-impregnated ear tags in the 1980s.

First reports of resistance in horn flies to pyrethroids appeared in Georgia,[34] but soon resistance was evident in Louisiana[35] and Florida.[36] Differences in susceptibility of resistant and susceptible flies were detected by topical application of insecticides to flies, exposing flies to treated petri dishes, or exposing flies to treated cloths. In general, resistance was 10- to 40-fold for permethrin, fenvalerate, and flucythrinate used in ear tags. The resistance spectrum of pyrethroid-resistant flies included DDT, several other pyrethroids, but not carbamate or organophosphorus insecticides.[37]

Generally, resistance does not appear until the 3rd year of use of ear tags. Resistant strains have been documented from Florida, Alabama, Kentucky, Louisiana, Texas, Oklahoma, Kansas, Nebraska, California, and Hawaii.[38] In a comprehensive review of the resistance problem in horn flies,[39] resistance to DDT, toxaphene, methoxychlor, ronnel, stirofos, cypermethrin, deltamethrin, fenvalerate, flucythrinate, and permethrin was presented. A behavioral response in resistant horn flies to pyrethroids has been documented.[40]

B. Other Species

Recently, the house fly was shown to be resistant to the pyrethroids in Canada[41,42] and in the U.S.[43]

The face fly✦, *Musca autumnalis* DeGeer, was shown to have some resistance (< fourfold) to methoxychlor but to none of a variety of organophosphorus or pyrethroid insecticides generally used to control this species.[44]

IV. OVERVIEW AND CURRENT TECHNOLOGY

It is inevitable that with the continued use of insecticides and acaricides to control arthropod pests of livestock, selection would be such that certain species would develop strains resistant to the treatments.

Relatively few species with strains that are resistant to insecticides and acaricides are found in the U.S. and Canada. Resistance reported in *Amblyomma americanum*, *Boophilus annulatus*, *Dermacentor variabilis*, and *Haematopinus eurysternus* requires verification. Where resistant strains have appeared there has been a shift to an alternative insecticide or acaricide that has provided satisfactory control.

The most important resistance problem in the U.S. is that of the horn fly to pyrethroid insecticides. The insecticide-impregnated ear tag technology is a significant advance in the control of horn flies. However, the rate at which selection for resistance to the insecticides used in ear tags occurred suggests that this technology may be lost if it is not used in control strategies that resolve or minimize the resistance problem. Even if new chemistries are found for use in ear tags, their use may be short-lived if the technology is not carefully used along with other technologies in an integrated pest management (IPM) program for the control of horn flies.

REFERENCES

1. **Brown, A. W. A.**, Insecticide resistance in arthropods, *WHO Monogr.*, 38, 1958.
2. **Schoof, H. F.**, Resistance in arthropods of medical and veterinary importance — 1946—58, *Misc. Publ. Entomol. Soc. Am.*, 1, 3, 1959.
3. **McDuffie, W. C.**, Current status of insecticide resistance in livestock pests, *Misc. Publ. Entomol. Soc. Am.*, 2, 49, 1960.
4. **Harris, R. L., Graham, O. H., and McDuffie, W. C.**, Resistance of livestock insects to insecticides in the United States, *Agric. Vet. Chem. Agric. Eng.*, 6, 78, 1965.
5. **Graham, O. H. and Harris, R. L.**, Recent developments in the control of some arthropods of public health and veterinary importance, *Bull. Entomol. Soc. Am.*, 12, 319, 1966.
6. **Brown, A. W. A.**, Pest resistance to pesticides, in *Pesticides in the Environment*, Vol. 1, Part 2, White-Stevens, R., Ed., Marcel Dekker, New York, 1971, 457.
7. **Brown, A. W. A. and Pal, R.**, Insecticide resistance in arthropods, *WHO Monogr.*, 38, 1971.
8. **Drummond, R. O.**, Resistance in ticks and insects of veterinary importance, in *Pesticide Management and Insecticide Resistance*, Watson, D. L. and Brown, A. W. A., Eds., Academic Press, New York, 1977, 303.
9. Food and Agriculture Organization of the United Nations, Report of the first session of the FAO working party of experts on resistance of pests to pesticides, Meeting Report PL/1965/18, Food and Agriculture Organization, Rome, 1967.
10. World Health Organization, Resistance of vectors and reservoirs of disease to pesticides, *WHO Tech. Rep.*, 585, 1976.
11. World Health Organization, Resistance of vectors of disease to pesticides, *WHO Tech. Rep.*, 655, 1980.

12. **Georghiou, G. P.,** The occurrence of resistance to pesticides in arthropods, an index of cases reported through 1980, Food and Agriculture Organization of the United Nations, Rome, 1981.

13. **Georghiou, G. P. and Saito, T., Eds.,** *Pest Resistance to Pesticides,* Plenum Press, New York, 1983.

14. **Knipling, E. F.,** Acquired resistance to phenothiazine by larvae of the primary screwworm, *J. Econ. Entomol.,* 35, 63, 1942.

15. **Lieux, D. R. and Mulrennan, J. A.,** Investigation of the biology and control of midges in Florida (Diptera: Tendipedidae), *Mosq. News,* 16, 201, 1956.

16. **Knipling, E. F.,** On the insecticide resistance problem, *Agric. Chem.,* 9, 46, 1954.

17. **Smith, C. N., Davis, A. N., Weidhaas, D. E., and Seabrook, E. L.,** Insecticide resistance in the salt-marsh sand fly *Culicoides furens, J. Econ. Entomol.,* 52, 352, 1959.

18. **Moore, B., Drummond, R. O., and Brundrett, H. M.,** Tests of insecticides for the control of goat lice in 1957 and 1958, *J. Econ. Entomol.,* 52, 980, 1959.

19. **Anthony, D. W.,** Tests with DDT, lindane and malathion for control of the long-nosed cattle louse *Linognathus vituli* (L.), *J. Econ. Entomol.,* 52, 782, 1959.

20. **Burns, E. C. and Wilson, B. H.,** Field resistance of horn flies to the organic phosphate insecticide ronnel, *J. Econ. Entomol.,* 56, 718, 1963.

21. **Rodriguez, J. L. and Riehl, L. A.,** Northern fowl mite tolerant to malathion, *J. Econ. Entomol.,* 56, 509, 1963.

22. **Harris, R. L., Frazar, E. D., and Graham, O. H.,** Resistance to ronnel in a strain of horn flies, *J. Econ. Entomol.,* 59, 387, 1966.

23. **Mount, G. A.,** Use of WHO tsetse fly kit for determining resistance in the stable fly, *J. Econ. Entomol.,* 58, 794, 1965.

24. **Nelson, W. A.,** Louse research and control in western Canada, *Entomol. Newsl.,* 44, 1, 1966.

25. **Fischang, W. J.,** Phosphate resistant roaches coming? NPCA's Dr. Spear says to Eastern PCO conferees, "It's probable", *Pest Cont.,* 28, 38, 1960.

26. **Georghiou, G. P. and Mulla, M. S.,** Resistance to chlorinated hydrocarbon insecticides in the eye gnat, *Hippelates collusor, J. Econ. Entomol.,* 54, 695, 1961.

27. **Mulla, M. S.,** Resistance in the eye gnat *Hippelates collusor* to soil insecticides, *J. Econ. Entomol.,* 55, 130, 1962.

28. **Jamnback, H. and West, A. S.,** Decreased susceptibility of blackfly larvae to *p,p'*-DDT in New York State and eastern Canada, *J. Econ. Entomol.,* 63, 218, 1970.

29. **Georghiou, G. P.,** Differential susceptibility and resistance to insecticides of coexisting populations of *Musca domestica, Fannia canicularis, F. femoralis,* and *Ophyra leucostoma, J. Econ. Entomol.,* 60, 1338, 1967.

30. **Bland, R. G.,** Toxicity of ronnel, dimethoate, and malathion to little house fly adults, *J. Econ. Entomol.,* 59, 1435, 1966.

31. **Hall, R. D., Townsend, L. H., Jr., and Turner, E. C., Jr.,** Laboratory and field tests to compare the effectiveness of organophosphorous, carbamate, and synthetic pyrethroid acaricides against northern fowl mites, *J. Econ. Entomol.,* 71, 315, 1978.

32. **Arthur, F. H. and Axtell, R. C.,** Susceptibility of northern fowl mites in North Carolina to five acaricides, *Poultry Sci.,* 62, 428, 1983.

33. **Sheppard, C.,** Stirofos resistance in a population of horn flies, *J. Ga. Entomol. Soc.,* 18, 370, 1983.

34. **Sheppard, D. C.,** Fenvalerate and flucythrinate resistance in a horn fly population, *J. Agric. Entomol.,* 1, 305, 1984.

35. **Quisenberry, S. S., Lockwood, J. A., Byford, R. L., Wilson, H. K., and Sparks, T. C.,** Pyrethroid resistance in the horn fly, *Haematobia irritans* (L.) (Diptera: Muscidae), *J. Econ. Entomol.,* 77, 1095, 1984.

36. **Schmidt, C. D., Kunz, S. E., Petersen, H. D., and Robertson, J. L.,** Resistance of horn flies (Diptera: Muscidae) to permethrin and fenvalerate, *J. Econ. Entomol.,* 78, 402, 1985.

37. **Byford, R. L., Quisenberry, S. S., Sparks, T. C., and Lockwood, J. A.,** Spectrum of insecticide cross-resistance in pyrethroid-resistant populations of *Haematobia irritans* (Diptera: Muscidae), *J. Econ. Entomol.,* 78, 768, 1985.

38. **Kunz, S. E.,** Horn fly resistance, *Anim. Nutr. Health,* 40, 40, 1985.

39. **Sparks, T. C., Quisenberry, S. S., Lockwood, J. A., Byford, R. L., and Roush, R. T.,** Insecticide resistance in the horn fly, *Haematobia irritans, J. Agric. Entomol.,* 2, 217, 1985.

40. **Lockwood, J. A., Byford, R. L., Story, R. N., Sparks, T. C., and Quisenberry, S. S.,** Behavioral resistance to the pyrethroids in the horn fly, *Haematobia irritans* (Diptera: Muscidae), *Environ. Entomol.,* 14, 873, 1985.

41. **Harris, C. R., Turnbull, S. A., Whistlecraft, J. W., and Surgeoner, G. A.,** Multiple resistance shown by field strains of house fly, *Musca domestica* (Diptera: Muscidae), to organochlorine, organophosphorus, carbamate, and pyrethroid insecticides, *Can. Entomol.,* 114, 447, 1982.

42. **MacDonald, R. S., Surgeoner, G. A., Solomon, K. R., and Harris, C. R.,** Effect of four spray regimes on the development of permethrin and dichlorvos resistance, in the laboratory, by the house fly (Diptera: Muscidae), *J. Econ. Entomol.,* 76, 417, 1983.

43. **Horton, D. L., Sheppard, D. C., Nolan, M. P., Jr., Ottens, R. J., and Joyce, J. A.,** House fly (Diptera: Muscidae) resistance to permethrin in a Georgia caged layer poultry operation, *J. Agric. Entomol.,* 2, 196, 1985.

44. **Knapp, F. W., Herald, F., and Schwinghammer, K. A.,** Comparative toxicity of selected insecticides to laboratory-reared and field-collected face flies (Diptera: Muscidae), *J. Econ. Entomol.,* 78, 860, 1985.

Chapter 20

USE OF THE STERILE INSECT TECHNIQUE (SIT) FOR SCREWWORMS AND OTHER ARTHROPOD PESTS OF LIVESTOCK*

I. INTRODUCTION

The success of the sterile insect technique (SIT) for eradication of the screwworm*, *Cochliomyia hominivorax* (Coquerel), has stimulated scientists to devote considerable energy and thought to the use of insects to eradicate or control their own kind. Knipling[1] proposed four possible ways of using insects for their own destruction: (1) release of sexually sterile insects, (2) use of chemosterilants to produce sexual sterility in the natural population of insects, (3) release of adults infested with pathogens that would destroy larval progeny by contaminating the environment, and (4) release of insects with genetic deficiencies, such as inability to fly or diapause, or deficiencies in immature stages, that would render progeny unable to survive in nature.

The use of SIT and other genetic techniques to control insects has been the subject of articles and reviews which have focused on various genetic anomalies or induced genetic conditions. Approaches discussed included the use of recessive lethal genes,[2] chemical sterilization,[3] cytoplasmic incompatability,[4] conditional lethal traits,[5] chromosome rearrangements,[6] and a wide variety of genetic methods.[7]

Insect population suppression and management with a variety of techniques was the subject of an outstanding book by Knipling[8] which thoroughly reviews the theory and practice of autocidal control by release of insects that are sexually sterile, carry deleterious genes, or are treated so that they transfer a lethal or sterilizing agent to mates in the natural population. The use of genetic techniques to control insects of veterinary importance was briefly reviewed by Dame.[9]

We will present the highlights of the SIT program that has eradicated screwworms from the U.S. We shall review the pilot projects that have evaluated the use of SIT to eradicate the horn fly*, *Haematobia irritans* (Linnaeus), and the stable fly*, *Stomoxys calcitrans* (Linnaeus), and the progress on the SIT pilot project to eradicate heel flies, *Hypoderma* spp. Also, we shall briefly discuss research on the sterile hybrid cattle tick, *Boophilus* spp.

II. SCREWWORM ERADICATION PROGRAM

The screwworm, an obligate, myiasis-producing parasite of warm-blooded animals, including man, is limited in its distribution to the tropic, subtropic, and temperate regions of the Americas. Female flies lay eggs on wounds, cuts, and other abrasions of living animals, and larvae feed on living tissue. Such infestations attract other ovipositing flies and the resultant massive infestations may lead to the death of the animal. Because the screwworm does not diapause, sufficient cold weather eliminates flies during the winter. At one time, screwworm flies generally overwintered in south Texas and limited areas of other states along the border with Mexico. During the summer, infestations could be found as far north as the Dakotas as the result of movement of infested animals or migration of flies. In 1933, screwworms were found in Georgia and a population that overwintered in Florida that year provided a continuing source of infestation for the southeastern states.[10]

---

* Common names of insects and acarines, as listed in *Common Names of Insects and Related Organisms* (published by the Entomological Society of America), are marked with a ♦ the first time they are cited preceding the scientific name.

Table 1
KEY PUBLICATIONS OF RESEARCH
ASSOCIATED WITH THE STERILE
INSECT TECHNIQUE FOR THE
ERADICATION OF SCREWWORMS

Topic of publication	Ref.
Taxonomic and biological differentation of *Cochliomyia hominivorax* (= *americana*) from *C. macellaria*	17, 18
Rearing of screwworm larvae in vitro	19
Radiation sterilization of screwworms	20, 21
Eradication of screwworms from Curacao, Netherlands Antilles	22, 23
Development of liquid rearing media for screwworm larvae	24
Development of a chemically defined attractant for screwworm flies	25
Development of the SWASS attractant-toxicant system to suppress screwworm flies	26, 27

Because of its importance to man and his livestock, the screwworm has been the subject of research for many years. In their annotated bibliography of the screwworm, Snow et al.[11] list 621 references. The use of chemicals and other technologies to control screwworm larvae and adults is discussed in Chapter 7. In this section, we will focus on the highlights of the research that led up to, have contributed to, and continue to contribute to the screwworm eradication program. This highly successful program has been the subject of a number of review articles[12-16] which can be consulted for further detailed information. Certain research activities which are landmarks in the development of knowledge that led up to and were used to implement and improve the eradication program are presented in Table 1.

A. Early Research and Field Tests

In 1938, Drs. E. F. Knipling, R. C. Bushland, and A. W. Lindquist discussed possibilities of the use of sterilized males for eradication of screwworms.[75] After World War II, Bushland conducted the original experiments on the effects of x-rays on survival and fertility of screwworms.[20,21] Following field trials on Sanibel Island, Fla., the first large-scale trial of the sterile insect technique was made on the Island of Curacao in the Netherlands Antilles. Sterile flies released by air at the rate of 3 flies per hectare per week on the 44,000-ha island eradicated screwworms in three to four generations or 4 months.[22,23]

B. Southeastern States

After the success of the Curacao program, attention was focused on the problem of the screwworms that overwintered on some 12.9 million ha of the Florida penninsula.[28] The southeastern program was unofficially started in December 1957 with a pilot rearing facility used to rear flies for distribution in a limited area of Florida to take advantage of an unusually cold winter that caused a decrease in the geographical area occupied by overwintering screwworms. The official program started in July 1958 with the opening of a screwworm rearing facility at Sebring, Fla., with the capacity to rear 50 million flies per week. The overwintering area and a buffer area (to prevent migration of fertile flies north of the overwintering area) were treated with a minimum of four flies per hectare per week. In June 1959, the last screwworm infestation was recorded. The cost of the entire program was ca. $7 million which was about one third of the annual estimated losses in livestock to screwworms in the Southeast.[29]

C. Southwestern States and Mexico

Livestock producer groups in the southwestern states urged their state and national representatives to have congress authorize funds for a southwestern program. The goal was to eradicate screwworms from some 12.9 million ha in Texas and other western states and establish a 160-km wide barrier zone along the Mexico-U.S. border to prevent reinfestation of flies from Mexico.

During the winter of 1961 to 1962, 20 million flies per week, reared at Kerrville, Tex., were distributed in south Texas to take advantage of an unusually severe winter that eliminated screwworms from most of Texas. A screwworm rearing facility at Moore Field, near Mission, Tex., began producing 100 million flies per week in August 1962. Progress of eradication was measured by recording the numbers of samples sent by the public to Mission for identification that contained screwworm larvae. There was a dramatic decrease in the number of screwworm cases (those samples that contained screwworm larvae) from 1962 to 1964.[14] In 1964, a barrier zone along the Texas-Mexico border was established. Screwworms were declared eradicated from Texas and New Mexico in 1964 and from Arizona and California in 1966 as a result of the absence of continuously breeding populations. Screwworms were officially declared eradicated from the U.S. in 1966, and the federal government became responsible for maintenance of a 3100-km-long barrier zone from Texas to California. However, there were still screwworm cases found in the U.S. because of invasion of flies from Mexico. A statistical review of the program from 1962 through 1969 contained a summary of screwworm cases in the U.S. and Mexico and reported that >43 billion sterile flies were released in 8 years.[30] Numbers of screwworm cases in the U.S. were low from 1966 to 1971, but, in 1972, large numbers of screwworm cases were found in areas of the U.S. that had been repopulated with screwworms.

In 1972, a formal agreement between the governments of Mexico and the U.S. established a joint Mexico-U.S. Commission for the Eradication of Screwworms. The goal of this commission was to eradicate screwworms from Mexico as far south as the Isthmus of Tehuantepec. The commission constructed a new screwworm fly rearing facility at Tuxtla Gutierrez, Chiapas, Mexico, that was capable of rearing in excess of 500 million flies per week.

During the period of 1971 through 1975, screwworms were eradicated from Puerto Rico, Vieques, and the Virgin Islands[31] as the result of treating animals and releasing >1.8 billion sterile flies. During 1972 to 1976, all of the procedures and techniques used in the program were reevaluated. There were changes in the strains of flies reared and in the procedures for rearing and distributing those flies. A wind-oriented trap that was more efficient and selective than the standard fly trap was developed[32] that used the screwworm fly attractant, swormlure.[25] Further research led to the development of the screwworm adult suppression system (SWASS) to attract and kill adult screwworms, especially female flies.[26] A massive publicity program in Texas called "SOS-Stamp Out Screwworm-Mission 77" realerted producers to find and treat screwworm-infested animals. The rearing facility at Tuxtla Gutierrez began to produce flies for distribution in Mexico in 1976. As a result, the number of screwworm cases in the U.S. was reduced from 29,671 in 1976 to only 457 in 1977 — a reduction of 98.5%.[33]

The success of the program since 1977 has been attributed to improved quality of sterile flies and their handling, use of SWASS, more sterile flies available, better aerial distribution of flies, and increased cooperation by livestock owners to prevent or treat wounds.[34] In 1983, there were no screwworm cases reported from the U.S. In 1984, the program successfully eliminated screwworm flies from all of northern Mexico south to the 20th parallel. A 400-km-wide barrier zone maintained at the Isthmus of Tehuantepec is needed to prevent reinfestation of flies from the Yucatan Peninsula of Mexico and Central America. An animal treatment program is in effect in order to prevent the movement of infested animals into the eradicated area. The success of the program has stimulated the development of plans for a program to use the sterile insect technique to eradicate screwworms south to the Darien Gap in Panama.[35]

In a Symposium on Eradication of the Screwworm from the United States, 11 brief papers summarized the research and program activities of the screwworm eradication program.[36] These papers should be required reading for anyone wishing to learn about the technology and the strategy of the program.

III. THE HORN FLY SIT PILOT PROJECT

Kunz and Eschle[37] suggested that an eradication effort based on integrated use of insecticides to lower natural populations of horn flies with subsequent release of laboratory-reared, sterile adults was technically feasible.

After initial findings that horn flies could be sterilized by gamma radiation,[38] critical tests showed dosages of 2.0 to 2.5 krad used to irradiate pupae or adults resulted in sterility of males and infecundity of females. Irradiated males are competitive with normal males.[39,40]

A. West Texas Test

In a semi-isolated area in west Texas, laboratory-reared horn flies, exposed as pupae to 2 krads, released at a ratio of ten sterile to one fertile fly, caused a downward trend in reproduction which was decreased by 98% during the last 3 weeks of a 16-week test period.[41] This test allowed for the accumulation of data on rearing and the effects of handling and radiation on flies[42] and on methods of estimating sterility in field populations.[43]

In a separate study, the release of sterile horn flies onto a nonisolated herd of cattle in east Texas caused a downward trend in reproduction and ca. 90% control near the end of the study.[44]

B. The Hawaiian Program

A large pilot test on the Puu-O-Hoku Ranch on Molokai, Ha., was initiated to determine if the use of an insect growth regulator, methopene, plus the release of sterile horn flies could eliminate a native population of horn flies. Methoprene was added to the drinking water of the cattle in order to inhibit the emergence of horn fly adults from the manure of the treated cattle.[45,46] The water treatment did not affect the released sterile horn flies as would conventional adulticides. Horn flies were mass reared[47,48] and sterilized as adults with 2.5 krad. Sterile flies (both sexes) were released on the cattle at the rate of ca. 1.6×10^6 flies per week. The numbers of horn fly eggs per manure pat and percentage hatch of these eggs were steadily reduced, until at week 14 of the test, there was no hatch of the few eggs found, and by week 16, no eggs were found. Release of sterile flies was discontinued at week 21, and no horn flies were observed until week 30 when infested cattle were moved into the area.[49]

Throughout the island of Molokai, fly populations were reduced by an average of 83% by the methoprene treatment and selective applications of methoxychlor to cattle. Unfortunately, a pathogen so devastated the rearing of horn flies that the sterile male portion of the project could not be implemented.[50]

IV. THE STABLE FLY SIT PILOT PROJECT

The stable fly can be sterilized by exposure of pupae or adults to radiation[51] or treating adults with chemosterilants.[52] Stable fly adults, sterilized by immersion as pupae in metepa or methiotepa, and released into a natural population at a ratio of one sterile per one fertile fly, caused an increase in the sterility of the egg masses and a marked decrease in the population of flies.[53] The SIT was proposed[54] as an economically feasible method to provide long- or short-term control of stable flies. Procedures were developed for the mass rearing of stable flies.[55]

This research led to a large pilot test on St. Croix, U.S. Virgin Islands, in order to evaluate the use of the sterile male technique to supplement chemical, biological, and physical control measures for the stable fly. Data were obtained on the effect of radiation and marking flies with fluorescent pigments on the sterility and survival of stable flies.[56,57]

The treatment of larval breeding sites with a spray of methoxychlor, release of 1×10^5 sterile flies per day for 18 months (sterilized as adults by exposure to 2.5 krad), and release of a fly pupal parasite, *Spalangia endius* Walker, at selected sites, reduced the stable fly population on the island by 99.9%.[58-60] Although no larval breeding was observed, the few fertile flies that were found during the last 6 months of the project apparently came from either isolated breeding sites or immigrated from islands 40 km away. They also may have been introduced on imported animals since the fertile flies were found near the airport and boat docks.[61]

V. THE HEEL FLY SIT PILOT PROJECT

The common cattle grub♦, *Hypoderma lineatum* (Villers), and the northern cattle grub♦, *H. bovis* (Linnaeus), are found in the U.S. and Canada. Knipling[62] first suggested that the release of a few sterile male heel flies, in the year following the use of systemic insecticides to essentially eliminate the natural population of heel flies, should eradicate the flies. This thesis was further developed by Graham and Drummond[63] and Graham et al.,[64] who noted that adult heel flies that eclosed from pupae of *H. lineatum* exposed to 5 krad were sterile, and sterile males successfully mated normal females.[65]

A four-phase pilot study in Canada included treatment of cattle with systemics, continuing treatment plus release of sterile males, no treatment but continuing release of sterile males, and discontinued sterile male release.[66] After 3 years of phase 1 and 3 years of phase 2, a native population of *H. lineatum* was eliminated from 5000 cattle on a 22,500-ha ranch.

In 1982, Agriculture Canada and ARS/USDA initiated a 5-year, cooperative large-scale pilot test in Glacier County, Montana and Alberta, Canada.[67] Cattle were treated with systemic insecticides to reduce the populations of both species of cattle grubs and, in certain limited areas inside the treatment area, sterile male heel flies of both species were released. In order to obtain the heel flies, calves (naturally infested with cattle grub larvae) were held in a large indoor arena in Browning, Mon. As cattle grub larvae exited from the backs of these cattle they were collected from the inside of fabric screens that had been glued to the cattle's backs. The collected larvae were allowed to pupate, and these pupae were subjected to irradiation of 5 krad for *H. lineatum* and 8 krad for *H. bovis*. A brief interim report on the 1st year of the test[68] indicated that, in the U.S., the first systemic treatment reduced cattle grub populations by nearly 99% and sterile male flies were released at 14 semiweekly intervals so as to provide estimated ratios of five to nine sterile flies to every one fertile fly. Further results of the test are not available at the time of this writing.

VI. RESEARCH ON THE STERILE HYBRID *BOOPHILUS*

Interspecific crosses between the cattle tick♦, *Boophilus annulatus* (Say), and the southern cattle tick♦, *B. microplus* (Canestrini), produced viable hybrids in which the males were sterile and the females were fertile.[69] Normal females mated to hybrid males laid normal-sized egg masses that did not hatch. Hybrid females mated to fertile males produced additional sterile males and fertile females which laid eggs that had reduced hatch. These females, when mated to fertile males, produced additional sterile male progeny and fertile female progeny.[70] This pattern continued for three generations, but some fertility of males was observed in the progeny of the fourth generation of backcrosses.[71]

A theoretical model[72] indicated that sterile hybrids could be used effectively to eradicate low levels of native *Boophilus* ticks and that eradication could be achieved within a 2-year period. A more descriptive, computer-simulated model showed that the release of sterile hybrid ticks on a weekly schedule would eradicate *Boophilus* in a period of some 18 months.[73]

Although the effectiveness of this sterile hybrid technique has not been demonstrated, research is underway in order to obtain data on the problems and logistics of the use of this technique. Hybrid males, as a result of the cross between *B. annulatus* males and *B. microplus* females, were found to have longer survival times and greater mating frequencies than hybrid males as a result of the cross between *B. microplus* males and *B. annulatus* females, and parthenogenesis of hybrid females was of little consequence.[74]

VII. OVERVIEW AND CURRENT TECHNOLOGY

The screwworm program is an excellent example of how the innovative thinking of scientists led to the basic research which discovered applicable information. This information was expanded and developed into a technology to solve a very important practical problem. The implementation of the sterile insect program to eradicate screwworms involved cooperation between members of a U.S. Department of Agriculture (USDA) research organization, Entomology Research Division (now Agricultural Research Service [ARS]), a USDA eradication organization, Animal Disease Eradication Division (now Animal and Plant Health Inspection Service), state and federal legislatures, livestock boards, livestock producer groups, state universities, extension services, private foundations such as Southwest Animal Health Research Foundation, sportsmen, and the general public. Later, cooperation included agreements between the governments of Mexico and the U.S. to extend the program into Mexico. The success of the program has stimulated planning for the eradication of screwworms from Central America to a barrier zone in Panama.

The sterile male technique was appropriate for use against the screwworm because billions of flies could be reared relatively inexpensively for sterilization and release, and density of natural populations was low. Other factors that favored the extensive eradication program were that the species had limited geographical distribution, was difficult to control by conventional means, and was of economic significance. Also, government infrastructures existed that provided personnel who were trained, skilled, and experienced in both eradication and research, and the public fully supported the program.

The three pilot projects discussed do not each have all of the factors that were listed above for the screwworm program. Critical problems with the stable fly, horn fly, and heel flies are that these pests are widely distributed and the task of excluding them from an area when they have been eradicated would be extremely difficult. Also, stable flies and horn flies both suck blood, and the release of millions of these flies in the short term may not be feasible, especially with the stable fly which attacks a wide variety of hosts, including man. Also, both of these species diapause. The major problem with the use of SIT for cattle grubs is the lack of an in vitro rearing technique for the larvae. The present technique of collecting larvae from cattle cannot provide enough flies and is very expensive.

REFERENCES

1. **Knipling, E. F.,** Use of insects for their own destruction, *J. Econ. Entomol.,* 53, 415, 1960.
2. **LaChance, L. E. and Knipling, E. F.,** Control of insect populations through genetic manipulations, *Ann. Entomol. Soc. Am.,* 55, 515, 1962.
3. **Smith, C. N.,** Prospects for vector control through sterilization procedures, *Bull. WHO,* 29, 99, 1963.
4. **Knipling, E. F., Laven, H., Craig, G. B., Pal, R., Kitzmiller, J. B., Smith, C. N., and Brown, A. W. A.,** Genetic control of insects of public health importance, *Bull. WHO,* 38, 421, 1968.
5. **Klassen, W., Creech, J. F., and Bell, R. A.,** The potential for genetic suppression of insect populations by their adaptations to climate, *U.S. Dep. Agric. Misc. Publ.,* 1178, 1970.
6. **Whitten, M. J.,** Insect control by genetic manipulation of natural populations, *Science,* 171, 682, 1971.
7. **Smith, R. H. and von Borstel, R. C.,** Genetic control of insect populations, *Science,* 178, 1164, 1972.
8. **Knipling, E. F.,** The Basic Principles of Insect Population Suppression and Management, *U.S. Dep. Agric. Agric. Handb.,* 512, 1979.
9. **Dame, D. A.,** Control of insects of veterinary importance by genetic techniques, *Prev. Vet. Med.,* 2, 515, 1984.
10. **Dove, W. E. and Parman, D. C.,** Screw worms in the southeastern states, *J. Econ. Entomol.,* 28, 765, 1935.
11. **Snow, J. W., Siebenaler, A. J., and Newell, F. G.,** Annotated bibliography of the screwworm, *Cochliomyia hominivorax* (Coquerel), ARM-S-14, U.S. Department of Agriculture, Washington, D.C., 1981.
12. **Knipling, E. F.,** The eradication of the screw-worm fly, *Sci. Am.,* 203, 54, 1960.
13. **Bushland, R. C.,** Male sterilization for the control of insects, in *Advances in Pest Control Research,* Vol. 3, Metcalf, R. L., Ed., Interscience, New York, 1960, 1.
14. **Baumhover, A. H.,** Eradication of the screwworm fly an agent of myiasis, *J. Am. Med. Assoc.,* 196, 240, 1966.
15. **Bushland, R. C.,** Screwworm research and eradication, *Bull. Entomol. Soc. Am.,* 21, 23, 1975.
16. **Bushland, R. C.,** Eradication and suppression of the screwworm fly by the sterile male technique, in *Systems for Stimulating the Development of Fundamental Research,* Knipling, E. F., Ed., National Academy Science, Washington, D.C., 1978, 10.
17. **Cushing, E. C. and Patton, W. S.,** Studies on the higher Diptera of medical and veterinary importance, *Cochliomyia americana* sp. nov., the screw-worm fly of the new world, *Ann. Trop. Med. Parasitol.,* 27, 539, 1933.
18. **Laake, E. W., Cushing, E. C., and Parish, H. E.,** Biology of the primary screw worm fly, *Cochliomyia americana,* and a comparison of its stages with those of *C. macellaria, U.S. Dep. Agric. Tech. Bull.,* 500, 1936.
19. **Melvin, R. and Bushland, R. C.,** The nutritional requirements of screwworm larvae, *J. Econ. Entomol.,* 33, 850, 1940.
20. **Bushland, R. C. and Hopkins, D. E.,** Experiments with screw-worm flies sterilized by X-rays, *J. Econ. Entomol.,* 44, 725, 1951.
21. **Bushland, R. C. and Hopkins, D. E.,** Sterilization of screw-worm flies with X-rays and gamma-rays, *J. Econ. Entomol.,* 46, 648, 1953.
22. **Bushland, R. C., Lindquist, A. W., and Knipling, E. F.,** Eradication of screw-worms through release of sterilized males, *Science,* 122, 287, 1955.
23. **Baumhover, A. H., Graham, A. J., Bitter, B. A., Hopkins, D. E., New, W. D., Dudley, F. H., and Bushland, R. C.,** Screw-worm control through release of sterilized flies, *J. Econ. Entomol.,* 48, 462, 1955.
24. **Gingrich, R. E., Graham, A. J., and Hightower, B. G.,** Media containing liquefied nutrients for mass-rearing larvae of the screw-worm, *J. Econ. Entomol.,* 64, 678, 1971.
25. **Jones, C. M., Oehler, D. D., Snow, J. W., and Grabbe, R. R.,** A chemical attractant for screwworm flies, *J. Econ. Entomol.,* 69, 389, 1976.
26. **Coppedge, J. R., Broce, A. B., Tannahill, F. H., Goodenough, J. L., Snow, J. W., and Crystal, M. M.,** Development of a bait system for suppression of adult screwworms, *J. Econ. Entomol.,* 71, 483, 1978.
27. **Coppedge, J. R., Goodenough, J. L., Broce, A. B., Tannahill, F. H., Snow, J. W., Crystal, M. M., and Petersen, H. Del Var,** Evaluation of the screwworm adult suppression system (SWASS) on the island of Curacao, *J. Econ. Entomol.,* 71, 579, 1978.
28. **Knipling, E. F.,** Possibilities of insect control or eradication through the use of sexually sterile males, *J. Econ. Entomol.,* 48, 459, 1955.
29. **Baumhover, A. H., Husman, C. N., Skipper, C. C., and New, W. D.,** Field observations on the effects of releasing sterile screw-worms in Florida, *J. Econ. Entomol.,* 52, 1202, 1959.
30. **Eddy, G. W. and DeVaney, J. A.,** A brief statistical review of the United States-Mexico screw-worm eradication program, *Bull. Entomol. Soc. Am.,* 16, 159, 1970.

31. **Williams, D. L., Gartman, S. C., and Hourrigan, J. L.,** Screwworm eradication in Puerto Rico and the Virgin Islands, *World Anim. Rev.,* 21, 31, 1977.
32. **Broce, A. B., Goodenough, J. L., and Coppedge, J. R.,** A wind oriented trap for screwworm flies, *J. Econ. Entomol.,* 70, 413, 1977.
33. **Snow, J. W. and Whitten, C. J.,** Status of the screwworm (Diptera: Calliphoridae) control program in the southwestern United States during 1977, *J. Med. Entomol.,* 15, 518, 1979.
34. **Whitten, C. J.,** The sterile insect technique in the control of the screwworm, IAEA-SM-255/7, International Atomic Energy Agency Special Report, Vienna, 1982, 79.
35. **Snow, J. W., Whitten, C. J., Salinas, A., Ferrer, J., and Sudlow, W. H.,** The screwworm, *Cochliomyia hominivorax* (Diptera: Calliphoridae), in Central America and proposed plans for its eradication south to the Darien Gap in Panama, *J. Med. Entomol.,* 22, 353, 1985.
36. **Graham, O. H. Ed.,** Symposium on eradication of the screwworm from the United States and Mexico, *Misc. Publ. Entomol. Soc. Am.,* 62, 1985.
37. **Kunz, S. E. and Eschle, J. L.,** Possible use of the sterile-male technique for eradication of the horn fly, in Sterility Principle for Insect Control or Eradication, IAEA-SM-138/27, International Atomic Energy Agency Special Report, Vienna, 1971, 145.
38. **Lewis, L. F. and Eddy, G. W.,** Some effects of gamma radiation on the horn fly, *J. Econ. Entomol.,* 57, 275, 1964.
39. **Chamberlain, W. F.,** Horn flies: emergence, survival, and sterility after ⁶⁰Co irradiation of pupae, *J. Econ. Entomol.,* 67, 381, 1974.
40. **Chamberlain, W. F. and Gingrich, A. R.,** Gamma irradiation of adult horn flies, *J. Econ. Entomol.,* 71, 422, 1978.
41. **Eschle, J. L., Kunz, S. E., Schmidt, C. D., Hogan, B. F., and Drummond, R. O.,** Suppression of a population of horn flies with the sterile-male technique, *Environ. Entomol.,* 2, 976, 1973.
42. **Schmidt, C. D., Eschle, J. L., Kunz, S. E., and Dreiss, J. M.,** Sterile-male technique for suppression of the horn fly: effects of irradiation, handling, and release on laboratory-reared flies, *Environ. Entomol.,* 3, 287, 1974.
43. **Kunz, S. E., Eschle, J. L., and Cunningham, J. R.,** Methods of estimating sterility in a field population of horn flies (Diptera: Muscidae), *J. Med. Entomol.,* 12, 513, 1975.
44. **Kunz, S. E., Graham, M. R., Hogan, B. F., and Eschle, J. L.,** Effect of releases of sterile horn flies into a native population of horn flies, *Environ. Entomol.,* 3, 159, 1974.
45. **Beadles, M. L., Miller, J. A., Chamberlain, W. F., Eschle, J. L., and Harris, R. L.,** The horn fly: methoprene in drinking water of cattle for control, *J. Econ. Entomol.,* 68, 781, 1975.
46. **Miller, J. A., Chamberlain, W. F., Beadles, M. L., Pickens, M. O., and Gingrich, A. R.,** Methoprene for control of horn flies: application to drinking water of cattle via a tablet formulation, *J. Econ. Entomol.,* 69, 330, 1976.
47. **Miller, J. A., Schmidt, C. D., and Eschle, J. L.,** Systems for large-scale rearing of the horn fly, *Haematobia irritans* (L.), *Am. Soc. Agric. Eng.,* Paper No. 75-4517, 1975.
48. **Miller, J. A., Schmidt, C. D., and Eschle, J. L.,** Mass rearing of horn flies on a host, AAT-S-8, U.S. Department of Agriculture, Washington, D.C., 1979.
49. **Eschle, J. L., Miller, J. A., and Schmidt, C. D.,** Insect growth regulator and sterile males for suppression of horn flies, *Nature (London),* 265, 325, 1977.
50. **Miller, J. A., Eschle, J. L., Hopkins, D. E., Wright, F. C., and Matter, J. J.,** Methoprene for control of horn flies: a suppression program on the Island of Molokai, Hawaii, *J. Econ. Entomol.,* 70, 417, 1977.
51. **Offori, E. D.,** Gamma irradiation of *Stomoxys calcitrans, J. Econ. Entomol.,* 63, 574, 1970.
52. **Harris, R. L.,** Chemical induction of sterility in the stable fly, *J. Econ. Entomol.,* 55, 882, 1962.
53. **LaBrecque, G. C., Meifert, D. W., and Rye, J., Jr.,** Experimental control of stable flies, *Stomoxys calcitrans* (Diptera: Muscidae), by releases of chemosterilized adults, *Can. Entomol.,* 104, 885, 1972.
54. **LaBrecque, G. C., Meifert, D. W., and Weidhaas, D. E.,** Potential of the sterile-male technique for the control or eradication of stable flies, *Stomoxys calcitrans* Linnaeus, IAEA-SM-186/55, International Atomic Energy Agency Special Report, Vienna, 1975, 449.
55. **Bailey, D. L., Whitfield, T. L., and LaBrecque, G. C.,** Laboratory biology and techniques for mass producing the stable fly, *Stomoxys calcitrans* (L.) (Diptera: Muscidae), *J. Med. Entomol.,* 12, 189, 1975.
56. **Williams, D. F., LaBrecque, G. C., and Patterson, R. S.,** Effect of gamma rays and/or fluorescent pigments on sterility and survival of the stable fly, *Fla. Entomol.,* 60, 297, 1977.
57. **Whitfield, T. L., LaBrecque, G. C., Patterson, R. S., and Meifert, D. W.,** Effect of gamma irradiation on sterility and longevity of stable flies, *J. Econ. Entomol.,* 71, 608, 1978.
58. **LaBrecque, G. C., Patterson, R. S., Williams, D. F., and Weidhaas, D. E.,** Control of the stable fly, *Stomoxys calcitrans* (Diptera: Muscidae), on St. Croix, U.S. Virgin Islands, using integrated pest management measures. I. Feasibility of sterile male releases, *J. Med. Entomol.,* 18, 194, 1981.

59. **Williams, D. F., Patterson, R. S., LaBrecque, G. C., and Weidhaas, D. E.,** Control of the stable fly, *Stomoxys calcitrans* (Diptera: Muscidae), on St. Croix, U.S. Virgin Islands, using integrated pest management measures. II. Mass rearing and sterilization, *J. Med. Entomol.,* 18, 197, 1981.

60. **Patterson, R. S., LaBrecque, G. C., Williams, D. F., and Weidhaas, D. E.,** Control of the stable fly, *Stomoxys calcitrans* (Diptera: Muscidae), on St. Croix, U.S. Virgin Islands, using integrated pest management measures. III. Field techniques and population control, *J. Med. Entomol.,* 18, 203, 1981.

61. **Patterson, R. S., LaBrecque, G. C., and Williams, D. F.,** Use of the sterile male technique as an adjunct to insecticidal and physical methods for stable fly control on the island of St. Croix, U.S.V.I., IAEA-SM-240/16, International Atomic Energy Agency Special Report, Vienna, 1980.

62. **Knipling, E. F.,** The potential role of the sterility method for insect population control with special reference to combining this method with conventional methods, ARS-33-98, U.S. Department of Agriculture, Washington, D.C., 1964.

63. **Graham, O. H. and Drummond, R. O.,** The potential of animal systemic insecticides for eradicating cattle grubs, *Hypoderma* spp., *J. Econ. Entomol.,* 60, 1050, 1967.

64. **Graham, O. H., Drummond, R. O., and Hoffman, R. A.,** Possibilities of the sterile-male technique for the control of livestock insects in the United States of America, in *Control of Livestock Insect Pests by the Sterile-Male Technique,* International Atomic Energy Agency, Vienna, 1968, 41.

65. **Drummond, R. O.,** Effects of gamma radiation on the fertility of the common cattle grub, *Hypoderma lineatum* (de Villers), *J. Rad. Biol.,* 7, 491, 1963.

66. **Weintraub, J.,** Pilot test of serile insect releases for warble fly control, in Research Highlights — 1977, Croome, G. C. R., Ed., Agriculture Canada Research Station, Lethbridge, Alberta, 1978, 48.

67. **Kunz, S. E., Drummond, R. O., and Weintraub, J.,** A pilot test to study the use of the sterile insect technique for eradication of cattle grubs, *Prev. Vet. Med.,* 2, 523, 1984.

68. **Weintraub, J. and Scholl, P. J.,** The joint Canada-U.S.A. pilot project on warble grub control, in Research Highlights — 1983, Sears, L. J. L. and Wilson, D. B., Eds., Agriculture Canada Research Station, Lethbridge, Alberta, 1984, 30.

69. **Graham, O. H., Price, M. A., and Trevino, J. L.,** Cross-mating experiments with *Boophilus annulatus* and *B. microplus* (Acarina: Ixodidae), *J. Med. Entomol.,* 9, 531, 1972.

70. **Thompson, G. D., Osburn, R. L., Davey, R. B., Drummond, R. O., and Price, M. A.,** Hybrid sterility in cattle ticks (Acari: Ixodidae), *Experientia,* 37, 127, 1981.

71. **Thompson, G. D., Osburn, R. L., Davey, R. B., and Price, M. A.,** The dynamics of hybrid sterility between *Boophilus annulatus* and *B. microplus* (Acari: Ixodidae) through successive generations, *J. Med. Entomol.,* 18, 413, 1981.

72. **Osburn, R. L. and Knipling, E. F.,** The potential use of sterile hybrid *Boophilus* ticks (Acari: Ixodidae) as a supplemental eradication technique, *J. Med. Entomol.,* 19, 637, 1982.

73. **Weidhaas, D. E., Haile, D. G., George, J. E., Osburn, R. L., and Drummond, R. O.,** A basic model for use in computer simulations of *Boophilus* tick biology and control, AAT-S-32, U.S. Department of Agriculture, Washington, D.C., 1983.

74. **Davey, R. B., Osburn, R. L., and Castillo, C.,** Longevity and mating behavior in males and parthenogenesis in females in hybridized *Boophilus* ticks (Acari: Ixodidae), *J. Med. Entomol.,* 20, 614, 1983.

75. **Bushland, R. C.,** personal communication.

Chapter 21

BIOCONTROL OF ARTHROPOD PESTS OF LIVESTOCK*

I. INTRODUCTION

The technologies developed and used for the control of arthropod pests of livestock primarily involve the use of insecticides or acaricides — the major focus of the book. Other possibilities for developing alternative technologies include biological control of these pests. Specific aspects of biological control of arthropod pests are reviewed in this chapter. There is considerable current research activity on biological control of arthropod pests of livestock. Biological control of arthropod pests of livestock includes the use of breeds of livestock that are innately resistant to the pests or the enhancement of the natural immunity of livestock to these pests. That subject is addressed in Chapter 22. In this chapter we shall focus on "conventional" biocontrol agents.

Biocontrol of arthropod pests in general has been the subject of a number of broad reviews. The book by Clausen[1] contains a literature review of more than 2600 references and presents some limited information on parasites and predators of ticks, blow flies, eye gnats, mosquitoes, horn flies, house flies, stable flies, face flies, flesh flies, and black flies. Biological control of arthropod pests of livestock was reviewed by Legner and Poorbaugh,[2] Legner et al.,[3] Bay et al.,[4] Laird,[5] Undeen,[6] and Lacey and Undeen.[7] All of these reviews broadly included information on parasites, predators, competitors, and pathogens, including *Bacillus thuringiensis* (BT).

Because the use of BT as a control material has been reviewed in several previous chapters, we will not discuss this agent in this chapter. We will limit ourselves to other biocontrol technologies, specifically the use of parasites, predators, and competitors, which have been tested in the field against three broad groups of arthropod pests of livestock: flies that breed in poultry or bovine manure, other flies, and ticks.

II. BIOCONTROL OF FLIES THAT BREED IN POULTRY MANURE

Moon,[8] in a broad discussion on biological control through interspecific competition in a neutral resource, listed chicken manure as a site for potential biocontrol of flies by interspecific competition. Several papers in the proceedings of a workshop on the Status of Biological Control of Filth Flies[9] addressed the biological control of flies that breed in poultry manure.

A. Pupal Parasites

Pioneering research by Legner and associates in California[10] showed that release in the summer of *Spalangia endius* Walker, *S. cameroni* Perkins, *S. nigroaenea* Curtis, and *Muscidifurax raptor* Girault and Sanders caused an increase in the numbers of parasitized pupae of *Fannia femoralis* Stein, but not *Ophyra leucostoma* (Wiedemann). Inoculative releases of *S. endius*, *M. raptor*, and *Tachinaephagus zealandicus* Ashmead in the winter increased parasitism rates of the house fly♦, *Musca domestica* Linnaeus, but not *Fannia* spp.[11]

Daily inoculative releases of *S. endius* suppressed populations of house flies in commercial poultry facilities.[12,13] The release of *Pachycrepoideus vindemiae* (Rondani) caused an increase in the mortality of house fly pupae.[14] Release of *M. raptor* significantly increased

---

* Common names of insects and acarines, as listed in *Common Names of Insects and Related Organisms* (published by the Entomological Society of America), are marked with a ♦ the first time they are cited preceding the scientific name.

the rate of parasitism in house fly pupae and reduced house fly populations in a narrow caged-layer house, but not in a high-rise caged-layer house.[15] Release of *S. endius* produced 100% parasitism of house fly pupae.[16] Releases of *M. raptor* were not as successful as those of *S. endius* for control of house flies.[17] Weekly releases of *M. raptor* resulted in a higher rate of parasitism of pupae and a decreased population of house flies when compared with data from farms without parasite releases.[18]

A recent guide to pupal parasites of muscoid flies in manure[19] presented a key to identify the parasites and contained 306 annotated references. A larger number of species of parasites of the house fly were collected from manure in confined animal production facilities than in pastures.[20] Thus, these confined systems are more suitable candidates for augmentative release of parasites for fly control than pasture situations. The integration of appropriate removal and handling of manure, use of parasites and predators, plus selective use of insecticides, mostly adulticides, to control house flies and other pests in manure in poultry houses is discussed in Chapter 16.

B. Competitors

The fact that populations of house fly larvae were reduced in manure that was infested with larvae of the black soldier fly♦, *Hermetia illucens* (Linnaeus), suggested that this species could be used as a biocontrol organism.[21-23] Control of house flies by soldier flies was presumed to be the result of competition and modification of the breeding medium. Recently the production of an oviposition-deterring allomone by soldier fly larvae was suggested as another regulating mechanism.[24]

C. Predators

Because larvae of the black garbage fly, *Ophyra leucostoma* (Wiedemann), preyed on larvae of the house fly and other flies that breed in poultry manure,[25] this species was suggested[26] as a potential biocontrol agent. Larvae of the black dump fly, *Ophyra aenescens* (Wiedemann), in poultry manure replaced house fly larvae that were killed with Larvadex® treatment and remained dominant after treatment was discontinued. Although this predaceous species may also be a potential biocontrol agent,[27] when adults of the black dump fly become numerous, this species can become a problem itself.

Populations of a predaceous mite, *Macrocheles muscaedomestica* (Scopoli), if not eliminated by insecticides applied to poultry manure, would suppress populations of the house fly.[28] A large number of predaceous mites, beetles, and flies were found in poultry manure.[29] Scheduling of manure removal affected both the numbers of predators and their effect on fly larvae.[30] The use of adulticides for fly control and minimum treatment of poultry manure to allow for control by natural predators was an effective technique to control flies.[31-35]

D. Cockerels

Cockerels confined to the floor under hens held in caged-layer cages provided complete control of house fly larvae and pupae[36] and mixed sexed pullets were also effective.[37] Further tests indicated that cockerels could control house flies, but there were a number of cockerel management practices that needed to be followed for the technique to be successful.[38] This control methodology was not sufficiently practical to become an established technique.

III. BIOCONTROL OF FLIES THAT BREED IN CATTLE MANURE

There are two facets to the biocontrol of arthropod pests in cattle manure. One involves parasites, predators, and competitors of the pest flies, principally the horn fly♦, *Haematobia irritans* (Linnaeus), and the face fly♦, *Musca autumnalis* DeGeer, that breed in undisturbed cattle manure. The second involves the organisms that are associated with a wider variety of pests, principally the house fly and the stable fly[*], *Stomoxys calcitrans* (Linnaeus), and a number of other species of filth flies that breed in manure of confined cattle. Moon[8] included cattle dung as another neutral resource as a site for biological control of flies by interspecific competition.

A. Range Cattle Manure

A variety of arthropods have been recovered from undisturbed cattle manure. For example, 151 species of insects, many of which were entomophagous, were collected from undisturbed cattle manure in California.[39] Several predators were found to attack face fly eggs and larvae[40] in undisturbed manure, and several native hymenopterous parasites were found to attack face fly pupae.[41,42] Parasites were found in only 0.5% of face fly pupae collected in the field.[43] The number of face flies that emerged from manure was directly affected by competition by larvae of other coprophagous Diptera.[44]

There was an inverse relationship between the numbers of horn flies and the numbers of all other insects that emerged from undisturbed cattle manure.[45] Competitors, predators, and other agents in range cattle manure reduced populations of the horn fly by some 90%.[46] Beetles, mostly staphylinids, hydrophilids, and histerids, caused considerable mortality of horn fly larvae in manure.[47]

1. Dung Beetles

Fincher[48] presented an excellent review of the possible benefits to be obtained from the introduction of dung-burying beetles, mostly scarabaeids, that remove cattle manure from the surface of pastures. Potential benefits included reduced pasture contamination by manure, recycling of tons of nitrogen normally lost to the atmosphere, reduced incidence of helminth parasites, and lowered populations of both horn flies and face flies on cattle. He reported that the dung beetle fauna of the U.S. was relatively limited, with only ten species capable of burying significant amounts of dung per day.

The native U.S. dung beetle population has been augmented by the release of four imported species: *Onthophagus gazella* Fabricius, *Onitis alexis* Klug, *Euoniticellus intermedius* Rice, and *Onthophagus taurus* Schreber, which was released in California but also has been discovered in southeastern states. Any effect of these beetles on populations of pest flies of grazing cattle has yet to be determined. Unfortunately, the dung-burying activities of dung beetles may not be compatible with the predaceous activities of staphylinids in manure.[49]

Although the numbers and kinds of biocontrol agents, except for a few staphylinid and hydrophilid predators, are limited in Canada, they provided a significant reduction of horn fly breeding in manure.[50] One imported dung beetle, *Onthophagus nuchicornis* (Linnaeus), was found, and the importation of exotic dung-burying beatles was encouraged.[51] Moon et al.[52] discussed the benefits, in terms of the control of face flies, that could be obtained from the introduction of a variety of dung-burying beetles.

The reader interested in the possible use of dung beetles for the control of biting flies that breed in undisturbed bovine manure must read the literature from Australia on the ambitious research program to find, colonize, import, rear, and release dung beetles to control the buffalo fly, *Haematobia irritans exigua* (de Meijere), and the bush fly, *Musca vetustissima* Walker.

2. Parasitic Nematodes

Of special note in the U.S. was the limited research[53] on control of the face fly with a nematode parasite, *Heterotylenchus autumnalis* Nickle, which apparently was transported to North America with the face fly.[54] This nematode affects reproduction of the female flies[55] and appeared to be an important natural control mechanism in certain locations.[56]

3. Predaceous Mites

Production of house flies from intact dairy cattle manure that was infested with the predaceous mites, *Macrocheles muscaedomestica* (Scopoli) and *Glyptholaspis confusa* (Foa), was less than production of flies from manure treated with dicofol to kill the mites.[57] In his review of mites as biological control agents of dung-breeding flies, Krantz[58] noted that most coprophilous macrochelid mites were found in pasture and range dung. He reported that Australian scientists released *M. peregrinus* Kranz in Australia in 1980 and 1981, and that it had become established and extended its range. Its effect on pest flies had not been determined.

4. The Red Imported Fire Ant

It is of interest to note that in the southern U.S., the presence of the red imported fire ant♦, *Solenopsis invicta* Buren, causes a significant reduction in numbers of horn flies emerging from manure pats,[59] but also may interfere with the effectiveness of dung-burying beetles.[60,61] *S. invicta* also was an effective predator of stable fly pupae and larvae.[62]

B. Confined Cattle Manure

As discussed in Chapter 18, the large amounts of cattle manure and other wastes that accumulate at feedlots and dairies are ideal environments for the breeding of flies. The high concentration of flies and their potential for creating problems makes it mandatory that some measures be instituted to control fly pests, especially house flies and stable flies. Several papers in the proceedings of a workshop on the Status of Biological Control of Filth Flies[9] present an overview of the current status of the biological control of flies that breed in confined cattle manure. A large variety of parasites, predators, and competitors are found in manure of confined cattle.[63]

1. Pupal Parasites

Sustained releases of *S. endius* controlled house flies in a small dairy calf barn[64] and a nonisolated field population of house flies, stable flies, and *Physiphora aeneae* (Fabricius).[65,66] Sustained releases of *S. endius* failed to control house flies or stable flies in feedlots,[67] although some parasitic activity was noted. Hymenopterous parasites of manure-breeding flies are commercially available in the U.S. However, control afforded by the release of these parasites is variable and often disappointing.

2. Predaceous Mites

Outdoor piles of manure produced fewer house flies than piles that had mites killed with dicofol, and adding *Macrocheles muscaedomestica* and *Glyptholaspis confusa* to manure held in indoor cages resulted in fewer horn flies than collected from manure with no mites.[57]

Krantz[58] noted that the macrochelid fauna of "domestic" manure was much less than the fauna of "pastoral" dung pads. Considerable knowledge is necessary before these mites could be used as a practical control technology. Anderson[68] focused on the need for pesticide-resistant macrochelids and uropodids so that they can continue to control pest flies after insecticide treatments of manure.

IV. BIOCONTROL OF FLIES OTHER THAN MANURE-BREEDING FLIES

A laboratory-reared braconid, *Alysia ridibunda* Say, that parasitized blowfly larvae, especially *Sarcophaga* spp., was released and quickly reached large numbers in nature. These large numbers caused an immediate increase in parasitism of blow fly larvae in the field, but did not attack larvae of the screwworm♦, *Cochliomyia hominivorax* (Coquerel), and, after 1 year, *A. ridibunda* had practically disappeared from the area.[69]

The release of a parasite, *Phanurus emersoni* Girault, of horse fly eggs reduced the population of horse flies in the release area.[70] *Stictia carolina* (Fabricius) and *Bembix texana* Cresson, two wasp predators of horse flies, reduced tabanid populations on cattle herds if numbers of wasps exceeded two or more per animal.[71] Although a number of pupae of *Tabanus nigrovittatus* Macquart were parasitized by a parasitic wasp, *Trichopria* sp., the species seemed to provide little biological control of the horse fly.[72] Cattle grazing may have consumed sufficient forage around swampy areas to decrease emergent vegetation which was the site of oviposition by female horse and deer flies and thus reduced the populations of flies the next year.[73]

V. BIOCONTROL OF TICKS

Because most species of ticks spend a considerable portion of their life cycles off of their hosts in the environment, they should be available as hosts for a variety of biocontrol organisms. The subject of chemical and "nonchemical" control of ticks has been reviewed by Wilkinson,[74] Sutherst,[75] and Matthewson.[76]

The use of grasses as a biological control agent for ticks was first presented by De Jesus,[77] who determined that gordura grass, *Melinis minutiflora* Beauv., also called molasses grass, repelled and trapped larvae of the southern cattle tick♦, *Boophilus microplus* (Canestrini). Gamba grass, *Andropogon gayanus,* also reduced tick populations.[78] Tropical legumes of the genus *Stylosanthes* entrapped and killed larval ticks.[79,80] Other studies[81] indicated that these legumes also repelled ticks, so that in mixed stands with grasses, the ticks could ascend other grasses and not be controlled by the legumes.

Cole[82] noted that releases of millions of *Hunterellus hookeri* Howard in Montana did not control the Rocky Mountain wood tick♦, *Dermacentor andersoni* Stiles, and ca. 100,000 females released on Martha's Vineyard, Massachusetts, did not reduce the population of the American dog tick,♦ *D. variabilis* (Say). Another encyrtid wasp, *Ixodiphagus texanus* Howard, was shown to overwinter in *D. variabilis.*[83]

Of special interest in the U.S. is the effect of predation on the lone star tick♦, *Amblyomma americanum* (Linnaeus), by the red imported fire ant. Whenever fire ants invade an area, the local population of lone star ticks is greatly reduced. The ants kill engorged female ticks and also attack eggs and engorged larvae.[84-86] The fire ant♦, *S. geminata* (Fabricius), also preyed on engorged females of the southern cattle tick in Mexico.[87]

Ticks are the hosts for a large number of pathogenic bacteria and fungi.[88] Several of 158 fungal extracts applied to ticks prevented the females from laying eggs.[89] However, they appear to be of little practical use for tick control.

VI. OVERVIEW AND CURRENT TECHNOLOGY

It is obvious that there has been considerable interest in the use of biological organisms to control arthropod pests of livestock. Some advances toward the development of a technology of biocontrol have taken place in the use of parasites, predators, and competitors to control flies that breed in the manure of livestock. Releases of pupal parasites of house flies have controlled house flies in poultry facilities. Competition of larvae of the black soldier fly with house fly larvae may be developed into a control technology. Practical use has been made of allowing predaceous mites to survive in poultry manure to prey on house fly larvae.

Considerable interest has been shown in the use of dung-burying beetles to control horn flies and face flies that breed in undisturbed manure. The Australian experience has been that, despite the fact that a number of imported beetles have survived and been able to destroy and bury tons of manure, there is no evidence of reduction of populations of the buffalo fly and the bush fly. Predaceous mites have been imported into Australia to see if they can be efficient biocontrol organisms.

Manure produced by confined livestock is an excellent site for the breeding of flies. The production of hymenopterous parasites of the house fly has become a commercial enterprise, but the release of these parasites has failed to consistently control flies around confined livestock. Lack of quality control of the parasites, inadequate data on the extent of fly breeding, and inability to measure the amount of control obtained have been problems associated with this technology.

Biocontrol of ticks is also of interest but anti-tick grasses, parasites, fungi and other potential biocontrol organisms are yet only in the stage of laboratory discovery and evaluation.

Obviously, much has been learned about the complex relationship between potential biocontrol organisms and arthropod pests of livestock. Although there is considerable research activity at the present time, much needs to be done before biocontrol can be used as a practiced control technology.

REFERENCES

1. **Clausen, C. P., Ed.,** Introduced parasites and predators of arthropod pests and weeds: a world review, *U.S. Dep. Agric. Agric. Handb.,* 480, 1978.
2. **Legner, E. F. and Poorbaugh, J. H., Jr.,** Biological control of vector and noxious synanthropic flies: a review, *Calif. Vector Views,* 19, 81, 1972.
3. **Legner, E. F., Sjogren, R. D., and Hall, I. M.,** The biological control of medically important arthropods, *Crit. Rev. Environ. Control.,* 4, 85, 1974.
4. **Bay, E. C., Berg, C. O., Chapman, H. C., and Legner, E. F.,** Biological control of medical and veterinary pests, in *Theory and Practice of Biological Control,* Huffaker, C. B. and Messinger, P. S., Eds., Academic Press, New York, 1976, 457.
5. **Laird, M.,** Biocontrol in veterinary entomology, *Adv. Vet. Sci. Comp. Med.,* 24, 145, 1980.
6. **Undeen, A. H.,** Biological control of the Psychodidae, Ceratopogonidae, and Simuliidae (Diptera), including new data on the effect of *Bacillus thuringiensis* var. *israelensis* on Simuliidae, in *Comparative Pathobiology,* Vol. 7, Cheng, T. C., Ed., Plenum Press, New York, 1984, 143.
7. **Lacey, L. A. and Undeen, A. H.,** Microbial control of black flies and mosquitoes, *Annu. Rev. Entomol.,* 31, 265, 1986.
8. **Moon, R. D.,** Biological control through interspecific competition, *Environ. Entomol.,* 9, 723, 1980.
9. **Patterson, R. S., Koehler, P. G., Morgan, P. B., and Harris, R. L., Eds.,** Status of biological control of filth flies, in U.S. Department of Agriculture Science and Education Administration, U.S. Department of Agriculture, Washington, D.C., 1981.
10. **Legner, E. F. and Brydon, H. W.,** Suppression of dung-inhabiting fly populations by pupal parasites, *Ann. Entomol. Soc. Am.,* 59, 638, 1966.
11. **Olton, G. S. and Legner, E. F.,** Winter inoculative releases of parasitoids to reduce houseflies in poultry manure, *J. Econ. Entomol.,* 68, 35, 1975.
12. **Morgan, P. B., Patterson, R. S., LaBrecque, G. C., Weidhaas, D. E., and Benton, A.,** Suppression of a field population of houseflies with *Spalangia endius, Science,* 189, 388, 1975.
13. **Morgan, P. B., Patterson, R. S., LaBrecque, G. C., Weidhaas, D. E., Benton, A., and Whitfield, T.,** Rearing and release of the house fly pupal parasite *Spalangia endius* Walker, *Environ. Entomol.,* 4, 609, 1975.
14. **Pickens, L. G. and Miller, R. W.,** Using frozen host pupae to increase the efficiency of a parasite-release program, *Fla. Entomol.,* 61, 153, 1978.
15. **Rutz, D. A. and Axtell, R. C.,** Sustained releases of *Muscidifurax raptor* (Hymenoptera: Pteromalidae) for house fly *(Musca domestica)* control in two types of caged-layer poultry houses, *Environ. Entomol.,* 8, 1105, 1979.
16. **Morgan, P. B., Weidhaas, D. E., and Patterson, R. S.,** Host-parasite relationship: augmentative releases of *Spalangia endius* Walker used in conjunction with population modeling to suppress field populations of *Musca domestica* L. (Hymenoptera: Pteromalidae and Diptera: Muscidae), *J. Kans. Entomol. Soc.,* 54, 496, 1981.
17. **Morgan, P. B., Weidhaas, D. E., and Patterson, R. S.,** Programmed releases of *Spalangia endius* and *Muscidifurax raptor* (Hymenoptera: Pteromalidae) against estimated populations of *Musca domestica* (Diptera: Muscidae), *J. Med. Entomol.,* 18, 158, 1981.

18. **Rutz, D. A. and Axtell, R. C.**, House fly *(Musca domestica)* control in broiler-breeder poultry houses by pupal parasites (Hymenoptera: Pteromalidae): indigenous parasite species and releases of *Muscidifurax raptor*, *Environ. Entomol.*, 10, 343, 1981.

19. **Rueda, L. M. and Axtell, R. C.**, Guide to common species of pupal parasites (Hymenoptera: Pteromalidae) of the house fly and other muscoid flies associated with poultry and livestock manure, *N.C. Agric. Res. Serv. Tech. Bull.*, 278, 1985.

20. **Rueda, L. M. and Axtell, R. C.**, Comparison of hymenopterous parasites of house fly, *Musca domestica* (Diptera: Muscidae), pupae in different livestock and poultry production systems, *Environ. Entomol.*, 14, 217, 1985.

21. **Furman, D. P., Young, R. D., and Catts, E. P.**, *Hermetia illucens* (Linnaeus) as a factor in the natural control of *Musca domestica* Linnaeus, *J. Econ. Entomol.*, 52, 917, 1959.

22. **Axtell, R. C. and Edwards, T. D.**, *Hermetia illucens* control in poultry manure by larviciding, *J. Econ. Entomol.*, 63, 1786, 1970.

23. **Sheppard, C.**, House fly and lesser fly control utilizing the black soldier fly in manure management systems for caged laying hens, *Environ. Entomol.*, 12, 1439, 1983.

24. **Bradley, S. W. and Sheppard, D. C.**, House fly oviposition inhibition by larvae of *Hermetia illucens*, the black soldier fly, *J. Chem. Ecol.*, 10, 853, 1984.

25. **Anderson, J. R. and Poorbaugh, J. H.**, Biological control possibility for house flies, *Calif. Agric.*, 18, 2, 1964.

26. **Anderson, J. R.**, The behavior and ecology of various flies associated with poultry ranches in northern California, *Proc. 32nd Annu. Conf. Calif. Mosq. Control Assoc.*, 30, 1964.

27. **Nolan, M. P., III and Kissam, J. B.**, *Ophyra aenescens:* a potential bio-control alternative for house fly control in poultry houses, *J. Agric. Entomol.*, 2, 192, 1985.

28. **Axtell, R. C.**, Integrated house fly control: populations of fly larvae and predaceous mites, *Macrocheles muscaedomesticae*, in poultry manure after larvicide treatment, *J. Econ. Entomol.*, 61, 245, 1968.

29. **Peck, J. H. and Anderson, J. R.**, Arthropod predators of immature Diptera developing in poultry droppings in northern California, *J. Med. Entomol.*, 6, 163, 1969.

30. **Peck, J. H. and Anderson, J. R.**, Influence of poultry-manure-removal schedules on various Diptera larvae and selected arthropod predators, *J. Econ. Entomol.*, 63, 82, 1970.

31. **Anderson, J. R.**, A preliminary study of integrated fly control on northern California poultry ranches, *Proc. 33rd Annu. Conf. Calif. Mosq. Control Assoc.*, 42, 1965.

32. **Rodriguez, J. G., Singh, P., and Taylor, B.**, Manure mites and their role in fly control, *J. Med. Entomol.*, 7, 335, 1970.

33. **Axtell, R. C.**, Integrated fly-control program for caged-poultry houses, *J. Econ. Entomol.*, 63, 400, 1970.

34. **Axtell, R. C.**, Fly control in caged-poultry houses: comparison of larviciding and integrated control programs, *J. Econ. Entomol.*, 63, 1734, 1970.

35. **Wicht, M. C., Jr. and Rodriguez, J. G.**, Integrated control of muscid flies in poultry houses using predator mites, selected pesticides and microbial agents, *J. Med. Entomol.*, 7, 687, 1970.

36. **Rodriguez, J. L., Jr. and Riehl, L. A.**, Results with cockerels for house fly control in poultry droppings, *J. Econ. Entomol.*, 52, 542, 1959.

37. **LaBrecque, G. C. and Smith, C. N.**, Tests with young poultry for the control of house fly larvae under caged laying hens, *J. Econ. Entomol.*, 53, 696, 1960.

38. **Rodriguez, J. L. and Riehl, L. A.**, Control of flies in manure of chickens and rabbits by cockerels in southern California, *J. Econ. Entomol.*, 55, 473, 1962.

39. **Poorbaugh, J. H., Anderson, J. R., and Burger, J. F.**, The insect inhabitants of undisturbed cattle droppings in northern California, *Calif. Vector Views*, 15, 17, 1968.

40. **Valiela, I.**, An experimental study of the mortality factors of larval *Musca autumnalis* DeGeer, *Ecol. Monogr.*, 39, 199, 1969.

41. **Thomas, G. D. and Wingo, C. W.**, Parasites of the face fly and two other species of dung-inhabiting flies in Missouri, *J. Econ. Entomol.*, 61, 147, 1968.

42. **Turner, E. C., Jr., Burton, R. P., and Gerhardt, R. R.**, Natural parasitism of dung-breeding Diptera: a comparison between native hosts and an introduced host, the face fly, *J. Econ. Entomol.*, 61, 1012, 1968.

43. **Hayes, C. G. and Turner, E. C., Jr.**, Field and laboratory evaluation of parasitism of the face fly in Virginia, *J. Econ. Entomol.*, 64, 443, 1971.

44. **Moon, R. D.**, Effects of larval competition on face fly, *Environ. Entomol.*, 9, 325, 1980.

45. **Blume, R. R., Kunz, S. E., Hogan, B. F., and Matter, J. J.**, Biological and ecological investigations of horn flies in central Texas: influence of other insects in cattle manure, *J. Econ. Entomol.*, 63, 1121, 1970.

46. **Kunz, S. E., Hogan, B. F., Blume, R. R., and Eschle, J. L.**, Some bionomical aspects of horn fly populations in central Texas, *Environ. Entomol.*, 1, 565, 1972.

47. **Thomas, G. D. and Morgan, C. E.,** Field-mortality studies of the immature stages of the horn fly in Missouri, *Environ. Entomol.,* 1, 453, 1972.

48. **Fincher, G. T.,** The potential value of dung beetles in pasture ecosystems, *J. Ga. Entomol. Soc.,* 16, 316, 1981.

49. **Roth, J. P.,** Compatibility of coprophagous scarabs and fimicolous staphylinids as biological control agents of the horn fly, *Haematobia irritans* (L.) (Diptera: Muscidae), *Environ. Entomol.,* 12, 124, 1983.

50. **MacQueen, A. and Beirne, B. P.,** Influence of other insects on production of horn fly, *Haematobia irritans* (Diptera: Muscidae), from cattle dung in south-central British Columbia, *Can. Entomol.,* 107, 1255, 1975.

51. **MacQueen, A. and Beirne, B. P.,** Dung burial activity and fly control potential of *Onthophagus nuchicornis* (Coleoptera: Scarabaeinae) in British Columbia, *Can. Entomol.,* 107, 1215, 1975.

52. **Moon, R. D., Loomis, E. C., and Anderson, J. R.,** Influence of two species of dung beetles on larvae of face fly, *Environ. Entomol.,* 9, 607, 1980.

53. **Jones, C. M. and Perdue, J. M.,** *Heterotylenchus autumnalis,* a parasite of the face fly, *J. Econ. Entomol.,* 60, 1393, 1967.

54. **Stoffolano, J. G., Jr.,** Distribution of the nematode *Heterotylenchus autumnalis,* a parasite of the face fly, in New England with notes on its origin, *J. Econ. Entomol.,* 61, 861, 1968.

55. **Treece, R. E. and Miller, T. A.,** Observations on *Heterotylenchus autumnalis* in relation to the face fly, *J. Econ. Entomol.,* 61, 454, 1968.

56. **Thomas, G. D., Puttler, B., and Morgan, C. E.,** Further studies of field parasitism of the face fly by the nematode *Heterotylenchus autumnalis* in central Missouri, with notes on the gonadotrophic cycles of the face fly, *Environ. Entomol.,* 1, 759, 1972.

57. **Axtell, R. C.,** Effect of Macrochelidae (Acarina: Mesostigmata) on house fly production from dairy cattle manure, *J. Econ. Entomol.,* 56, 317, 1963.

58. **Krantz, G. W.,** Mites as biological control agents of dung-breeding flies, with special reference to the Macrochelidae, in *Biological Control of Pests by Mites,* Special Publication No. 3304, University of California Agricultural Experiment Station, Berkeley, 1983, 91.

59. **Schmidt, C. D.,** Influence of fire ants on horn flies and other dung-breeding Diptera in Bexar County, Texas, *Southwest. Entomol.,* 9, 174, 1984.

60. **Summerlin, J. W., Olson, J. K., Blume, R. R., Aga, A., and Bay, D. E.,** Red imported fire ant: effects on *Onthophagus gazella* and the horn fly, *Environ. Entomol.,* 6, 440, 1977.

61. **Summerlin, J. W., Petersen, H. D., and Harris, R. L.,** Red imported fire ant (Hymenoptera: Formicidae): effects on the horn fly (Diptera: Muscidae) and coprophagous scarabs, *Environ. Entomol.,* 13, 1405, 1984.

62. **Summerlin, J. W. and Kunz, S. E.,** Predation of the red imported fire ant on stable flies, *Southwest. Entomol.,* 3, 260, 1978.

63. **Legner, E. F. and Olton, G. S.,** Worldwide survey and comparison of adult predator and scavenger insect populations associated with domestic animal manure where livestock is artificially congregated, *Hilgardia,* 40, 225, 1970.

64. **Morgan, P. B., Patterson, R. S., and LaBrecque, G. C.,** Controlling house flies at a dairy installation by releasing a protelean parasitoid, *Spalangia endius* (Hymenoptera: Pteromalidae), *J. Ga. Entomol. Soc.,* 2, 39, 1976.

65. **Morgan, P. B. and Patterson, R. S.,** Sustained releases of *Spalangia endius* to parasitize field populations of three species of filth breeding flies, *J. Econ. Entomol.,* 70, 450, 1977.

66. **Morgan, P. B.,** Sustained releases of *Spalangia endius* Walker (Hymenoptera: Pteromalidae) for the control of *Musca domestica* L. and *Stomoxys calcitrans* (L.) (Diptera: Muscidae), *J. Kans. Entomol. Soc.,* 53, 367, 1980.

67. **Petersen, J. J., Meyer, J. A., Stage, D. A., and Morgan, P. B.,** Evaluation of sequential releases of *Spalangia endius* (Hymenoptera: Pteromalidae) for control of house flies and stable flies (Diptera: Muscidae) associated with confined livestock in eastern Nebraska, *J. Econ. Entomol.,* 76, 283, 1983.

68. **Anderson, J. R.,** Mites as biological control agents of dung-breeding pests: practical considerations and selection for pesticide resistance, in *Biological Control of Pests by Mites,* Special Publication No. 3304, University of California Agricultural Experiment Station, Berkeley, 1983, 99.

69. **Lindquist, A. W.,** The introduction of an indigenous blowfly parasite, *Alysia ridibunda* Say, into Uvalde County, Texas, *Ann. Entomol. Soc. Am.,* 33, 103, 1940.

70. **Parman, D. C.,** Experimental dissemination of the tabanid egg parasite *Phanurus emersoni* Girault and biological notes on the species, *U.S. Dep. Agric. Circ.,* 18, 1928.

71. **Roberts, L. W. and Wilson, B. H.,** Predation on horse flies by two bembicine wasp species in certain areas of southern Louisiana, *J. Econ. Entomol.,* 60, 412, 1967.

72. **Magnarelli, L. A. and Anderson, J. F.,** Parasitism of *Tabanus nigrovittatus* immatures (Diptera: Tabanidae) by *Trichopria* sp. (Hymenoptera: Diapriidae), *J. Med. Entomol.,* 17, 481, 1980.

73. **Easton, E. R.,** Reduction of horse and deer flies on the cottonwood range and livestock experiment station as a result of grazing, *J. Econ. Entomol.,* 75, 292, 1982.

74. **Wilkinson, P. R.,** Ecological aspects of pest management of ixodid ticks, in *Recent Advances in Acarology,* Vol. 2, Rodriguez, J. G., Ed., Academic Press, New York, 1979, 25.

75. **Sutherst, R. W.,** Management of arthropod parasitism in livestock, in *Tropical Parasitoses and Parasitic Zoonoses,* Dunsmore, J. C., Ed., World Association for the Advancement of Veterinary Parasitology, Perth, 1983, 41.

76. **Matthewson, M. D.,** The future of tick control: a review of the chemical and non-chemical options, *Prev. Vet. Med.,* 2, 559, 1984.

77. **De Jesus, Z.,** The repellent and killing effects of gordura grass on the larvae of the cattle tick, *Boophilus australis, Philipp. J. Anim. Ind.,* 1, 193, 1934.

78. **Thompson, K. C., Roa, E. J., and Romero, N. T.,** Anti-tick grasses as the basis for developing practical tropical tick control packages, *Trop. Anim. Health Prod.,* 10, 179, 1978.

79. **Sutherst, R. W., Jones, R. J., and Schnitzerling, H. J.,** Tropical legumes of the genus *Stylosanthes* immobilize and kill cattle ticks, *Nature (London),* 295, 320, 1982.

80. **Zimmerman, R. H., Garris, G. I., and Beaver, J. S.,** Potential of *Stylosanthes* plants as a component in an integrated pest management approach to tick control, *Prev. Vet. Med.,* 2, 579, 1984.

81. **Norval, R. A. I., Tebele, N., Short, N. J., and Clatworthy, J. N.,** A laboratory study on the control of economically important tick species with legumes of the genus *Stylosanthes, Zimbabwe Vet. J.,* 14, 26, 1983.

82. **Cole, M. M.,** Biological control of ticks by the use of hymenopterous parasites, a review, EBL/43.65, World Health Org., 1965.

83. **Logan, T. M., Bowman, J. L., and Hair, J. A.,** Parthenogenesis and overwintering behavior in *Ixodiphagus texanus* Howard, *J. Agric. Entomol.,* 2, 272, 1985.

84. **Harris, W. G. and Burns, E. C.,** Predation on the lone star tick by the imported fire ant, *Environ. Entomol.,* 1, 362, 1972.

85. **Burns, E. C. and Melancon, D. G.,** Effect of imported fire ant (Hymenoptera: Formicidae) invasion on lone star tick (Acarina: Ixodidae) populations, *J. Med. Entomol.,* 14, 247, 1977.

86. **Fleetwood, S. C., Teel, P. D., and Thompson, G.,** Impact of imported fire ant on lone star tick mortality in open and canopied pasture habitats of east central Texas, *Southwest. Entomol.,* 9, 158, 1984.

87. **Butler, J. F., Camino, M. L., and Perez, T. O.,** *Boophilus microplus* and the fire ant *Solenopsis geminata,* in *Recent Advances in Acarology,* Vol. 1, Rodriguez, J. G., Ed., Academic Press, New York, 1979, 469.

88. **Hoogstraal, H.,** XXI. Pathogens of Acarina (Ticks), *Bull. WHO,* 55(Suppl. 1), 337, 1977.

89. **Connole, M. D.,** Effect of fungal extracts on the cattle tick, *Boophilus microplus, Aust. Vet. J.,* 45, 207, 1969.

Chapter 22

RESISTANCE OF LIVESTOCK TO ARTHROPOD PESTS*

I. INTRODUCTION

Although the major theme of this book is the review of the technology of the use of chemicals to control arthropod pests of livestock, it is appropriate that the last two chapters focus on "nonchemical" methods of control. One facet of the biological control of arthropod pests of livestock is the selection and use of breeds of animals that are naturally resistant to these pests. A part of that same facet is the artificial stimulation or enhancement of the immune response of livestock so that susceptible animals could become temporarily or permanently resistant to the pests.

The immune response of animals to arthropod pests has been the focus of a large number of recent review articles. These many review articles are justified because of the rapid changes in the field of immunology in the last 15 years and the need to bring into focus the areas where advances have been made and where additional research is necessary. These reviews contain extensive literature citations which we will not list. We will list only the review papers and other limited pertinent references of unusual interest to our subject.

Nelson et al.[1] reviewed the life histories of ectoparasites, spacial distribution on hosts, feeding mechanisms, effects of host nutrition, and endocrine state on the ectoparasites and toxins produced by ectoparasites. Nelson et al.[2] reviewed the literature through 1975 and presented considerable information on hematological, serological, and clinical responses of hosts to ectoparasites, arthropod antigens, immunosuppression and tolerance, histopathology, susceptibility, and resistance. These authors noted that the wide use of effective pesticides may have allowed for parasite-susceptible animals to be maintained in the herd, which, in turn, increased the need for protection by pesticides in order to keep these susceptible animals in the herd.

Allen and Nelson[3] limited their review to *Sarcoptes, Demodex,* the sheep ked♦, *Melophagus ovinus* (Linnaeus), Anoplura, and Ixodidae that cause a demonstrable immune response in hosts because of their prolonged infestation or feeding times. They did not review short-term or fast-feeding arthropods, such as biting flies, fleas, and mosquitoes, for they noted that, although these pests may cause irritation, the host's immunological responses to them do not protect the host from these pests nor do they cause direct harm to these arthropods. They stressed the importance of salivary gland antigens (especially in ticks) and the function of cutaneous hypersensitivity reactions in immune responses.

Wikel[4] focused on the immunological responses of hosts to lice, fleas, mosquitoes, sheep keds, mites, and ticks. He stated "Our knowledge of the immunologic aspects of most host-arthropod relationships is at best superficial". He stressed the fact that the antibody- and cell-mediated immune responses of hosts included several components, such as complement, vasoactive amines, and prostaglandins, and that information from the field of mammalian immunology and immunoparasitology could be applied to the understanding of arthropod-host systems. A more recent review by Wikel[5] gives an indication of the dynamics in research in arthropod-host responses since 34 of the 123 references cited (27%) were published after 1980.

The relationship of the nutrition of animals to their responses to ectoparasites was reviewed by Nelson,[6] who concluded that standard recommendations of vitamin intake may not be

* Common names of insects and acarines, as listed in *Common Names of Insects and Related Organisms* (published by the Entomological Society of America), are marked with a ♦ the first time they are cited preceding the scientific name.

adequate for animals to defend themselves against ectoparasites and that malnutrition in an animal may not become apparent until it is stressed by an ectoparasite.

There has been recent interest and progress in immunological studies on responses of sheep to sheep keds, chickens to the northern fowl mite♦, *Ornithonyssus sylviarum* (Canestrini and Fanzago), and cattle to cattle grub larvae and ticks.

II. THE SHEEP KED

The early increase in ked numbers on lambs was followed by a later decline which was the result of a physiological response of the host, and lambs infested with larger numbers of keds developed resistance sooner than lambs infested with smaller numbers of keds.[7] The nature of the acquired resistance was such that it could be broken by stressors, such as pituitary-adrenal system stimulators.[8] Resistance to keds was the result of constriction of the blood supply to the outer dermis which diminished the food supply available to the keds.[9] The addition or deletion of vitamin A in the diet of lambs and sheep affected their resistance to keds, and such antibiosis or nutritional resistance was probably different from the previously demonstrated acquired resistance.[10] There was some cross-resistance in sheep to keds and to the Rocky Mountain wood tick♦, *Dermacentor andersoni* Stiles. This resistance was evident in the decreased survival of males and of the weights of engorged females.[11] The resistance of sheep to keds was shown to be cutaneous, locally mediated, and characterized by increasing numbers of eosinophils.[9,12] Finally, the nature of the acquired resistance in sheep to keds was postulated[13] to be a chronic inflammatory response combined with cell-mediated immune-effector elements.

III. THE NORTHERN FOWL MITE

Matthysse et al.[14] determined that certain strains of white leghorn chickens were less suitable hosts than other strains and that chickens develop circulating, precipitating and skin-sensitizing antibodies to northern fowl mites. An immediate-type skin sensitivity may provide some functional immunity, and immunocompetence varied with strain, sex, and individual chicken. Noting that it was well documented that larger populations of northern fowl mites were found on male chickens than on females, Hall et al.[15] slightly increased resistance in roosters with intramuscular injections of estradiol cypionate. Hens had a greater susceptibility to mite infestation at the onset of sexual maturity.

Antibody response in chickens to a crude mite antigen increased as the numbers of mites on the chickens increased.[16] Chickens with the heaviest mite populations had earlier and greater immune responses, which remained high even as mite populations decreased. In a further study, hens previously infested with northern fowl mites were shown to develop a resistance that was related to the intensity of the previous infestation.[17]

Cockerels from a strain of chickens that had a high plasma corticosterone response to social stress had lower populations of northern fowl mites than cockerels from a strain with a low response.[18] There were significant differences in mite populations among 16 inbred lines of chickens as well as a positive relationship between the size of the mite population and body weight of the chicken.[19] There were significant differences in infestation levels among seven lines of chickens, and certain lines had genetic factors from the Giant Jungle Fowl that appeared to provide for resistance to mites.[20] In selective mating trials with roosters and hens that had light or heavy populations of northern fowl mites, F_1 progeny exhibited some differences in susceptibility due to the selective breeding of parents.[21] It was suggested that selection for resistance to northern fowl mites was possible but would require long-term, well-controlled experiments with a wide genetic base.

IV. CATTLE GRUB LARVAE

There are both innate and acquired elements of resistance of cattle to larvae of the common cattle grub,♦ *Hypoderma lineatum* (Villers), and the northern cattle grub♦, *H. bovis* (Linnaeus). Certain cattle have more cattle grub larvae in their backs than others, there is a greater mortality of larvae in backs of certain cattle than others, and older cattle have fewer cattle grub larvae than younger animals.[22] The innate resistance in calves and yearlings was impaired by a vitamin A deficiency.[23]

Cattle grub larvae were killed with systemics while in the backs of cattle, and the next year, although cattle were not retreated, the previously treated cattle had fewer cattle grub larvae in their backs than untreated animals.[24] Thus the killing of cattle grub larvae in the backs of cattle was interpreted as having increased the resistance of the cattle to the subsequent infestation and that the degree of resistance appeared to be related to the number of larvae killed in the backs of the cattle. In contrast,[25] when first instar cattle grub larvae were killed in cattle with systemics, there was a significant difference in numbers of larvae that appeared in backs of treated and untreated cattle that year. The next year none of the treated or untreated cattle were treated, and there was no significant difference in numbers of larvae found in backs of previously treated and untreated calves.

Research has been conducted on the treatment of cattle with larval antigens to elicit an immune response in order to control first instar cattle grub larvae before they reach the backs of cattle. In early research, antigens were used in the same manner that animal systemic insecticides were used, i.e., given as a massive treatment after cattle had been infested with larvae. Crude antigens made from homogenized first instar *H. lineatum* larvae injected intramuscularly into calves did not prevent *H. lineatum* larvae from reaching cattle's backs, but provided a highly significant reduction in numbers of *H. bovis* larvae.[26] A similarly prepared and administered antigen gave a 60% reduction in hypodermal larvae.[27] A crude antigen of first instar *H. lineatum* larvae and the antigen plus the adjuvant, sodium alginate, did not control cattle grub larvae.[28] The dynamics of antibody production by uninfested and infested cattle in response to larval antigens indicated a direct relationship between the level of antibody production and previous infestation.[29] A crude antigen of the soluble extract of whole esophageal first instar *H. lineatum* larvae, but not a metabolic antigen derived from in vitro culture of such larvae, injected into calves previously injected with known numbers of larvae caused a >60% reduction in numbers of *H. lineatum* and *H. bovis* larvae that appeared in the animals' backs and survived to pupate.[30] In other studies with artificially infested cattle,[31] the resistance in calves increased as the number of cattle grub larvae administered was increased, and the onset of resistance was more rapid in older cattle injected with higher initial numbers of larvae than in cattle injected with lower initial numbers. Further studies on both humoral and cellular responses of previously infested and uninfested cattle to an infestation of first instar *H. lineatum* larvae showed that resistance was not related to the number and intensity of previous infestations and involved a cellular component of the immune system.[32]

Chapters by Beesley[33] and Boulard and Troccon[34] reviewed research on the *Hypoderma*-host relationship and the use of an antibody titer to define dynamics of host immunity to cattle grubs. An enzyme-linked immunosorbent assay (ELISA) to detect humoral antibodies to *H. bovis*[35] provided a means for making a clear diagnosis of infestation. The detection of infested cattle, which should be the only ones treated with systemic insecticides, would greatly increase the efficiency of the current warble fly eradication program in the U.K.[36]

Crude antigens from first instar *H. lineatum* larvae were injected into previously infested and uninfested cattle, and fraction 4, which contains Hypodermin A, was found to elicit the most intense skin reaction in cattle and was selected for further vaccination trials, but protection against infestation was not determined.[37] Crude antigens from first instar *H.*

lineatum larvae injected into previously uninfested cattle elicited elevated antibody activity, and, upon challenge with larvae, the previously uninfested cattle were changed, by this immunization, to the immunological equivalent, in terms of antibody activity and response to infestation, of previously infested cattle.[38]

V. TICKS

A. Reviews

The resistance of cattle to ticks has been the subject of a great deal of research, especially in Australia where the southern cattle tick♦, *Boophilus microplus* (Canestrini), is an important pest of cattle. In their selected bibliography, McGowan and Barker[39] included only papers which "offered detailed methodologies, innovative concepts, and . . . historically significant contributions" and still listed 252 references. Allen[40] focused on the research on resistance in guinea pigs to ticks and in cattle to *B. microplus* and concluded that resistance to ticks is "dependent apparently on the acquisition of a cutaneous hypersensitivity to tick salivary antigens". Willadsen[41] discussed the expression of resistance, various types of immune responses (such as antibody formation and complement activation, delayed or immediate hypersensitivity and cellular reactions), as well as the nature of antigens and possible artificial immunization of animals. Oberem[42] stressed the knowledge that had been gained on the nature of the immunological response, including humoral, cellular, and hypersensitivity factors and their interactions. He noted that response is affected by a variety of external factors, such as stress, photoperiod, reproductive status, drugs, infestation with other parasites, and nature of the antigenic challenge. Wikel[43] discussed the host's immune response to ticks and mites and noted that "our knowledge of many aspects of the relationships described . . . is limited". Brown[44] reviewed the immunology of acquired resistance and focused on the action of host basophils on the feeding success of ticks.

The resistance of cattle to *B. microplus* has been used as one of the criterion for the selection of cattle breeds and crossbreeds for general use in Australia, but general acceptance of tick-resistant breeds by cattle producers in tropical Australia has been limited.[45]

B. Ticks and Small Mammals

In the U.S. and Canada, because of the absence of *Boophilus* spp., research on tick-host systems has focused on three-host species, predominantly the Rocky Mountain wood tick♦, *Dermacentor andersoni* Stiles, and the lone star tick♦, *Amblyomma americanum* (Linnaeus). Expression of resistance of guinea pigs to *D. andersoni* was shown to involve a generalized cutaneous basophil hypersensitivity response to a salivary gland antigen.[46-49] Such an antigen, derived from partially engorged female ticks and administered to previously uninfested guinea pigs, induced a degree of resistance to subsequent infestations.[50]

Feeding of immature *A. americanum* on previously infested guinea pigs[51] caused increased mortality of ticks and a marked infiltration of basophils and eosinophils to feeding sites in sensitized guinea pigs. Guinea pigs, resistant to ticks as a result of feeding of larvae of *D. andersoni* or *A. americanum*, were also variably resistant to infestations of the American dog tick♦, *D. variabilis* (Say), and the blacklegged tick♦, *Ixodes scapularis* Say.[52] Resistance to feeding of *A. americanum* and the brown dog tick♦, *Rhipicephalus sanguineus* (Latreille), could be passively transferred from immune guinea pigs to naive guinea pigs by transfer of serum or peritoneal exudate cells.[53] T cell and IgG_1 antibodies were responsible for the ability of the immune serum to transfer resistance to naive guinea pigs, and the degree of resistance was correlated with the degree of expression of the resulting cutaneous basophil response.[54] The immune reaction in guinea pigs was generally cross reactive to several tick genera.[55] Basophils must be present for the expression of immunity,[56] and a basophil-derived mediator, other than histamine, was required for the immune cutaneous basophil resistance of guinea pigs to ticks.[57] Gel electrophoresis of immunoprecipitated tick salivary gland proteins indicated that one, or possibly two, crucial antigens were responsible for inducing the immune response in guinea pigs to *A. americanum.*[58] An antigen from tick salivary gland extract injected into guinea pigs induced levels of immunization equal to natural challenge.[59] A 20,000-mol wt protein appeared responsible for the response. Primary tissue culture cells of larvae of *A. americanum* administered to naive guinea pigs induced resistance to *A. americanum* and *D. andersoni.*[60]

Extracts of homogenates of males of the Gulf Coast tick♦, *A. maculatum* Koch, injected into rabbits caused an increase in passive hemagglutination antibody titers, in the size of tick feeding lesions and a decrease in weights of nymphs and adults fed on immunized rabbits.[61] Extracts of midguts of the American dog ticks, but not of whole ticks, injected into rats caused delayed attachment, reduced engorgement weights, and a decreased egg production. These effects were the result of an ingested antibody specific for digestive tract antigens.[62]

Cottontail rabbits, *Sylvilagus floridanus* Allen, developed a resistance to infestations of the rabbit tick♦, *Haemaphysalis leporispalustris* (Packard), that was correlated with the development of skin-sensitizing antibodies.[63] Rabbits resistant to the rabbit tick were also resistant to the American dog tick.[64] Interestingly, the snowshoe hare, *Lepus americanus* Erxleben, did not develop resistance to multiple infestations of the rabbit tick.[65]

C. Ticks and Cattle

In the U.S., resistance in Brahman, Hereford and Hereford × Brahman crossbred cattle was manifested in the reduction of numbers of females engorging, engorgment weights, and weights of egg masses of female *A. americanum.*[66] When Jersey and Hereford calves were injected with an antigen from an extract of homogenized whole adult *A. americanum,* numbers and weights of female ticks that fed on immunized calves were less than those fed on nonimmunized calves, and males feeding on immunized calves died prematurely or became immobilized in feeding exudates.[67]

Feeding of *D. andersoni* on Hereford cows and calves stimulated the production of precipitating antibodies to a salivary gland antigen which indicated the presence of an antigen-reactive cell population.[68] Because there appeared to be no differences in numbers of female *D. andersoni* attached to several breeds of cattle, there was little indication that selection for tick resistance would readily be accomplished, so Wilkinson[69] proposed that a more feasible approach might be artificial sensitization of existing herds to increase resistance. However, an extract of *D. variabilis* in an adjuvant injected into yearling steers did not increase their resistance to feeding of *D. andersoni* or to tick paralysis.[70]

Holstein calves infested with *A. americanum* adults developed an immunity characterized by decreased weight of ticks and egg masses associated with a local cutaneous basophil response and peripheral blood basophilia.[71] Brahman and Brahman × Hereford crossbred calves, infested one to three times with *A. americanum* adults, developed a resistance that was manifested in decreased percentages of females that engorged and in the weights of these females and their egg masses. Infested calves had skin reactions and peripheral blood lymphocytes that reacted to salivary gland extracts from *D. andersoni* as well as *A. americanum* and the Cayenne tick♦, *A. cajennense* (Fabricius).[72]

VI. OVERVIEW AND CURRENT TECHNOLOGY

There has been considerable interest in the last 15 years on research to understand the immunological nature of the reaction of hosts to arthropod pests. A number of reviews have shown that rapid advances in immunological research in general have been brought to focus on the arthropod pest-host immunological relationship.

While researchers have characterized aspects of the immunological basis of the host-reaction of sheep to sheep keds, there is no indication of efforts to utilize this knowledge to develop a new control technology for the pest.

Research done on the response of chickens to the northern fowl mite is encouraging because of the evidence that there is an immunological aspect to the response. Preliminary studies indicated that the capability to acquire resistance is inherited. It seems that the short generation time span in poultry should benefit efforts to identify and select lines of chickens that are most capable of developing resistance to the northern fowl mite.

It is obvious that in the last several years considerable progress has been made in the acquisition of knowledge on the *Hypoderma*-cattle immunological relationship. Further studies, conducted in the light of greater knowledge of the immune response in general, could lead to a vaccine that may provide for the immunological control of cattle grub larvae.

There is also considerable interest in the response of hosts to ticks. Although no specific control measures have been developed, there is a reasonable expectation that with continued research on tick-host relationships and input from ''basic'' immunology, practical tick control technology may come from manipulation and enhancement of the host immune response.

We look for rapid advances in knowledge about the arthropod pest-host relationship and a practical control technology available for cattle grubs and ticks in the next few years.

REFERENCES

1. **Nelson, W. A., Keirans, J. E., Bell, J. F., and Clifford, C. M.,** Host-ectoparasite relationships, *J. Med. Entomol.,* 12, 143, 1975.
2. **Nelson, W. A., Bell, J. F., Clifford, C. M., and Keirans, J. E.,** Interaction of ectoparasites and their hosts, *J. Med. Entomol.,* 13, 389, 1977.
3. **Allen, J. R. and Nelson, W. A.,** Immunological responses to ectoparasites, *Fortsch. Zool.,* 27, 169, 1982.
4. **Wikel, S. K.,** Immune responses to arthropods and their products, *Annu. Rev. Entomol.,* 27, 21, 1982.
5. **Wikel, S. K.,** Immunomodulation of host responses to ectoparasite infestation — an overview, *Vet. Parasitol.,* 14, 321, 1984.
6. **Nelson, W. A.,** Effects of nutrition of animals on their ectoparasites, *J. Med. Entomol.,* 21, 621, 1984.
7. **Nelson, W. A.,** Development in sheep of resistance to the ked *Melophagus ovinus* (L.). I. Effects of seasonal manipulation of infestations, *Exp. Parasitol.,* 12, 41, 1962.
8. **Nelson, W. A.,** Development in sheep of resistance to the ked *Melophagus ovinus* (L.). II. Effects of adrenocorticotrophic hormone and cortisone, *Exp. Parasitol.,* 12, 45, 1962.
9. **Nelson, W. A. and Bainborough, A. R.,** Development in sheep of resistance to the ked *Melophagus ovinus* (L.). III. Histopathology of sheep skin as a clue to the nature of resistance, *Exp. Parasitol.,* 13, 118, 1963.
10. **Nelson, W. A. and Hironaka, R.,** Effect of protein and vitamin A intake of sheep on numbers of the sheep ked, *Melophagus ovinus* (L.), *Exp. Parasitol.,* 18, 274, 1966.
11. **Nelson, W. A., Weintraub, J., and Hironaka, R.,** Effects of vitamin A deficiency and ked resistance on the feeding of *Dermacentor andersoni* on sheep, *Exp. Parasitol.,* 22, 240, 1968.
12. **Nelson, W. A. and Kozub, G. C.,** *Melophagus ovinus* (Diptera: Hippoboscidae): evidence of local mediation in acquired resistance of sheep to keds, *J. Med. Entomol.,* 17, 291, 1980.
13. **Baron, R. W. and Nelson, W. A.,** Aspects of the humoral and cell-mediated immune responses of sheep to the ked *Melophagus ovinus* (Diptera: Hippoboscidae), *J. Med. Entomol.,* 22, 544, 1985.
14. **Matthysse, J. G., Jones, C. J., and Purnasiri, A.,** Development of northern fowl mite populations on chickens, effects on the host, and immunology, *Search Agric.,* 4, 1, 1974.
15. **Hall, R. D., Gross, W. B., and Turner, E. C., Jr.,** Preliminary observations on northern fowl mite infestations on estrogenized roosters and in relation to initial egg production in hens, *Poultry Sci.,* 57, 1088, 1978.

16. **DeVaney, J. A. and Ziprin, R. L.,** Detection and correlation of immune responses in white leghorn chickens to northern fowl mite, *Ornithonyssus sylviarum* (Canestrini and Fanzago), populations, *Poultry Sci.,* 59, 34, 1980.

17. **DeVaney, J. A. and Ziprin, R. L.,** Acquired immune response of white leghorn hens to populations of northern fowl mite, *Ornithonyssus sylviarum* (Canestrini and Fanzago), *Poultry Sci.,* 59, 1742, 1980.

18. **Hall, R. D. and Gross, W. B.,** Effect of social stress and inherited plasma corticosterone levels in chickens on populations of the northern fowl mite, *Ornithonyssus sylviarum, J. Parasitol.,* 61, 1096, 1975.

19. **Eklund, J., Loomis, E., and Abplanalp, H.,** Genetic resistance of white leghorn chickens to infestation by the northern fowl mite, *Ornithonyssus sylviarum, Arch. Geflugelk.,* 44, 195, 1980.

20. **DeVaney, J. A., Gyles, N. R., and Lancaster, J. L., Jr.,** Evaluation of Arkansas rous sarcoma regressor and progressor lines and Giant Jungle Fowl for genetic resistance to the northern fowl mite, *Poultry Sci.,* 61, 2327, 1982.

21. **DeVaney, J. A.,** Influence of northern fowl mite populations of parent chickens on their F_1 progeny, *Poultry Sci.,* 63, 589, 1984.

22. **Scharff, D. K.,** Cattle grubs — their biologies, their distribution, and experiments in their control, *Mont. State Coll. Agric. Exp. Stn. Bull.,* 471, 1950.

23. **Gingrich, R. E.,** Differentiation of resistance in cattle to larval *Hypoderma lineatum, Vet. Parasitol.,* 7, 243, 1980.

24. **Knapp, F. W., Brethour, J. R., Harvey, T. L., and Roan, C. C.,** Field observations of increasing resistance of cattle to cattle grubs, *J. Econ. Entomol.,* 52, 1022, 1959.

25. **Drummond, R. O.,** The common cattle grub in cattle in southwestern Texas, *J. Econ. Entomol.,* 59, 1105, 1966.

26. **Khan, M. A., Connell, R., and Darcel, C. le Q.,** Immunization and parenteral chemotherapy for the control of cattle grubs *Hypoderma lineatum* (De Vill.) and *H. bovis* (L.) in cattle, *Can. J. Comp. Med.,* 24, 177, 1960.

27. **Sharma, R. M. and Chhabra, R. C.,** Further observations on the therapeutic control of *Hypoderma lineatum, Ind. J. Res.,* 2, 124, 1965.

28. **Khan, M. A.,** Efficacy of homologous antigens and coumaphos: comparative effect against the cattle grubs *Hypoderma* spp. and a discussion of coumaphos toxicity, *Vet. Rec.,* 83, 345, 1968.

29. **Robertson, R. H.,** Antibody production in cattle infected with *Hypoderma* spp., *Can. J. Zool.,* 58, 245, 1980.

30. **Baron, R. W. and Weintraub, J.,** Immunization of cattle against warbles, in Research Highlights 1981, Sears, L. J. L., Krogman, K. K., and Atkinson, T. G., Eds., Agriculture Canada Research Station, Lethbridge, Alberta, 1982, 24.

31. **Weintraub, J.,** Characteristics of host resistance to warble grub infestations, in Research Highlights 1979, Croome, G. C. R. and Wilson, D. G., Eds., Agriculture Canada Research Station, Lethbridge, Alberta, 1980, 63.

32. **Gingrich, R. E.,** Acquired resistance to *Hypoderma lineatum:* comparative immune response of resistant and susceptible cattle, *Vet. Parasitol.,* 9, 233, 1982.

33. **Beesley, W. N.,** Parasite: host relationships, in *Warble Fly Control in Europe,* Boulard, C. and Thornberry, H., Eds., A. A. Balkema, Rotterdam, 1984, 107.

34. **Boulard, C. and Troccon, J. L.,** Attempts to reduce adverse reactions following hypodermosis chemotherapy, in *Warble Fly Control in Europe,* Boulard, C. and Thornberry, H., Eds., A. A. Balkema, Rotterdam, 1984, 111.

35. **Sinclair, I. J. and Wassall, D. A.,** Enzyme-linked immunosorbent assay for the detection of antibodies to *Hypoderma bovis* in cattle, *Res. Vet. Sci.,* 34, 251, 1983.

36. **Tarry, D. W.,** Eradication of the cattle warble fly, *Vet. Annu.,* 25, 94, 1985.

37. **Pruett, J. H. and Barrett, C. C.,** Induction of intradermal skin reactions in the bovine by fractionated proteins of *Hypoderma lineatum, Vet. Parasitol.,* 16, 137, 1984.

38. **Pruett, J. H. and Barrett, C. C.,** Kinetic development of humoral anti-*Hypoderma lineatum* antibody activity in the serum of vaccinated and infested cattle, *Southwest. Entomol.,* 10, 39, 1985.

39. **McGowan, M. J. and Barker, R. W.,** A selected bibliography of tick-host resistance and immunological relationships, *Bull. Entomol. Soc. Am.,* 26, 17, 1980.

40. **Allen, J. R.,** The immune response as a factor in management of acari of veterinary importance, in *Recent Advances in Acarology,* Vol. 2, Rodriguez, J. G., Ed., Academic Press, New York, 1979, 15.

41. **Willadsen, P.,** Immunity to ticks, *Adv. Parasitol.,* 18, 293, 1980.

42. **Oberem, P. T.,** The immunological basis of host resistance to ticks — a review, *J. S. Afr. Vet. Assoc.,* 55, 215, 1984.

43. **Wikel, S. K.,** Tick and mite toxicosis and allergy, *Handb. Nat. Toxins,* 2, 371, 1984.

44. **Brown, S. J.,** Immunology of acquired resistance to ticks, *Parasitol. Today,* 1, 166, 1985.

45. **Seifert, G. W.,** Selection of beef cattle in Northern Australia for resistance to the cattle tick *(Boophilus microplus):* research and application, *Prev. Vet. Med.,* 2, 553, 1984.

46. **Wikel, S. K. and Allen, J. R.,** Acquired resistance to ticks. I. Passive transfer of resistance, *Immunology,* 30, 311, 1976.

47. **Wikel, S. K. and Allen, J. R.,** Acquired resistance to ticks. II. Effects of cyclophosphamide on resistance, *Immunology,* 30, 479, 1976.

48. **Wikel, S. K. and Allen, J. R.,** Acquired resistance to ticks. III. Cobra venom factor and the resistance response, *Immunology,* 32, 457, 1977.

49. **Wikel, S. K., Graham, J. E., and Allen, J. R.,** Acquired resistance to ticks. IV. Skin reactivity and *in vitro* lymphocyte responsiveness to salivary gland antigen, *Immunology,* 34, 257, 1978.

50. **Wikel, S. K.,** The induction of host resistance to tick infestation with a salivary gland antigen, *Am. J. Trop. Med. Hyg.,* 30, 284, 1981.

51. **Brown, S. J. and Knapp, F. W.,** Response of hypersensitized guinea pigs to the feeding of *Amblyomma americanum* ticks, *J. Parasitol.,* 83, 213, 1981.

52. **McTier, T. L., George, J. E., and Bennett, S. N.,** Resistance and cross-resistance of guinea pigs to *Dermacentor andersoni* Stiles, *D. variabilis* (Say), *Amblyomma americanum* (Linnaeus), and *Ixodes scapularis* Say, *J. Parasitol.,* 67, 813, 1981.

53. **Brown, S. J. and Askenase, P. W.,** Cutaneous basophil responses and immune resistance of guinea pigs to ticks: passive transfer with peritoneal exudate cells or serum, *J. Immunol.,* 127, 2163, 1981.

54. **Brown, S. J., Graziano, F. M., and Askenase, P. W.,** Immune serum transfer of cutaneous basophil-associated resistance to ticks: mediation by 7SIgG₁ antibodies, *J. Immunol.,* 129, 2407, 1982.

55. **Brown, S. J. and Askenase, P. W.,** Immune rejection of ectoparasites (ticks) by T cell and IgG₁ antibody recruitment of basophils and eosinophils, *Fed. Proc. Fed. Am. Soc. Exp. Biol.,* 42, 1744, 1983.

56. **Brown, S. J., Galli, S. J., Gleich, G. J., and Askenase, P. W.,** Ablation of immunity to *Amblyomma americanum,* by anti-basophil serum: Cooperation between basophils and eosinophils in expression of immunity to ectoparasites (ticks) in guinea pigs, *J. Immunol.,* 129, 790, 1982.

57. **Brown, S. J. and Askenase, P. W.,** Rejection of ticks from guinea pigs by anti-hapten-antibody-mediated degranulation of basophils at cutaneous basophil hypersensitivity sites: role of mediators other than histamine, *J. Immunol.,* 134, 1160, 1985.

58. **Brown, S. J. and Askenase, P. W.,** Analysis of host components mediating immune resistance to ticks, in *Acarology VI,* Vol. 2, Griffiths, D. A. and Bowman, C. E., Eds., Ellis Harwood, Chichester, U.K., 1984, 1040.

59. **Brown, S. J., Shapiro, S. Z., and Askenase, P. W.,** Characterization of tick antigens inducing host immune resistance. I. Immunization of guinea pigs with *Amblyomma americanum*-derived salivary gland extracts and identification of an important salivary gland protein antigen with guinea pig anti-tick antibodies, *J. Immunol.,* 133, 3319, 1984.

60. **Wikel, S. K.,** Resistance to ixodid tick infestation induced by administration of tick-tissue culture cells, *Ann. Trop. Med. Parasitol.,* 79, 513, 1985.

61. **McGowan, M. J., Homer, J. T., O'Dell, G. V., McNew, R. W., and Barker, R. W.,** Performance of ticks fed on rabbits inoculated with extracts derived from homogenized ticks *Amblyomma maculatum* Koch (Acarina: Ixodidae), *J. Parasitol.,* 66, 42, 1980.

62. **Ackerman, S., Floyd, M., and Sonenshine, D. E.,** Artificial immunity to *Dermacentor variabilis* (Acari: Ixodidae): vaccination using tick antigens, *J. Med. Entomol.,* 17, 391, 1980.

63. **McGowan, M. J., Camin, J. H., and McNew, R. W.,** Field study of the relationship between skin-sensitizing antibody production in the cottontail rabbit, *Sylvilagus floridanus,* and infestation by the rabbit tick, *Haemaphysalis leporispalustris* (Acari: Ixodidae), *J. Parasitol.,* 65, 692, 1979.

64. **McGowan, M. J., McNew, R. W., Homer, J. T., and Camin, J. H.,** Relationship between skin-sensitizing antibody production in the Eastern cottontail, *Sylvilagus floridanus,* and infestations by the rabbit tick, *Haemaphysalis leporispalustris,* and the American dog tick, *Dermacentor variabilis* (Acari: Ixodidae), *J. Med. Entomol.,* 19, 198, 1982.

65. **McGowan, M. J.,** Relationship between skin-sensitizing antibody production in the snowshoe hare, *Lepus americanus,* and infestations by the rabbit tick, *Haemaphysalis leporispalustris* (Acari: Ixodidae), *J. Parasitol.,* 71, 513, 1985.

66. **Strother, G. R., Burns, E. C., and Smart, L. I.,** Resistance of purebred Brahman, Hereford, and Brahman × Hereford crossbred cattle to the lone star tick, *Amblyomma americanum* (Acarina: Ixodidae), *J. Med. Entomol.,* 5, 559, 1974.

67. **McGowan, M. J., Barker, R. W., Homer, J. T., McNew, R. W., and Holscher, K. H.,** Success of tick feeding on calves immunized with *Amblyomma americanum* (Acari: Ixodidae) extract, *J. Med. Entomol.,* 18, 328, 1981.

68. **Wikel, S. K. and Osburn, R. L.,** Immune responsiveness of the bovine host to repeated low-level infestations with *Dermacentor andersoni, Ann. Trop. Med. Parsitol.,* 76, 405, 1982.

69. **Wilkinson, P. R.,** The potential for selection of cattle resistant to tick paralysis and attachment of Rocky mountain wood ticks, in Research Highlights 1981, Sears, L. J. L., Krogman, K. K., and Atkinson, A. G., Eds., Agriculture Canada Research Station, Lethbridge, Alberta, 1982, 25.

70. **Wilkinson, P. R. and Allen, J. R.,** A test of the efficacy of immunizing cattle against Rocky Mountain wood ticks, *J. Entomol. Soc. B.C.,* 80, 37, 1983.
71. **Brown, S. J., Barker, R. W., and Askenase, P. W.,** Bovine resistance to *Amblyomma americanum* ticks: an acquired immune response characterized by cutaneous basophil infiltrates, *Vet. Parasitol.,* 16, 147, 1984.
72. **George, J. E., Osburn, R. L., and Wikel, S. K.,** Acquisition and expression of resistance by *Bos indicus* and *Bos indicus* × *Bos taurus* calves to *Amblyomma americanum* infestation, *J. Parasitol.,* 71, 174, 1985.

APPENDIX

List of Organic Chemicals Reviewed

This appendix contains a list of the chemical names of some of the chemicals used as insecticides and acaricides in this book. We have not included in this appendix the large number of petroleum oils, plant oils, plant extracts, and basic chemicals that were used as control materials as presented in the early publications. The list is restricted to the more complex organic chemicals that were synthesized in the 1940s and later. Whenever an insecticide or acaricide had a common name that was approved for use in publications of the Entomological Society of America that name is preceded by an open diamond ($^\diamond$) and the chemical name is not given. These chemical names can be found in lists of names of commercial and experimental organic insecticides that are published periodically by the Entomological Society of America. The chemical nomenclature of the insecticides and acaricides that do not have approved common names are presented in accordance with the principles followed by *Chemical Abstracts*.

Chemical	Chemical name
$^\diamond$Acephate	
$^\diamond$Aldrin	
$^\diamond$Allethrin	
American Cyanamid CL-38064	O-(p-Ethylsulfamoyl)phenyl O,O-dimethyl phosphorothioate
American Cyanamid 12503	O,O-Diethyl O-[6-(3(2-phenyl)-pyridazinonyl)] phosphorothioate
$^\diamond$Amitraz	
$^\diamond$Apholate	
Aramite®	2-(p-$tert$-Butylphenoxy)-1-methylethyl 2-chloroethyl sulfite
$^\diamond$Azinphosmethyl	
$^\diamond$*Bacillus thuringiensis* Berliner (BT)	
B. thuringiensis subsp. *israelensis* (BTI)	
Barthrin	(6-Chloro-1,3-benzodioxol-5,5-yl)methyl 2,2-dimethyl-3-(2-methyl-1-propenyl)-cyclopropanecarboxylate
Bayer 21/200	O,O-Dimethyl O-3-chloro-4-methyl-2-oxo-2H-1-benzopyran-7-yl phosphorothioate
Bayer 22408	Naphthaloximido-O,O-diethyl phosphorothioate
Bayer 37341 (= Bayer 9017)	O,O-Diethyl O-[4-(methylthio)-3,5-xylyl] phosphorothioate
Bayer 37342 (= Bayer 9018)	O,O-Dimethyl O-[4-(methylthio)-3,5-xylyl] phosphorothioate
Bay-62863	Methyl-2,3-dihydro-2-methyl-7 benzofuranyl carbamate
Bay Vi-7533	2-Chloro-N[[[4-(trifluoromethoxy)phenyl]amino]carbonyl]benzamide
$^\diamond$Bendiocarb	
$^\diamond$Benzene hexachloride (BHC)	
$^\diamond$BHC (benzene hexachloride)	
Bomyl®	Dimethyl 3-[(dimethoxyphosphinyl) oxy]-2-pentenedioate
$^\diamond$Bromophos	
Butazolidin	Monosodium 4-butyl-1,2-diphenyl-3,5-pyrazolidinedone
$^\diamond$Butonate	
$^\diamond$Butoxy polypropylene glycol	
BW-11Z70	1,1-bis (p-Ethoxyphenyl)-2-nitropropane
$^\diamond$Carbaryl	
$^\diamond$Carbon disulfide (carbon bisulfide)	
$^\diamond$Carbon tetrachloride	
$^\diamond$Carbophenothion	
CGA-13353	Ethyl 3-methyl-4-[4-(phenylmethyl)phenoxy]-2-butenoate
CGA-19255	6-Azido-N-cyclopropyl-N'-ethyl-1,3,5-triazine-2,4-diamine
CGA-34296	2-{[4-Azido-6-(cyclopropylamino)-1,3,5-triazine-2-yl]-amino}propanenitrile
$^\diamond$Chlordane	

◇Chlordimeform
◇Chlorfenvinphos
◇Chlorphoxim
◇Chlorpicrin
◇Chlorpyrifos
Chlorthion   *O*-3-Chloro-4-nitrophenyl *O,O*-dimethyl phosphorothioate
Closantel   *N*-[5-Chloro-4-[(4-chlorophenyl)cyanomethyl]-2-methylphenyl]-2-hydroxy-3,5-diiodobenzamide

◇Coumaphos
◇Crotoxyphos
◇Crufomate
Cyclethrin   *dl*-2-(2-Cyclopentenyl)-4-hydroxy-3-methyl-2-cyclopenten-1-one esters of *cis* and *trans dl*-chrysanthemummonocarboxylic acids

◇Cyhexatin
◇Cypermethrin
Cythioate   *O,O*-Dimethyl *O*-[4-(aminosulfonyl)phenyl]phosphorothioate
DDD (◇TDE)
◇DDT
Decamethrin (◇deltamethrin)
◇Deet
◇Deltamethrin
◇Diazinon
◇Dicapthon
◇Dichlofenthion
◇Dichlorvos
◇Dicofol
◇Dieldrin
◇Diflubenzuron
Dilan   2-Nitro 1,1-bis(*p*-chlorophenyl)propane and butane mixture (1:2 ratio)

◇Dimethoate
◇Dimethrin
◇Dimetilan
Dinitro-*o*-cresol   4,6-Dinitro-*o*-cresol
Dinitroorthocyclohexylphenyl   2-Cyclohexyl-4,6-dinitrophenol
◇Dioxathion
Dition®   2-(2,4-Dihydroxyphenyl)-1-cyclohexene-1-carboxylic acid-w-lactone *O,O*-diethyl phosphorothioate
Dowco®-105   *O*-4-*tert*-Butyl-2-chlorophenyl *O*-methyl ethylphosphoramidothioate
Dowco®-109   *O*-4-*tert*-Butyl-2-chlorophenyl *O*-methyl methylphosphoramidothioate
Dowco®-175   2,4-Dichlorophenyl proplyl methyl phosphoramidothioate
Dri Die® 67   Silica and ammonium fluosilicate
Eli Lilly EL-979   4-Nitro-2-(1,1,2,2-tetrafluoroethyl)-6-(trifluoromethyl)-1*H*-benzimadozol-2-,01, sodium salt
Eli Lilly L-27   *N*-[2-Amino-3-nitro-5-(trifluoromethyl)phenyl]-2,2,3,3-tetrafluoropropanamide

◇Endosulfan
◇Endrin
◇EPN
Erythrosin B   Xanthene dye
◇Ethion
◇Famphur
◇Fenitrothion
◇Fenthion
◇Fenvalerate
◇Flucythrinate
Flumethrin   α-Cyano-(4-fluoro-3-phenoxy)benzyl-3-[2-(4-chlorophenyl)-ethenyl]-2,2-dimethyl cyclopropanecarboxylate

◇Formothion

GC-3582   2,2-Dichloro-1-(2,5-dichlorophenyl)vinyl diethyl phosphate

GC-8266 N-(1,1a,3,3a,4,5,5a,5b,6-Decachlorooctahydro-1,3,4-metheno-1H-cyclobuta[cd]pentalen-2-yl)ethyl N-carboxy-glycine

GC-9160   Ethyl 1,1a,3,3a,4,5,5,5a,5b,6-decachlorooctahydro-2-hydroxy-1,3,4-methano-2H-cyclobuta(cd)pentalene-2-levulinate

◇Heptachlor

Hooker HRS-1422   3,5-Diisoproplphenyl methylcarbamate

◇Hydroprene

◇Iodofenphos

◇Isobenzan

Isobornyl thiocyanoacetate   1,7,7-Trimethylbicyclo[2.2.1.] hept-2-yl *exo*-thiocyanoacetate

Isochlorthion O-4-Chloro-3-nitrophenyl O,O-dimethyl phosphorothioate

◇Isodrin

Ivermectin   At least 80% of 22,23-dihydro-5-O-demethylavermectin A$_{1a}$ and not more than 20% 22,23-dihydro-5-O-demethyl-25-de(1-methylpropyl)-25-(1-methylethyl)-avermectin A$_{1a}$

Larvadex® (CGA-72662) N-Cyclopropyl-1,3,5-triazine-2,4,6-triamine

Lethane A-70®   β,β′-Dithiocyano diethyl ether

Lethane B-72

Lethane-384®   2-(2-Butoxyethoxy)ethyl thiocyanate

◇Lindane

◇Malathion

Maretin® N-Hydroxynaphthalimide diethyl phosphate

◇Menazon

◇Metepa

◇Methidathion

◇Methiotepa

◇Methoprene

◇Methoxychlor

◇Methyl bromide

Methyl Trithion® S-{[(4-Chlorophenyl)thio]methyl}O,O-dimethyl phosphorodithioate

◇Mevinphos

MGK Repellent 11®   1,5a,6,9,9a,9b-Hexahydro-4a(4H)-dibenzofurancarboxaldehyde

MGK Repellent 264®   2-(2-Ethylhexyl)-3a,4,7,7a-tetrahydro-4,7-methano-1H-isoindole-1,3(2H)-dione

MGK Repellent 326®   di-n-Propyl 2,5-pyridinedicarboxylate

◇Mirex

Mobam® (MC-A-600)   Benzo[b]thien-4-yl methylcarbamate

◇Muscalure

◇Naled

Neotran®   di(4-Chlorophenoxy)methane

NIA-17370   [5-(phenylmethyl)-3-furanyl]methyl 2,2-dimethyl-3-(2-methyl-1-propenyl) cyclopropanecarboxylate

◇Nicotine

◇Nicotine sulfate

Nifluridide N-[2-Amino-3-nitro-5-(trifluoromethyl)phenyl)]-2,2,3,3-tetrafluoropropanamide
4-hydroxy-3-iodo-5-nitrobenzonitrile

Nitroxynil

◇Ovex

Paradichlorobenzene p-Dichlorobenzene

◇Parathion

◇Pentachlorophenol

◇Permethrin

Perthane®   1,1′-(2,2-Dichloroethylidene)bis[4-ethylbenzene]

Phenothiazine   Dibenzo-1,4-thiazine

◇Phosmet

◇Phosphamidon

◇Phoxim

Picloram   4-Amino-3,5,6-trichloropicolinic acid

◇Piperonyl butoxide

◇Piperonyl cyclonene

Pirazinon
◇Pirimiphos-methyl
Polybor 3®
◇Propetamphos
◇Propoxur
◇Propyl thiopyrophosphate
Pyramat
◇Pyrethrins
Pyrolan
Rafoxanide
◇Resmethrin
RO 06-9550
RO 08-4314
RO 20-3600

◇Ronnel
◇Rotenone
◇Schradan
Shell SD-4402

Shell SD-8211
Shell SD-8280
Shell SD-8436
Shell SD-8448
Shell 52-RL-71

Spencer S-6900

Stauffer HS-103
Stauffer N-2404
Stauffer R-1207
Stauffer R-2371
Stauffer R-20458
◇Stirofos
Strobane®
Sulfaquinoxalene®
Sulphenone
Tabutrex®
°TDE (DDD)
◇Temephos
◇Tepa
◇Tepp
◇Tetramethrin
Thanite®
Thiabendazole
Thiourea
◇Toxaphene
◇Trichlorfon
Tripene
Valone®
Vendex®
WARF antiresistant
Zytron®
◇2,4-D
2,4,5-T

O,O-Diethyl O-3-(2-propyl-6-methyl-4-pyrimidinyl)-thiophosphate

Disodium octaborate tetrahydrate

2-n-Propyl-4-methylpyrimidyl(6) dimethylcarbamate

3-Methyl-1-phenylpyrazol-5-yl dimethylcarbamate
3,5-Diiodo-3′-chloro-4′-(p-chlorophenoxy)salicylanilide

Methyl 10,11-epoxy-7-ethyl-3,11-dimethyl-2,6-tridacadienoate
10,11-Epoxy-3,7,10,11-tetramethyl-ethyl 2,6-dodecadienoic acid
4-[(6,7-Epoxy-3,7-dimethyl-2-nonenyl)oxy]-1,2-(methylenedioxy)-benzene

1,3,4,5,6,7,8,8-Octachloro-3a,4,7,7a-tetrahydro-4,7-methanophthalene

2-Chloro-1-(2,5-dichlorophenyl)vinyl dimethyl phosphate
2-Chloro-1-(2,4-dichlorophenyl)vinyl dimethyl phosphate
2-Chloro-1-(2,4-dibromophenyl)vinyl dimethyl phosphate
2-Chloro-2-(2,4,5-trichlorophenyl)vinyl diethyl phosphate
5,6,7,8,9,9-Hexachloro-1-4,2-3-diepoxy-1,2,3,4,4a,5,8,8a-octahydro-5,8-methanonaphthalene
O,O-Dimethyl phosphorodithioate S-ester with (N-formyl-2-mercapto-N-methylacetamide

(E)-S-[(3,7-dimethyl-2,6-octadienyl)oxy]-2-ethylpyridine
O-(2-Chloro-4-nitrophenyl) O-isopropyl ethyl phosphorothioate
3-Chloropropyl n-octyl sulfoxide
S-[bis(4-Chlorophenyl)dimethyl]diethyl phosphorothiolothionate
(E)-6,7,-Epoxy-1-(p-ethylphenoxy)-3,7-dimethyl-2-octene

Terpene polychlorinates (65% chlorine)
$N′$-2-Quinoxalinyl-sulfanilamide
p-Chlorophenyl phenyl sulfone and related sulfones
Dibutyl succinate

1,7,7-Trimethylbicyclo[2.2.1.] hept-2-yl *exo*-thiocyanoacetate
2-(4-Thiazolyl)benzinidazole
Thiocarbamide, NH_2CSNH_2

S-Ethyl (E,E)-11-methoxy-3,7,11-trimethyl-2,4-dodecadienthioate
2-iso-Valenyl-1,3-indandione
Hexabis (2-methyl-2-phenylpropyl)distannoxane
N,N-di-n-Butyl-p-chlorobenzenesulfonamide
O-2,4-Dichlorophenyl O-methyl isopropylphosphoramidothioate
(2,4-Dichlorophenoxy) acetic acid
(2,4,5-Trichlorophenoxy) acetic acid

INDEX

A

Poultry manure, 159—163
  biocontrol of flies in, 205—206
Pouron technique
  control of arthropod pests
    of horses, 119
    of sheep and goats, 127, 131, 132
  control of cattle grubs, 84
  control of face flies on cattle, 65
  control of horn flies on cattle, 31—32, 36
  control of lice on cattle, 94—95
  control of "small" biting and nuisance flies on
    cattle, 52
  control of ticks on cattle, 107—108
Precocene-2, 110
Predaceous mites, 206, 208, 209
Predators, 206
Propoxur, 44, 52, 116, 160, 168, 181
Propyl thiopyrophosphate, 162, 180
Prosimulium spp., 53
Protein-mineral blocks, 35
Protophormia terrae-novae, 71
Pruritus, 16
Psoregates
  bos, 99, 102
  ovis, 128
Psorophora spp., 5
Psoroptes
  cuniculi, 15, 118, 129
  equi, 115
  ovis, 11—12, 14—15
    control of, 99—100, 127—128
    eradication of, 16
Psoroptic scabs, 99—100, 102
Pulex irritans, 141, 146
Pupal parasites, 199, 205—206, 208
Pyramat, 64, 180
Pyrethrins
  area control of ticks and chiggers, 168
  control of arthropod pests
    of horses, 116, 117
    of poultry, 146, 147
    of sheep and goats, 125
    of swine, 140
  control of cattle grubs, 78
  control of flies in manure and around structures,
    180—183
  control of horn flies on cattle, 29—31
  control of horse flies and deer flies on cattle, 57, 58
  control of "small" biting and nuisance flies on
    cattle, 51
  control of stable flies and use of repellents on
    cattle, 44, 45
Pyrethroid
  area control of ticks and chiggers, 168
  control of arthropod pests of horses, 116, 120
  control of flies in manure and around structures,
    182—183
  control of horn flies on cattle, 32—33, 36
  control of horse flies and deer flies on cattle, 59
  control of lice on cattle, 95
  control of mites on cattle, 102

control of "small" biting and nuisance flies on
    cattle, 52, 53
control of stable flies and use of repellents on
    cattle, 45
control of ticks on cattle, 110
resistance to, 191, 192
Pyridine-adhesive mixture, 108
Pyrolan, 179—180

Q

Quarantine procedures, 12

R

R-1207, 44
Rabbit tick, 219
Rafoxanide, 131
Raillietia auris, 99, 102
Range cattle manure, 207—208
Repellents, see also specific agents
  control of arthropod pests
    of horses, 118
    of sheep and goats, 130
  control of face flies on cattle, 63—64
  control of horse flies and deer flies on cattle, 57—
    58
  control of screwworms on cattle and other
    livestock, 72
  control of "small" biting and nuisance flies on
    cattle, 51, 52
  control of stable flies and use of repellents on
    cattle, 43—47
Resin collars, 127
Resistant species, 189—192
Resmethrin, 58
Rhipicephalus sanguineus, 218
Ribbon spraying, 126
Rocky Mountain wood tick, 13
  control of, 105, 108, 110, 167—169, 209
  resistance to, 216, 218, 219
Ronnel
  control of arthropod pests
    of poultry, 151, 152
    of sheep and goats, 126—128, 130, 132
    of swine, 140
  control of cattle grubs, 80
  control of face flies on cattle, 64—67
  control of flies
    in manure and around structures, 177, 178, 180,
      182
    in poultry manure, 160, 162
  control of horn flies on cattle, 31
  control of lice on cattle, 94, 95
  control of screwworms on cattle and other
    livestock, 73
  control of "small" biting and nuisance flies on
    cattle, 53
  control of ticks on cattle, 107, 109
  effect on livestock production, 9
  resistance to, 191